Sports Medicine: Athletic Training and Rehabilitation Techniques

Sports Medicine: Athletic Training and Rehabilitation Techniques

Editor: Patrick Clinton

Callisto Reference
www.callistoreference.com

Callisto Reference,
118-35 Queens Blvd., Suite 400,
Forest Hills, NY 11375, USA

Visit us on the World Wide Web at:
www.callistoreference.com

ISBN: 978-1-63239-959-5 (Hardback)

Printed in China.

Cataloging-in-Publication Data

Sports medicine : athletic training and rehabilitation techniques / edited by Patrick Clinton.
p. cm.
Includes bibliographical references and index.
ISBN 978-1-63239-959-5
1. Sports medicine. 2. Athletes. 3. Physical education and training.
4. Medical rehabilitation. I. Clinton, Patrick.
RC1210 .S66 2018
617.102 7--dc23

Table of Contents

Preface

The world is advancing at a fast pace like never before. Therefore, the need is to keep up with the latest developments. This book was an idea that came to fruition when the specialists in the area realized the need to coordinate together and document essential themes in the subject. That's when I was requested to be the editor. Editing this book has been an honour as it brings together diverse authors researching on different streams of the field. The book collates essential materials contributed by veterans in the area which can be utilized by students and researchers alike.

Medicine has numerous branches and one of these branches is sports medicine. It is mainly concerned with the fitness and well-being of athletes. Sports medicine deals with the medical conditions that can be faced by sports persons or by people who exercise. Some of the common sports injuries encountered by athletes are muscle cramps, ACL tears, ankle sprains, shin splints, etc. This book provides significant information of this discipline to help develop a good understanding of sports medicine and related fields. Through this book, we attempt to further enlighten the readers about the new concepts in this field.

Each chapter is a sole-standing publication that reflects each author's interpretation. Thus, the book displays a multi-facetted picture of our current understanding of application, resources and aspects of the field. I would like to thank the contributors of this book and my family for their endless support.

Editor

1

Swimming performances in long distance open-water events with and without wetsuit

Sebastian Ulsamer[1], Christoph Alexander Rüst[1], Thomas Rosemann[1], Romuald Lepers[2] and Beat Knechtle[3*]

Abstract

Background: Existing literature showed improved swimming performances for swimmers wearing wetsuits competing under standardized conditions in races held in pools on short to middle distances. Data about the influence of wetsuits on swimming performances in long and ultra-long open-water swimming races are missing. It is unknown whether the benefit of wearing wetsuits is comparable in men and women. The aim of this study was to investigate the influence of wearing a wetsuit on open-water swimming performances at the 26.4 km 'Marathon Swim in Lake Zurich' in Lake Zurich, Switzerland, and the 3.8 km Lake Ontario Swim Team-Race (LOST-Race) in Lake Ontario, Canada.

Methods: Race times of the fastest female and male swimmers competing with and without wetsuit were compared using multi-level regression analyses and analysis of variance.

Results: In the 'Marathon Swim' in Lake Zurich, wearing a wetsuit had no effect on race time regarding the gender where athletes wearing a wetsuit were not faster than athletes without wetsuit. However, the ten fastest men wearing a wetsuit (410.6 ± 26.7 min) were faster (32.7%, $p < 0.01$) than the ten fastest women without wetsuit (544.9 ± 81.3 min). In the 'LOST-Race', the top ten men wearing a wetsuit (51.7 ± 2.5 min) were faster (13.2%, $p < 0.01$) than the top ten women wearing a wetsuit (58.5 ± 3.2 min). Additionally, the top ten men without wetsuit (52.1 ± 2.4 min) were faster (19.6%, $p < 0.01$) than the top ten women without wetsuit (62.3 ± 2.5 min). The top ten women wearing a wetsuit (58.5 ± 3.2 min) were faster (6.5%, $p < 0.01$) than top ten women without a wetsuit (62.3 ± 25 min).

Conclusions: These results suggest that wearing a wetsuit had a positive influence on swimming speed for both women and men but the benefit of the use of wetsuits seemed to depend on additional factors (*i.e.* race distance). Women seemed to benefit more from wearing wetsuits than men in longer open-water ultra-distance swimming races.

Keywords: Ultra-endurance, Swimming, Ironman, Neoprene suit, Swim performance

Background

Over the past decade the popularity of participation in ultra-endurance events such as ultra-marathon running [1-4], ultra-cycling [5], ultra-triathlons [6,7] and ultra-swimming [8-10] has considerably increased. For ultra-endurance swimmers, several events such as the 'Manhattan Island Swim' in New York [11], the 'Rottnest Channel Swim' in Australia [12], the 'Marathon Swim' in Lake Zurich in Switzerland [13] or the ‚English Channel Swim' between Dover and Calais [14] are held. Recent studies showed that women reduced the sex difference in open-water ultra-distance swimming [15,16] and were even able to outperform men [17].

Long-distance swimming splits are also included in other ultra-endurance events such as long-distance triathlons (*i.e.* Ironman triathlon) consisting of 3.8 km swimming, 180 km cycling and 42 km running [7]. The same 3.8 km swimming distance as held in Ironman competitions is covered by swimmers competing in the 'LOST-Race' (*i.e.* Lake Ontario Swim Team-Race), an open-water swimming race held in the Lake Ontario, Canada. The 'LOST-Race' is organized since 2008 by the Lake Ontario Swim Team [18]. When the race started in

* Correspondence: beat.knechtle@hispeed.ch
[3]Facharzt FMH für Allgemeinmedizin, Vadianstrasse 26, Gesundheitszentrum St. Gallen, St. Gallen, Switzerland
Full list of author information is available at the end of the article

2008, only eight swimmers participated but the number of swimmers increased continuously up to 94 starters in 2012 [19].

Generally, open-water ultra-swimmers are prohibited to wear wetsuits in open-water swimming events such as the, 'English Channel Swim', where the athletes have to cover a total distance of ~32 km [9]. In contrast to open-water ultra-distance swimming, participants at the 'Marathon Swim' in Lake Zurich, Switzerland, the longest open-water ultra-swim in Europe held in a lake covering a distance of ~26.4 km [13], are allowed to wear wetsuits when competing in the wetsuit category. These participants are separately ranked in a wetsuit category. Also the participants in the 'LOST-Race' are free to decide if they want to start in the wetsuit or in the non-wetsuit category [18].

In official Ironman competitions the permission of the use of wetsuits depends on the water temperature. Wetsuits are permitted when the water temperature is up to 24.5°C or colder but will be prohibited in water temperatures higher than 28.8°C. Athletes who choose wearing a wetsuit in water temperatures between 24.5°C and 28.8°C are allowed to participate but are not eligible for age-group awards or for qualifying slots for the Ironman World Championship [20].

When triathletes began wearing wetsuits during the swimming part of a triathlon race, anecdotal evidence as well as the empirical study of Parsons and Day [21] indicated that the swimming performance could be improved by wearing a wetsuit. Studies have been conducted since then investigating the influence of wearing a wetsuit on open-water swimming performance [22,23]. It has been shown that wearing wetsuits enhanced swimming performance by directly increasing buoyancy and holding the body in a more horizontal position, thereby allowing more effort to be expended in propulsive movement [23]. The performance gain while wearing a wetsuit was associated with an increased propulsion efficiency related to both a gain in buoyancy [24] and a reduction in drag [25]. It seemed that swimming performance improved more in inefficient swimmers with low buoyancy and swimming at low speed [26]. Wearing a wetsuit reduced drag during front crawl swimming [27,28] leading to a decreased energy cost of submaximal swimming and an increased distance per stroke [27]. Differences do also exist between fastskin and standard swim wetsuits regarding drag and buoyance where full-length fastskin swimsuits created less total hydrodynamic resistance than normal swimsuits while providing no additional buoyancy benefits [29]. Also a torso swim suit and a standard racing suit lead to differences in drag and performance. A torso suit reduced the energy demand of swimming whereas a standard racing suit reduced body drag [30]. Also the length of the swimming performance seems of importance where performance was not enhanced in rather short swimming distances [31].

Actually, literature about the effects of a wetsuit on long-distance and ultra-long-distance swimming performance is very small [22]. In all studies investigating the effect of wetsuits on swimming performance, participants were swimming in pools under standardized conditions or covered only short to middle distances of 400 m and 1,500 m or short swim times of 5 min to 30 min [21,22]. Studies on the effect of wearing wetsuits on swimming performance in open-water ultra-distance swimming are missing so far. According to Knechtle *et al.* [32] investigating predictor variables in an open-water ultra-endurance swimming event covering ~26.4 km, none of the known anthropometric variables in swimmers such as body fat, body height and length of the extremities showed a relationship with race time. Regarding the fact that there are rather few variables with potential influence on ultra-swimming performance, a positive effect of the use of a wetsuit on race time in an ultra-endurance open-water swimming contest would be of great interest.

In open-water ultra-distance swimming, Eichenberger *et al.* reported faster race times for male swimmers competing in the 'Marathon Swim' in Lake Zurich [10] compared to race times in female finishers and mentioned physiological and anthropometric differences as potential reasons for the sex difference in performance. Only the study of Toussaint *et al.* [24] compared the effects of wearing a wetsuit on the performance of male and female swimmers where changes in swimming times were equal in male and female swimmers swimming with and without wetsuits. As this study has been conducted under standardized conditions while swimming in a pool, no study investigated possible differences of the benefit of wearing wetsuits between male and female swimmers in long and ultra-long open-water swimming.

Therefore, the aim of the present study was to compare the performance of female and male open-water

Table 1 Number of participants in the 'Marathon Swim' in Lake Zurich (26.4 km) and in the 'LOST-Race' (3.8 km)

Distance	Total	Total with wetsuit	Total without wetsuit	Total men	Men with wetsuit	Men without wetsuit	Total women	Women with wetsuit	Women without wetsuit
26.4 km	300	80 (26.7%)	220 (73.3%)	189 (63.0%)	68 (36.0%)	121 (64.0%)	111 (37.0%)	12 (10.8%)	99 (89.2%)
3.8 km	284	202 (71.1%)	82 (28.9%)	173 (60.9%)	122 (70.5%)	51 (29.5%)	111 (39.1%)	80 (72.1%)	31 (27.9%)

swimmers competing with or without wearing a wetsuit in a long-distance (*i.e.* 3.8 km) and in an ultra-long-distance swimming (*i.e.* 26.4 km) event. We hypothesized that (*i*) swimmers wearing a wetsuit would finish the races in a shorter time than swimmers without wearing a wetsuit and (*ii*) women might be able to outperform men in the longer race distance (*i.e.* 26.4 km).

Methods

All procedures used in the study were approved by the Institutional Review Board of Kanton St. Gallen, Switzerland with a waiver of the requirement for informed consent of the participants given the fact that the study involved the analysis of publicly available data.

Data sampling

All data including race times and water temperatures was obtained from the official result lists published on the official homepages of the 'Marathon Swim' [33] in Lake Zurich, Switzerland, and the 'LOST-Race' [34] in Canada.

The 'Marathon Swim' in Lake Zurich

The 'Marathon Swim' in Lake Zurich takes place annually in Lake of Zurich in Switzerland at the beginning of August. The first edition of the race was in 1987. The use of wetsuits has been allowed since 2002 in a separate category and swimmers can compete in a wetsuit and a non-wetsuit category. The swimmers start together at 7:00 a.m. from Rapperswil and have to cross the length of the lake and finish in Zurich. The race covers a distance of ~26.4 km where the cut-off time is 12 h. The use of high-tech swimsuits and additional floating devices was prohibited in the non-wetsuit category. Each swimmer has to be accompanied by a support boat. The swimmers have to organize their own nutrition and support crew during the race. All athletes who ever successfully finished the 'Marathon Swim' in Lake Zurich between 2002 and 2012 were analysed regarding the association between wearing a wetsuit, sex and swimming speed.

The LOST-Race

The 'LOST-Race' is the abbreviation for the 'Lake Ontario Swim Team'-Race. This race is held annually 2008 in the middle of August. The race starts at 8.00 a.m. from the foot of Maple Grove Drive for 3.8 km to the Lighthouse Pier in downtown Oakville. This distance is equal to the swim split in an Ironman triathlon. The swimmers can compete in a wetsuit and a non-wetsuit category. All athletes who successfully finished in the 'LOST-Race' between 2008 and 2012 were analysed regarding the association between wearing a wetsuit, sex and swimming speed.

Data analysis

To examine the change in performance across years, race times of the annual top (*i.e.* swimmers with the

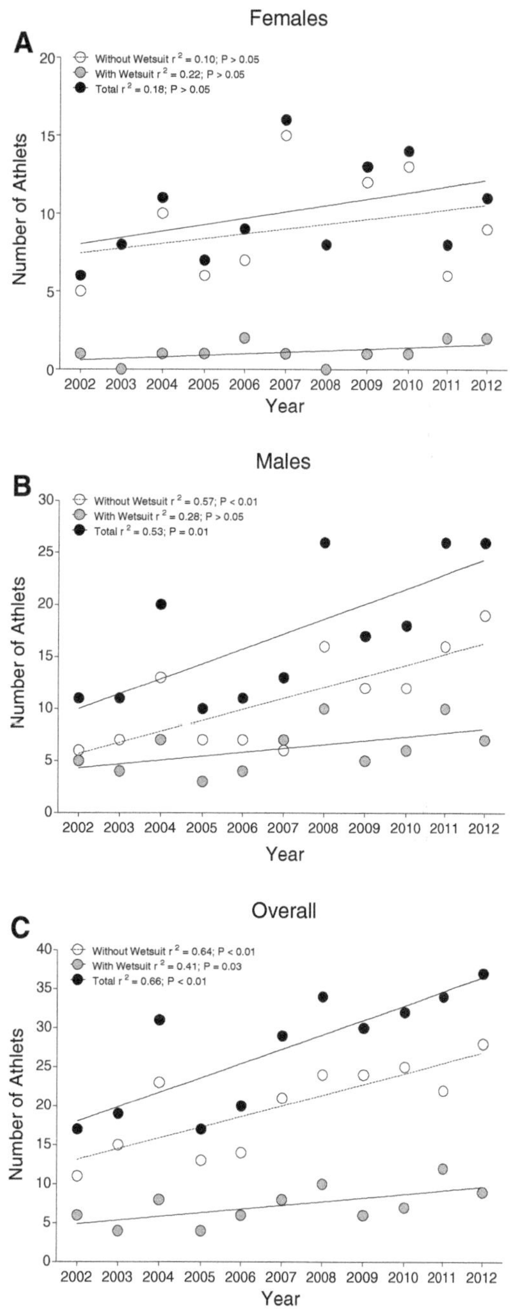

Figure 1 Annual number of finishers in the 'Marathon Swim' in Lake Zurich competing with and without wetsuit as well as total for women (Panel A), men (Panel B) and overall finishers (Panel C).

fastest race time) and annual top three (*i.e.* swimmers with the three fastest race times) female and male swimmers competing with and without wetsuit were determined for both races. Due to the low number of female finishers in the 'Marathon Swim' in Lake Zurich women could only be included in the analysis of the annual top swimmers. When in the 'LOST-Race' less than three athletes were recorded per category in a certain year, the specific year was excluded from analysis for that specific group. The mean race times of both the annual top and the annual top three athletes were pooled and performance was compared within swimsuit groups (*i.e.* wearing a wetsuit or not) between sexes and between wetsuit groups within sexes. Additionally, the overall (*i.e.* all finishers between 2002 and 2012) top ever, top three ever and top ten ever women and men competing with and without wetsuit were determined and compared within wetsuit groups between sexes and within sexes between wetsuit groups. As a last step, the interaction between wetsuit and sex on performance was determined for the annual top swimmers as well as for the top, top three and top ten swimmers ever.

Statistical analyses

Each set of data was tested for normal distribution and for homogeneity of variances prior to statistical analyses. Normal distribution was tested using a D'Agostino and Pearson omnibus normality test and homogeneity of variances was tested using a Levene's test. Trends in participation were analysed using regression analysis with 'straight line' and 'exponential growth equation' model, whereas for each set of data (*e.g.* each age group) both models where compared using Akaike's Information Criteria (AICc) to decide which model showed the highest probability of correctness. Single and multi-level regression analyses were used to investigate changes in performance of the finishers. A hierarchical regression model was used to avoid the impact of a cluster-effect on results in case one athlete finished more than once in the annual top or annual top three for the analysis of

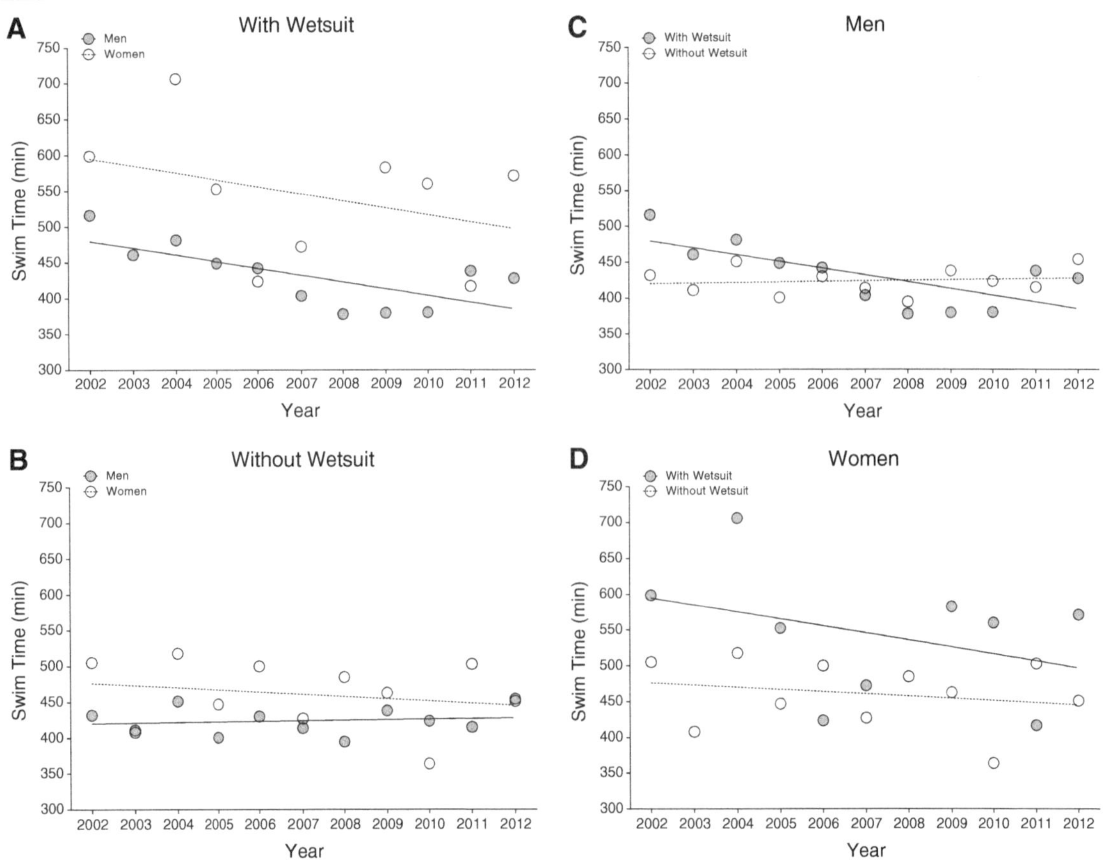

Figure 2 Race times of the annual fastest men and women competing with (Panel A) and without (Panel B) wetsuit 'Marathon Swim' in Lake Zurich and the comparison between race times with and without wetsuit for men (Panel C) and women (Panel D).

overall performance. Regression analyses of performance were corrected for age of athletes in 'Marathon Swim' in Lake Zurich to prevent a misinterpretation of an 'age-effect' as a 'time-effect'. To find significant differences between two groups, a Student's t-test was used with Welch's correction in case of unequal variances. To determine the interaction of sex and wetsuit on swimming performance, a two-way ANOVA (sex × wetsuit) was performed. Statistical analyses were performed using IBM SPSS Statistics (Version 19, IBM SPSS, Chicago, IL, USA) and GraphPad Prism (Version 5, GraphPad Software, La Jolla, CA, USA). Significance was accepted at $p < 0.05$ (two-sided for t-tests). Data in the text are given as mean ± standard deviation (SD).

Results

The 'Marathon Swim' in Lake Zurich

The participation trends in the 'Marathon Swim' in Lake Zurich are presented in Table 1. Between 2002 and 2012, a total of 300 swimmers, including 111 women (37%) and 189 men (63%), finished the race. Twelve women (10.8%) and 68 men (36.0%) started in the wetsuit category, 99 women (89.2%) and 121 men (64.0%) started without wearing a wetsuit. For women, no change in participation across years was recorded (Figure 1a), whereas for men, the number in finishers competing with wetsuit increased linearly (Figure 1b). Overall, the number of finishers competing with and without a wetsuit increased linearly (Figure 1c).

Figure 2 presents the race times of the annual fastest and Figure 3 of the annual three fastest finishers in the 'Marathon Swim' in Lake Zurich. Race times of the annual fastest and the annual three fastest men wearing a wetsuit and race times of the annual three fastest women without wetsuits decreased significantly across years (Table 2). There was no decrease in race times for the annual fastest men competing without a wetsuit and for the annual fastest women with and without a wetsuit over the last decade (Table 2).

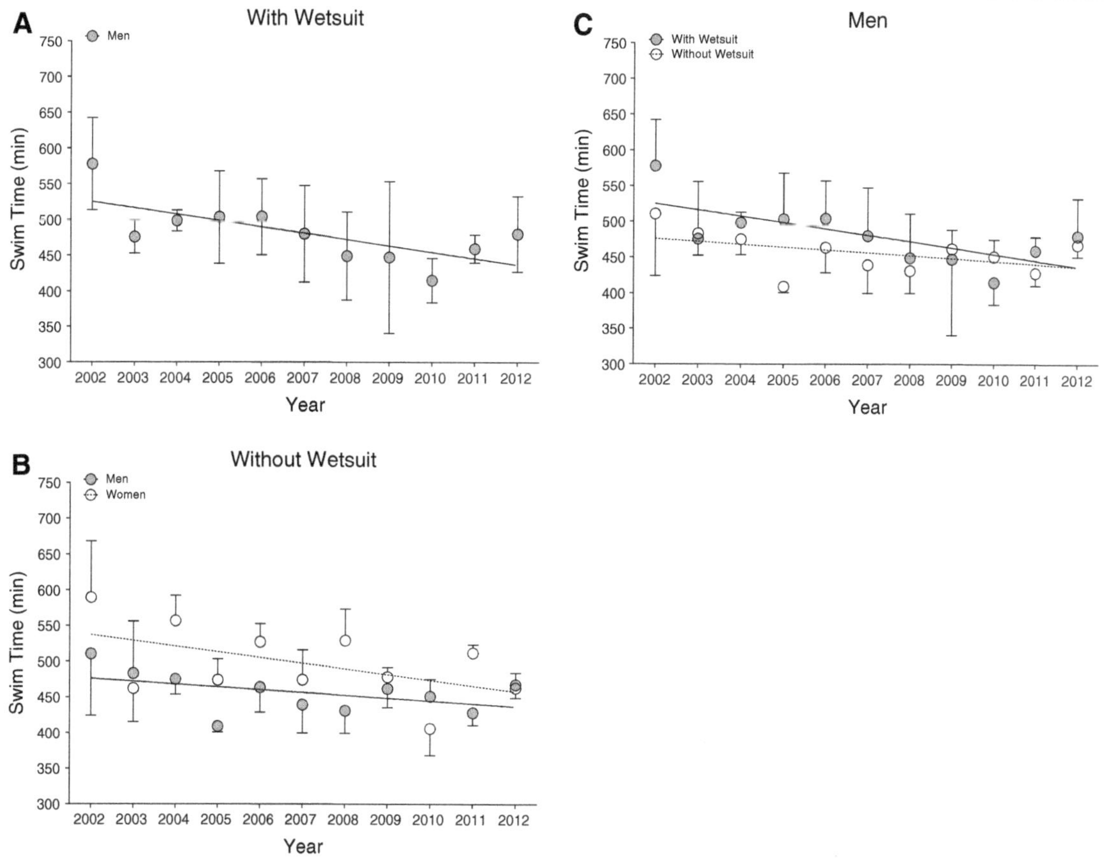

Figure 3 Race times of the annual top three men and women competing with (Panel A) and without (Panel B) wetsuit 'Marathon Swim' in Lake Zurich and the comparison between race times with and without wetsuit for men (Panel C).

Table 2 Multi-level regression analyses for change in performance across years for men and women (Model 1) with correction for multiple finishes (Model 2) and with correction for multiple finishes and age of the participants (Model 3)

Model	β	SE (β)	Stand. ß	T	P
Annual fastest men competing with wetsuit					
1	−9.425	3.189	−0.702	−2.955	0.016
2	−9.425	3.189	−0.702	−2.955	0.016
3	−9.058	3.376	−0.674	−2.683	0.028
Annual fastest men competing without wetsuit					
1	0.764	1.913	0.132	0.399	0.699
2	0.764	1.913	0.132	0.399	0.699
3	0.983	2.243	0.170	0.438	0.673
Annual fastest women competing with wetsuit					
1	−9.791	9.556	−0.361	−1.025	0.340
2	−9.791	9.556	−0.361	−1.025	0.340
3	−0.323	−0.935	0.386	−0.357	0.991
Annual fastest women competing without wetsuit					
1	−3.065	4.682	−0.213	−0.655	0.529
2	−3.065	4.682	−0.213	−0.655	0.529
3	0.204	0.670	0.522	0.231	0.710
Annual fastest three men competing with wetsuit					
1	−8.845	3.109	−0.455	−2.845	0.008
2	−8.845	3.109	−0.455	−2.845	0.008
3	−9.848	2.910	−0.507	−3.385	0.002
Annual fastest three men competing without wetsuit					
1	−3.945	2.366	−0.287	−1.668	0.105
2	−3.945	2.366	−0.287	−1.668	0.105
3	−4.117	2.500	−0.299	−1.647	0.110
Annual fastest three women competing with wetsuit					
1	−1.762	9.149	−0.061	−0.193	0.851
2	−1.762	9.149	−0.061	−0.193	0.851
3	−3.298	8.674	−0.114	−0.380	0.713
Annual fastest three women competing without wetsuit					
1	−7.956	2.994	−0.431	−2.657	0.012
2	−7.956	2.994	−0.431	−2.657	0.012
3	−6.875	3.035	−0.372	−2.265	0.031

Wearing a wetsuit had no effect on overall race time regarding the gender. Men in the wetsuit category finished the race within 534 ± 82 min while men competing without wetsuit had an average race time of 551 ± 89 min ($p > 0.05$, 3.1%). Women in the wetsuit category swam the 26.4 km in 572 ± 94 min while women competing without a wetsuit achieved an average race time of 589 ± 105 min ($p > 0.05$, 2.8%). However, race times for men wearing wetsuits were faster than race times for women wearing wetsuits. This finding was non-significant for the top three swimmers (379.4 ± 1.3 min *versus* 396.4 ± 28.8 min, 4.5%, $p > 0.05$) but significant for the top ten swimmers (410.6 ± 26.7 min *versus* 544.9 ± 81.3 min, 32.7%, $p < 0.01$) wearing wetsuits (Figure 4a). Male top three (401.6 ± 7.2 min *versus* 396.4 ± 28.8 min, 1.2%, $p > 0.05$) and male top ten (412.6 ± 9.02 min *versus* 434.2 ± 31.8 min, 5.2%, $p > 0.05$) swimmers competing without wearing wetsuits were not faster than female swimmers without wearing wetsuits (Figure 4b). Race times of the top three men in the wetsuit category were significantly ($p < 0.01$) faster (5.9%) than race times of the top three men without wetsuits. Race times of male top and male top three swimmers and race times of top ten swimmers in the wetsuit category and without wetsuits were similar (Figure 4c). The fastest (15%), the top three (10.3%, non-significant) and the top ten (25.5%, significant) race times of all women wearing wetsuits were slower than those of women competing without wetsuits (Figure 4d).

The LOST-Race

The participation trends in the 'LOST-Race' are shown in Table 1. In the years 2008 to 2012, 284 swimmers including 111 women (39.1%) and 173 men (60.9%) finished the race. Eighty women (72.1%) and 122 men (70.5%) started in the wetsuit category, 31 women (27.9%) and 51 men (29.5%) started without wearing a wetsuit. The number of finishers in the 'LOST-Race' increased significantly since the first event in the year 2008. The increase was consistent for female swimmers in the wetsuit category and without wetsuits (Figure 5a), male swimmers in the wetsuit category and without wetsuits (Figure 5b) and for the overall number of finishers (Figure 5c).

Figure 6 presents the race times of the annual fastest and Figure 7 of the annual three fastest finishers in the 'LOST-Race'. During the investigated years, race times of the annual top three male swimmers without wetsuits decreased significantly while race times of all other groups remained stable (Table 3).

Men in the wetsuit category finished the race within 73 ± 16 min. Men competing without wetsuits achieved an average race time of 73 ± 19 min ($p > 0.05$, 0.0%). Women in the wetsuit category finished within 79 ± 16 min while women competing without wetsuits finished within 80 ± 19 min ($p > 0.05$, 1.2%). Men in the wetsuit category swam the 3.8 km generally faster than women. This finding was consistent for the fastest swimmers (47.0 min *versus* 58.0 min) as well as for the top three swimmers (49.0 ± 2.0 min *versus* 54.7 ± 2.6 min, 11.6%, $p = 0.04$) and the top ten swimmers (51.7 ± 2.5 min *versus* 58.5 ± 3.2 min, 13.2%, $p < 0.01$) in the wetsuit category (Figure 8a). Also the male top (47.0 ± 0 min *versus* 58.0 ± 0 min), male top three (49.3 ±

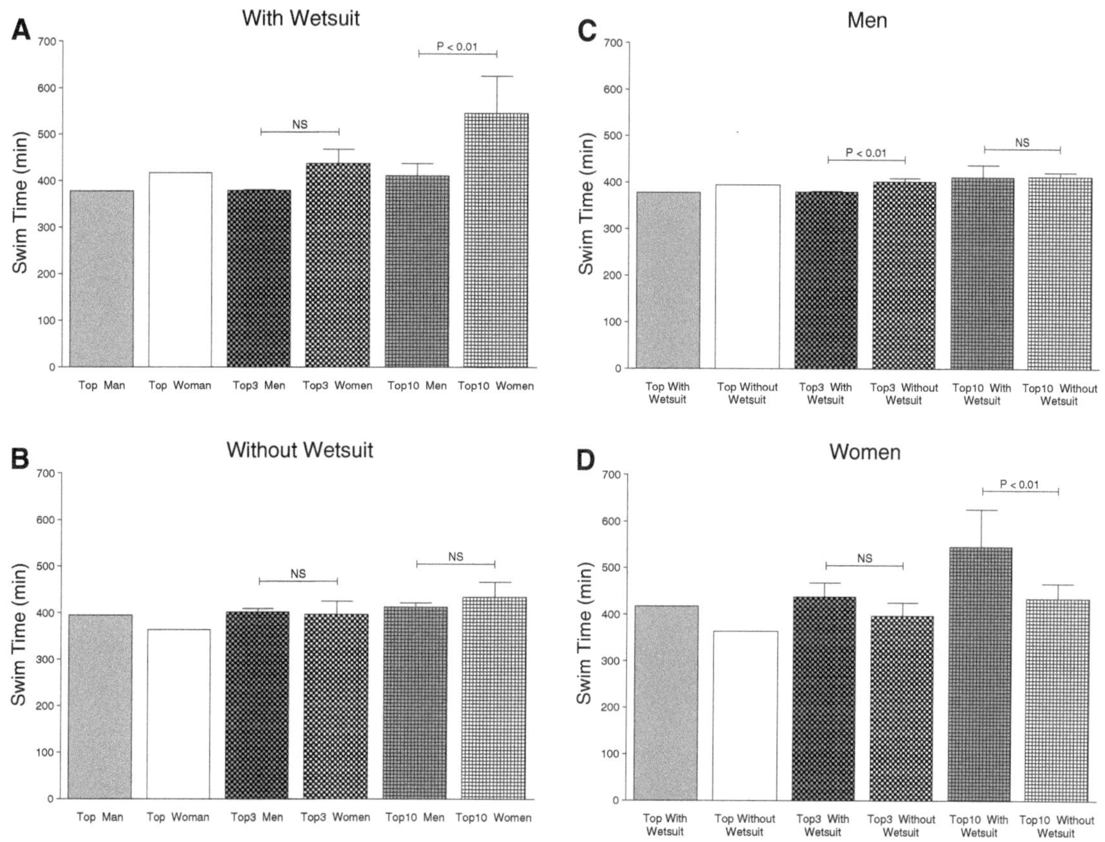

Figure 4 Race times of the top ever, top three ever and top ten ever men and women in the 'Marathon Swim' in Lake Zurich competing with (Panel A) and without (Panel B) wetsuit as well as the comparison between men (Panel C) and women (Panel D) competing with and without wetsuit.

2.5 min *versus* 59.3 ± 1.5 min, 20.3%, $p < 0.01$) and male top ten swimmers (52.1 ± 2.4 min *versus* 62.3 ± 2.5 min, 19.6%, $p < 0.01$) competing without wetsuit were faster than the female top swimmers (Figure 8b). When comparing race times of the fastest, the top three and the top ten male swimmers, equal race times for swimmers in the wetsuit category and swimmers competing without wetsuits were observed (Figure 8c). In contrast, the fastest female swimmers (52.0 ± 0 min *versus* 58.0 ± 0 min) as well as the top three (54.7 ± 2.5 min *versus* 59.3 ± 1.5 min, 8.5%, $p > 0.05$) and the top ten female swimmers (58.5 ± 3.2 min *versus* 62.3 ± 25 min, 6.5%, $p < 0.01$) competing in the wetsuit category were faster than swimmers without wetsuits (Figure 8d).

Discussion

The aim of the study was to compare for both male and female open-water swimmers the performance while competing with and without wearing a wetsuit in a long-distance (*e.g.* 3.8 km) and in an ultra-long-distance swimming (*e.g.* 26.4 km) event.

Swimmers wearing wetsuits were not faster than swimmers without wetsuits

The most important finding was that open-water swimmers competing while wearing a wetsuit were not generally faster in both the long and the ultra-long-distance swimming event than swimmers without wearing wetsuits depending upon whether the fastest, the three fastest or the ten fastest swimmers were considered. This finding contradicts existing literature [21,23] reporting better performances for swimmers competing while wearing wetsuits in short to middle distances between a standardized 500 m test track and 1,500 m.

In the 'Marathon Swim' in Lake Zurich, only the overall top three men wearing a wetsuit were swimming faster than swimmers without a wetsuit. Considering the overall fastest and the top ten as well as the annual fastest, the top three and the top ten male swimmers, race

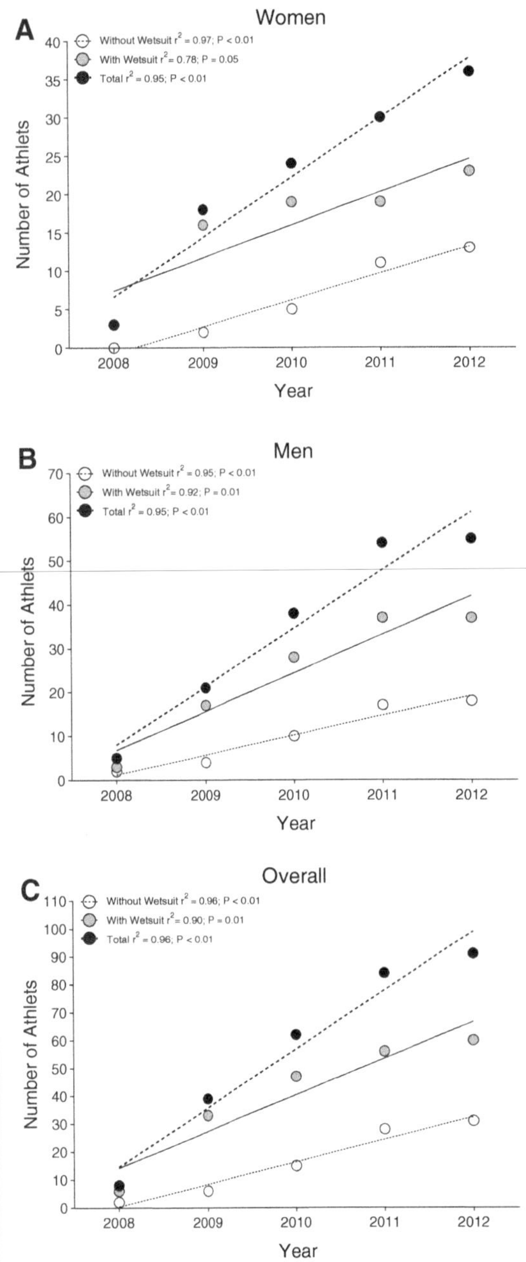

Figure 5 Annual numbers of finishers in the 'LOST-Race' competing with and without wetsuit and for women (Panel A), men (Panel B) and overall finishers (Panel C).

times were similar. Also in the 'LOST-Race', male swimmers wearing wetsuits were competing at the same speed like swimmers without a wetsuit. Female swimmers wearing a wetsuit performed significantly faster in 3.8 km while women wearing wetsuits swam significantly slower in 26.4 km than women without a wetsuit.

Our hypothesis that swimmers competing in a wetsuit would be faster in long and ultra-long-swimming distances was based on existing studies suggesting a positive effect of wearing a wetsuit on swimming performance [22,23,25,26]. All those studies were conducted in indoor pools with standardized water temperatures either covering short to middle distances on a standardized 500 m test track up to 1,500 m or standardized swimming times. It has been shown by Cordain and Kopriva [23] that wetsuits lift the body in a more horizontal position by providing higher buoyancy while swimming in indoor-pools. Thus less power is required for swimmers to maintain the swimming position leaving more energy to be expended for propulsion [23].

In Lake Zurich and Lake Ontario water temperatures were constantly over 20°C when the 'Marathon swim' [13] and the 'LOST-Race' [19] were held. Cordain and Kopriva [23] reported that swimmers competing in a pool with rather warm temperatures of ~26°-28°C complained about feeling too hot while swimming in a wetsuit. This problem was observed in a 1,500 m distance more often than in a 400 m distance [23]. Lowdon *et al.* [35] suggested a temperature of 17.7°C as for a positive effect of wetsuits on swimming race times because of their insulating features. Race times of the annual top three male swimmers without wetsuits on the 3.8 km long distance decreased significantly over the last years while race times of male top three swimmers wearing wetsuits remained unchanged. Thus, we assume that swimmers wearing wetsuits could have been disturbed by the reduced ability of the body to dissipate heat on that long distance when wearing wetsuits and therefore been unable to show an optimal performance.

In contrast, the race times of the annual top and top three swimmers on the ultra-long track decreased during the last decade and the top three male swimmers wearing wetsuits competing in the 26.4 km swam significantly faster than swimmers without wearing a wetsuit. Tipton *et al.* showed a decrease of body core temperature of 0.75°C per hour for swimmers performing in water with a temperature of 18°C without wetsuit [36]. We assume that even when wearing wetsuits while swimming in water of ~20°C for ~6-7 hours there will be a decrease of body core temperature leading to a better comfort and thus enabling to perform better.

Different clothing in ultra-endurance and Ironman-triathletes

The 'Marathon Swim' in Lake Zurich was initially introduced as a training event. Ultra-endurance swimmers still use it for preparation for more popular events like the 'English Channel Swim' [37]. Additionally, a lot of

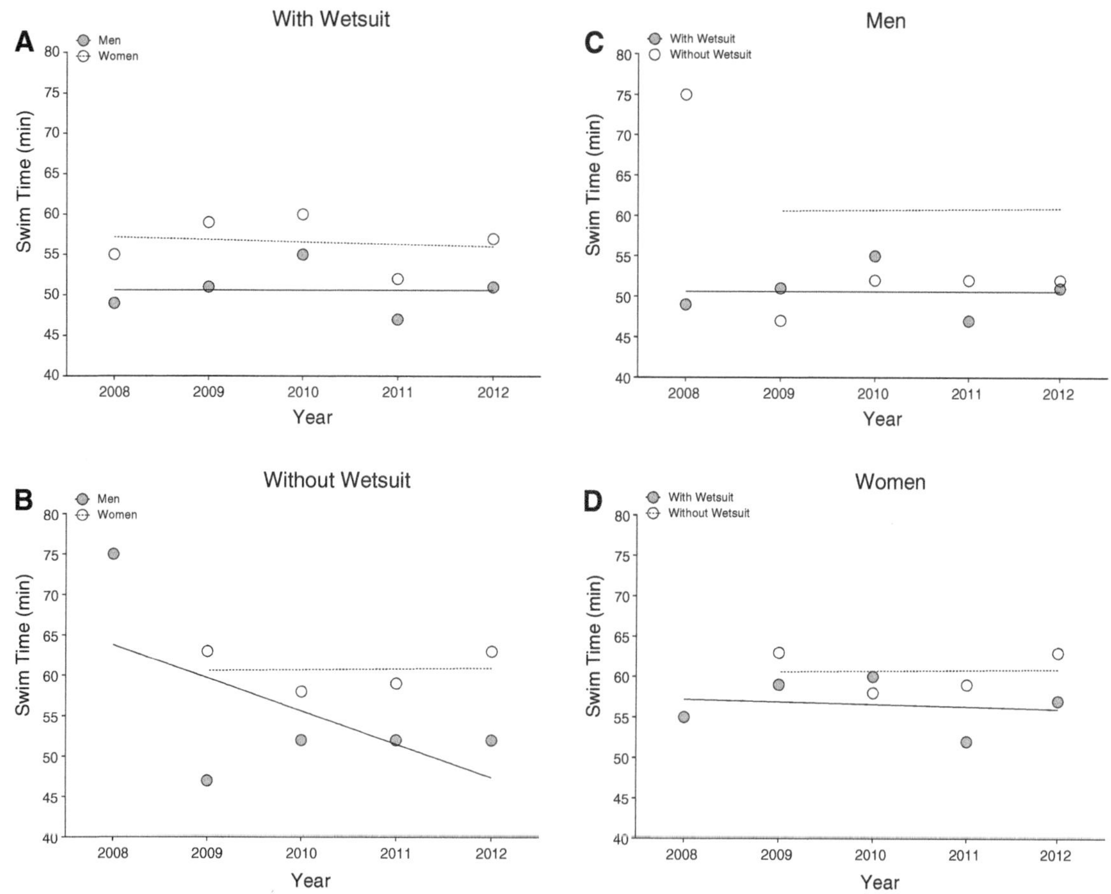

Figure 6 Race times of the fastest men and women competing with (Panel A) and without (Panel B) wetsuit in the 'LOST-Race' and the comparison of times for athletes competing with and without wetsuit for men (Panel C) and women (Panel D).

participants in the event are Ironman triathletes who were preparing for the swimming split of their competitions such as the 'Ironman Switzerland' and the 'Ironman 70.3' Rapperswil-Jona taking place in the Lake Zurich [38].

The use of wetsuits is not allowed in ultra-distance swimming events like the 'English Channel Swim'. In contrast, wearing a wetsuit is permitted in the most important Ironman competitions including the 'Ironman 70.3 Series' and the 'Ironman World Championship' as long as water temperature is 24.5°C or colder. Therefore, we suppose that most participants wearing a wetsuit when swimming in the 'Marathon Swim' in Lake Zurich were Ironman triathletes while ultra-endurance swimmers will rather swim without wetsuit when competing over the 26.4 km.

Knechtle *et al.* [37] compared the anthropometry of ultra-swimmers and Ironman athletes and showed that male and female ultra-swimmers have a higher body mass, a higher body mass index and a higher percentage of body fat than Ironman triathletes leading to a higher buoyancy and a better insulation against cold water temperatures. Leaner athletes thus were supposed to benefit more from wearing wetsuits than fatter swimmers [23]. On the other hand Knechtle *et al.* [37] suggested that other factors like training have a larger influence on swimming performance than anthropometric features. Triathletes have to prepare for three disciplines and as the swimming split in an Ironman triathlon is only 3.8 km and even in a Triple-Iron ultra-triathlon only 11.4 km, ultra-swimmers may be better trained for a swimming event covering 26.4 km [32]. It has been reported that female and male long-distance open-water swimmers competing in 'Marathon Swim' in Lake Zurich swam 16.2 ± 8.5 and 15.6 ± 13.3 km weekly, respectively, at a mean speed of 3.4 ± 0.6 and 3.5 ±

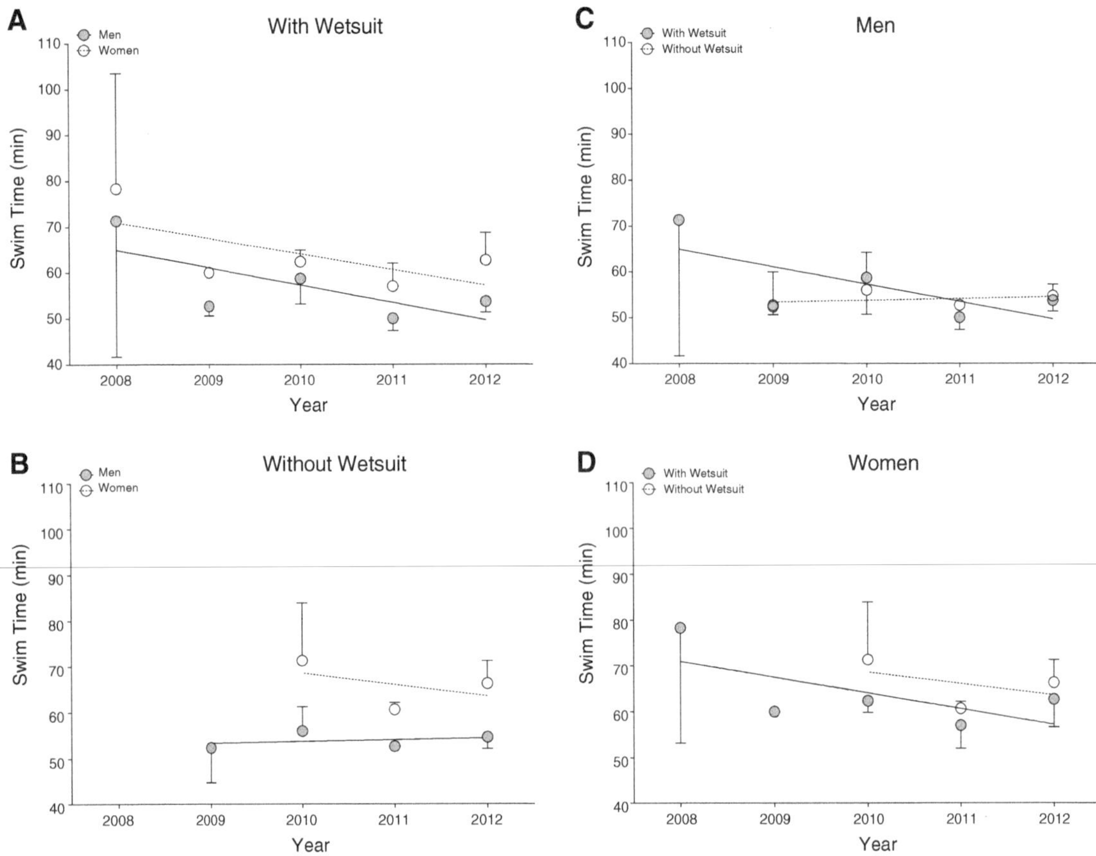

Figure 7 Race times of the top three men and women competing with (Panel A) and without (Panel B) wetsuit in the 'LOST-Race' and the comparison of times for athletes competing with and without wetsuit for men (Panel C) and women (Panel D).

0.5 km/h, respectively [32]. In contrast, female and male Ironman triathletes competing in 'Ironman Switzerland' swam 5.5 ± 2.4 and 6.7 ± 3.0 km weekly, respectively, at a mean speed of 2.1 ± 0.8 and 2.7 ± 0.6 km/h, respectively [39]. Most probably, also swimmers competing in a 3.8 km swim will train less that ultra-swimmers competing in a 26.4 km ultra-swim. The combination of better anthropometric features and better specialized training of ultra-swimmers for the event could have been the reason why the advantages of wearing a wetsuit have been compensated in this event.

Female athletes seemed to benefit more from wearing wetsuits than male swimmers

In the 'LOST-Race', female swimmers of all investigated performance levels were faster when wearing wetsuits than swimmers competing without wetsuits. In contrast, the race times of male swimmers were similar when competing with and without wetsuits. Swimming without wetsuits on the 3.8 km track resulted in a difference in race time of 19.6% in favour for male swimmers. In contrast, when wearing wetsuits, the top ten male swimmers performed only 11.9% faster than the top ten female athletes. This data is coinciding with the study of Lepers reporting a sex difference of 12% in the swimming split in an Ironman competition such as 'Ironman Hawaii' [40].

An explanation for the higher benefit of female swimmers from the use of wearing a wetsuit could be the anthropometric differences between the sexes. Male swimmers have a higher stroke volume and therefore a higher cardiac output than female athletes [41]. The vascularisation of the skeletal muscles is better in men because of the higher blood volume [41]. These factors result in a higher oxygen capacity for male swimmers. Furthermore, the maximum oxygen uptake is ~15-25% higher in men [41]. These factors in combination with higher androgen levels and a higher skeletal muscle mass lead to a higher strength and a higher endurance of male compared to female swimmers [10]. Wetsuits lift the

Table 3 Multi-level regression analyses for change in performance across years for men and women (Model 1) and with correction for multiple finishes (Model 2)

Model	*β*	SE (*β*)	Stand. ß	T	*P*
Annual fastest men competing with wetsuit					
1	0.000	1.083	0.000	0.000	1.000
2	0.000	1.083	0.000	0.000	1.000
Annual fastest men competing without wetsuit					
1	−4.100	3.272	−0.586	−1.253	0.299
2	−4.100	3.272	−0.586	−1.253	0.299
Annual fastest women competing with wetsuit					
1	−0.300	1.159	−0.148	−0.259	0.813
2	−0.300	1.159	−0.148	−0.259	0.813
Annual fastest women competing without wetsuit					
1	0.100	1.439	0.049	0.070	0.951
2	0.100	1.439	0.049	0.070	0.951
Annual fastest three men competing with wetsuit					
1	−3.800	2.419	−0.399	−1.571	0.140
2	−3.800	2.419	−0.399	−1.571	0.140
Annual fastest three men competing without wetsuit					
1	−4.717	2.040	-.555	−2.313	0.039
2	−4.717	2.040	-.555	−2.313	0.039
Annual fastest three women competing with wetsuit					
1	−3.433	2.193	-.398	−1.566	0.141
2	−3.433	2.193	-.398	−1.566	0.141
Annual fastest three women competing without wetsuit					
1	−0.775	2.191	−0.117	−0.354	0.732
2	−0.775	2.191	−0.117	−0.354	0.732

body in a more horizontal position by providing higher buoyancy. Therefore, less power is required to maintain the swimming-position leaving more energy to be expended in propulsion [23]. Because of the discussed physiological and anthropometrical features, female swimmers will be able to save more energy by using the floating features of wetsuits. Therefore, female swimmers might improve race times more than male swimmers. It is known that wetsuits lift the body in a more horizontal position by providing higher buoyancy. However, when we analyse the compression of the body due to the suit, one can expect that buoyancy could decrease as body mass is the same but body volume becomes lower. Regarding this aspect, buoyancy may decrease in both women and men. The reduction might be relatively higher in men with lower body fat then in women.

Female winners of the 'Marathon Swim' in Lake Zurich covering 26.4 km and wearing wetsuits were ~20.3% slower than male winners wearing wetsuits, while there was only a difference of ~8.0% between female and male winners without wearing a wetsuit. This finding contradicts our hypothesis that female swimmers would benefit more from wearing a wetsuit than male athletes. In the period from 2002 to 2012, a total number of only 12 female swimmers wearing a wetsuit finished the race leading to a mean of one annual female finisher wearing a wetsuit. Therefore, the statistical analyses concerning the sex difference in finishers wearing a wetsuit are most probably biased by the small number of female finishers. Future studies need to compare large groups of athletes to confirm the present findings.

Female swimmers have a lower skeletal muscle mass and a higher fat mass than male swimmers. This might lead to the assumption that female swimmers would present a more stable horizontal position in the water due to better buoyancy capability. On the other side, men have lower body fat and a higher skeletal muscle mass, so wetsuits might be more beneficial for male swimmers. Indeed, Cordain and Kopriva [23] suggested that the increase in performance by the increase in buoyancy might be of more benefit for leaner than for fatter subjects. This consideration might also be supported by the very recent finding that female open-water ultra-swimmers competing in the 46 km 'Manhattan Island Marathon Swim' with water temperatures <20°C were faster than male swimmers [17]. The increase in buoyancy might me more important than the reduction in drag. Toussaint *et al.* [24] showed that the effect of wetsuit on drag was not different between lighter female swimmer and heavier male swimmers. One might argue that men wearing a wetsuit might be faster than women in ~50 km at water temperatures <20°C.

Limitations of the study and implications for future research

This study was designed as a retrospective analysis of the performances in the 'Marathon Swim' in Lake Zurich and the 'LOST-Race'. We compared race times of swimmers wearing wetsuits with race times of swimmers competing without wearing wetsuits. This comparison could be biased by various factors like missing physiologic features [40], missing experience in ultra-endurance swimming and missing training volume [37]. A part of the participants in the 'Marathon Swim' in Lake Zurich are triathletes specialized in shorter swimming distances and therefore probably slower in this ultra-long distance. From the obtainable data we have no further information about the composition of the analysed groups. The resulting bias is a limitation of this study. Furthermore, the small number of female finishers in the 'Marathon Swim' in Lake Zurich might be a possible bias for the statistical analyses. Future studies would need to compare swimming performance in open-water ultra-distance swimming of distances of ~50 km at water temperatures <20°C. Men with

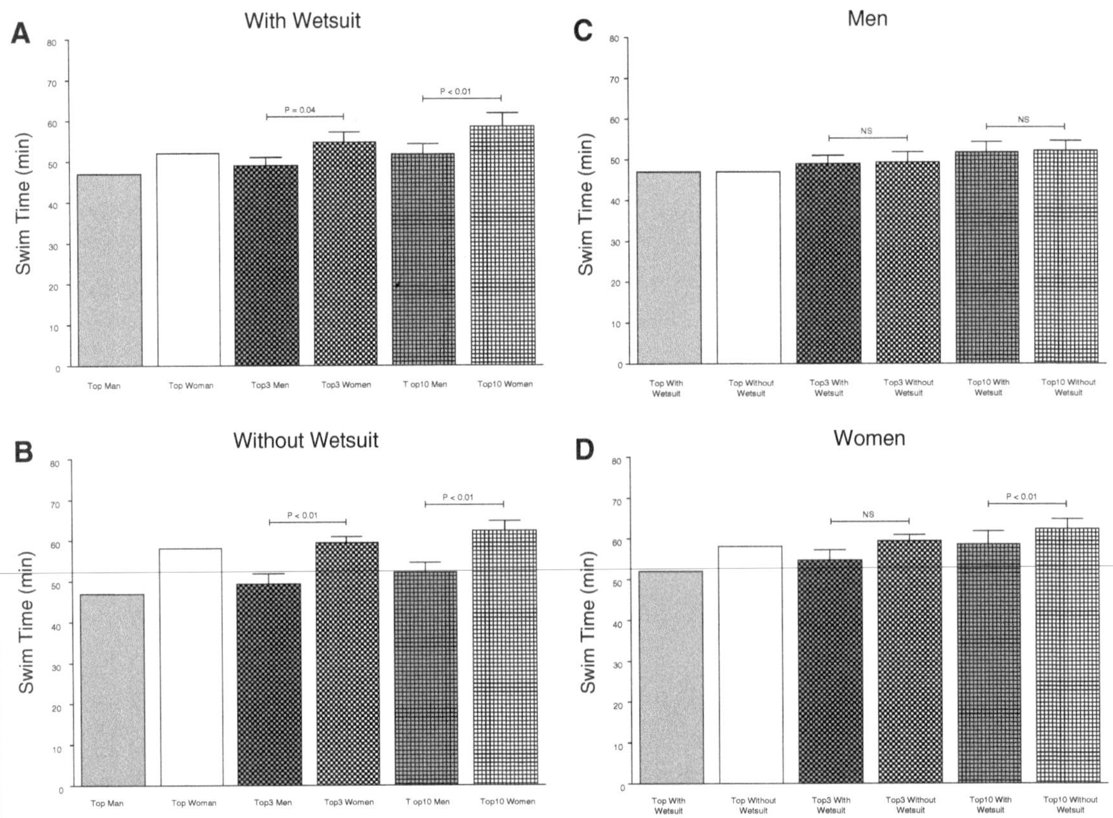

Figure 8 **Race times of the top ever, top three ever and top ten ever men and women in the 'LOST-Race' competing with (Panel A) and without (Panel B) wetsuit and the comparison between men (Panel C) and women (Panel D) competing with and without wetsuit.**

lower body fat might benefit from wearing a wetsuit under these conditions.

Conclusion

The present results suggest that swimmers competing in long and ultra-long-distance open-water swimming events could benefit from wearing wetsuits depending upon whether the fastest, the three fastest or the ten fastest swimmers were considered. This is consistent with existing literature reporting better performances in swimmers wearing wetsuits while swimming in indoor pools on short to middle distances. However, the present data suggest that the benefit of wearing wetsuits while competing in open-water swimming events may depend on various factors like water temperature and race distance as well as anthropometric and physiological features. Additionally, it depends upon the size of the analysed sample (*i.e.* the fastest, the three fastest or the ten fastest swimmers). The benefit of wearing wetsuits seemed also to be different in male and female swimmers. In order to obtain reliable information about the effect of wearing a wetsuit on swimming performance in long-distance and ultra-long-distance open-water swimming, additional studies should be conducted. It would be interesting to compare swimming times of the same male and female open-water ultra-distance swimmers once wearing wetsuits and once performing without wearing wetsuits. These studies should be conducted on different distances and with different water temperatures. As an additional procedure measurement of body temperature during the swim should be included. When the race conditions are known the obtained data could facilitate ultra-endurance swimmers and ironman swimmers the decision if wearing a wetsuit in a competition would be beneficial.

Competing interests
The authors declare that they have no competing interests.

Authors' contributions
SU collected the data and drafted the manuscript; CR performed the statistical analyses; TR and RL participated in the design of the study and

helped drafting the manuscript; and BK helped in interpretation of the results and drafting the manuscript. All authors read and approved the final manuscript.

Author details
[1]Institute of General Practice and for Health Services Research, University of Zurich, Zurich, Switzerland. [2]INSERM U1093, Faculty of Sport Sciences, University of Burgundy, Dijon, France. [3]Facharzt FMH für Allgemeinmedizin, Vadianstrasse 26, Gesundheitszentrum St. Gallen, St. Gallen, Switzerland.

References

1. Kim HJ, Lee YH, Kim CK: **Biomarkers of muscle and cartilage damage and inflammation during a 200 km run.** *Eur J Appl Physiol* 2007, **99:**443–447.
2. Knechtle B, Knechtle P, Rosemann T: **Low prevalence of exercise-associated hyponatremia in male 100 km ultra-marathon runners in Switzerland.** *Eur J Appl Physiol* 2011, **111:**1007–1016.
3. Lebus DK, Casazza GA, Hoffman MD, van Loan MD: **Can changes in body mass and total body water accurately predict hyponatremia after a 161-km running race?** *Clin J Sport Med* 2010, **20:**193–199.
4. Skenderi KP, Kavouras SA, Anastasiou CA, Yiannakouris N, Matalas AL: **Exertional Rhabdomyolysis during a 246-km continuous running race.** *Med Sci Sports Exerc* 2006, **38:**1054–1057.
5. Abou Shoak M, Knechtle B, Knechtle P, Rüst CA, Rosemann T, Lepers R: **Participation and performance trends in ultra cycling.** *Open Access J Sports Med* 2013, **4:**41–51.
6. Knechtle B, Knechtle P, Lepers R: **Participation and performance trends in ultra-triathlons from 1985 to 2009.** *Scand J Med Sci Sports* 2011, **21:**e82–e90.
7. Lepers R: **Analysis of Hawaii ironman performances in elite triathletes from 1981 to 2007.** *Med Sci Sports Exerc* 2008, **40:**1828–1834.
8. Fischer G, Knechtle B, Rüst CA, Rosemann T: **Male swimmers cross the English Channel faster than female swimmers.** *Scand J Med Sci Sports* 2013, **23:**e48–e55.
9. Eichenberger E, Knechtle B, Rüst CA, Knechtle P, Lepers R, Rosemann T: **No gender difference in peak performance in ultra-endurance swimming performance - analysis of the 'Zurich 12-h Swim' from 1996 to 2010.** *Chin J Physiol* 2012, **55:**346–351.
10. Eichenberger E, Knechtle B, Knechtle P, Rüst CA, Rosemann T, Lepers R, Senn O: **Sex difference in open-water ultra-swim performance in the longest freshwater lake swim in Europe.** *J Strength Cond Res* 2013, **27:**1362–1369.
11. NYC Swim: Website http://www.nycswim.org/Event/Event.aspx?Event_ID=2202, accessed September 09, 2013.
12. HBF Rottnest Channel Swim: Website http://www.rottnestchannelswim.com.au/, accessed September 09, 2013.
13. Sri Chinmoy Marathon Team Zürichsee-Schwimmen: http://ch.srichinmoyraces.org/main-ch, accessed September 09, 2013.
14. The Channel Swimming association: Website www.channelswimmingassociation.com, accessed September 09, 2013.
15. Rüst CA, Knechtle B, Rosemann T, Lepers R: **Women reduced the sex difference in open-water ultra-distance swimming La Traversée Internationale du Lac St-Jean, 1955–2012.** *Appl Physiol Nutr Metab* 2014, **39:**270–273.
16. Rüst CA, Lepers R, Rosemann T, Knechtle B: **Will women soon outperform men in open-water ultra-distance swimming in the 'Maratona del Golfo Capri-Napoli'?** *Springerplus* 2014, **3:**86.
17. Knechtle B, Rosemann T, Lepers R, Rüst CA: **Women outperform men in ultra-distance swimming - the 'Manhattan Island Marathon Swim' from 1983 to 2013.** *Int J Sports Physiol Perform* 2014. http://dx.doi.org/10.1123/ijspp.2013-0375.
18. L.O.S.T. Swimming (Lake Ontario Swim Team): Website http://lostswimming.com/?page_id=1544, accessed September 09, 2013.
19. L.O.S.T. Swimming (Lake Ontario Swim Team): Website http://lostswimming.com, accessed September 09, 2013.
20. Ironman World Championship: Website http://www.ironman.com/triathlon/events/ironman/world-championship/athletes/rules-and-regulations/swim-rules.aspx#ixzz2NRkj0H5O, accessed September 09, 2013.
21. Parsons L, Day SJ: **Do wet suits affect swimming speed?** *Br J Sports Med* 1986, **20:**129–131.
22. Tomikawa M, Shimoyama Y, Nomura T: **Factors related to the advantageous effects of wearing a wetsuit during swimming at different submaximal velocity in triathletes.** *J Sci Med Sport* 2008, **11:**417–423.
23. Cordain L, Kopriva R: **Wetsuits, body density and swimming performance.** *Br J Sports Med* 1991, **25:**31–33.
24. Toussaint HM, Bruinink L, Coster R, de Looze M, van Rossem B, van Veenen R, de Groot G: **Effect of a triathlon wet suit on drag during swimming.** *Med Sci Sports Exerc* 1989, **21:**325–328.
25. Tomikawa M, Nomura T: **Relationships between swim performance, maximal oxygen uptake and peak power output when wearing a wetsuit.** *J Sci Med Sport* 2009, **12:**317–322.
26. Chatard JC, Senegas X, Selles M, Dreanot P, Geyssant A: **Wet suit effect: a comparison between competitive swimmers and triathletes.** *Med Sci Sports Exerc* 1995, **27:**580–586.
27. Chatard JC, Wilson B: **Effect of fastskin suits on performance, drag, and energy cost of swimming.** *Med Sci Sports Exerc* 2008, **40:**1149–1154.
28. Toussaint HM, Truijens M, Elzinga MJ, van de Ven A, de Best H, Snabel B, de Groot G: **Effect of a Fast-skin 'body' suit on drag during front crawl swimming.** *Sports Biomech* 2002, **1:**1–10.
29. Benjanuvatra N, Dawson G, Blanksby BA, Elliott BC: **Comparison of buoyancy, passive and net active drag forces between Fastskin and standard swimsuits.** *J Sci Med Sport* 2002, **5:**115–123.
30. Starling RD, Costill DL, Trappe TA, Jozsi AC, Trappe SW, Goodpaster BH: **Effect of swimming suit design on the energy demands of swimming.** *Med Sci Sports Exerc* 1995, **27:**1086–1089.
31. Roberts BS, Kamel KS, Hedrick CE, McLean SP, Sharp RL: **Effect of a FastSkin suit on submaximal freestyle swimming.** *Med Sci Sports Exerc* 2003, **35:**519–524.
32. Knechtle B, Baumann B, Knechtle P, Rosemann T: **Speed during training and anthropometric measures in relation to race performance by male and female open-water ultra-endurance swimmers.** *Percept Mot Skills* 2010, **111:**463–474.
33. Sri Chinmoy Marathon Team Zürichsee-Schwimmen: Website http://ch.srichinmoyraces.org/veranstaltungen/zhlake/ accessed September 09, 2013.
34. L.O.S.T. Swimming (Lake Ontario Swim Team): Website www.lostswimming.com, accessed September 09, 2013.
35. Lowdon J, McKenzie D, Ridge B: **Effects of clothing and water temperature on swim performance.** *Aust J Sci Med Sport* 1992, **24:**33–38.
36. Tipton M, Eglin C, Gennser M, Golden F: **Immersion deaths and deterioration in swimming performance in cold water.** *Lancet* 1999, **354:**626–629.
37. Knechtle B, Baumann B, Knechtle B, Wirth A, Rosemann T: **A comparison of anthropometry between Ironman triathletes and ultra-swimmers.** *J Hum Kinet* 2010, **24:**57–64.
38. Ironman Zürich Switzerland: Website www.ironman.ch, accessed September 09, 2013.
39. Knechtle B, Wirth A, Baumann B, Knechtle P, Rosemann T, Oliver S: **Differential correlations between anthropometry, training volume, and performance in male and female Ironman triathletes.** *J Strength Cond Res* 2010, **24:**2785–2793.
40. Lepers R, Rüst CA, Stapley PJ, Knechtle B: **Relative improvements in endurance performance with age: evidence from 25 years of Hawaii Ironman racing.** *Age (Dordr)* 2013, **35:**953–962.
41. Lynch SL, Hoch AZ: **The female runner: gender specifics.** *Clin Sports Med* 2010, **29:**477–498.

2

Validity of treadmill- and track-based individual calibration methods for estimating free-living walking speed and VO_2 using the Actigraph accelerometer

Anthony Barnett[1,2*], Ester Cerin[1,3], Corneel Vandelanotte[4], Aya Matsumoto[5] and David Jenkins[6]

Abstract

Background: For many patients clinical prescription of walking will be beneficial to health and accelerometers can be used to monitor their walking intensity, frequency and duration over many days. Walking intensity should include establishment of individual specific accelerometer count, walking speed and energy expenditure (VO_2) relationships and this can be achieved using a walking protocol on a treadmill or overground. However, differences in gait mechanics during treadmill compared to overground walking may result in inaccurate estimations of free-living walking speed and VO_2. The aims of this study were to compare the validity of track- and treadmill-based calibration methods for estimating free-living level walking speed and VO_2 and to explain between-method differences in accuracy of estimation.

Methods: Fifty healthy adults [32 women and 18 men; mean (SD): 40 (13) years] walked at four pre-determined speeds on an outdoor track and a treadmill, and completed three 1-km self-paced level walks while wearing an Actigraph monitor and a mobile oxygen analyser. Speed- and VO_2-to-Actigraph count individual calibration equations were computed for each calibration method. Between-method differences in calibration equation parameters, prediction errors, and relationships of walking speed with VO_2 and Actigraph counts were assessed.

Results: The treadmill-calibration equation overestimated free-living walking speed (on average, by 0.7 $km \cdot h^{-1}$) and VO_2 (by 4.99 $ml \cdot kg^{-1} \cdot min^{-1}$), while the track-calibration equation did not. This was because treadmill walking, from which the calibration equation was derived, produced lower Actigraph counts and higher VO_2 for a given walking speed compared to walking on a track. The prediction error associated with the use of the treadmill-calibration method increased with free-living walking speed. This issue was not observed when using the track-calibration method.

Conclusions: The proposed track-based individual accelerometer calibration method can provide accurate and unbiased estimates of free-living walking speed and VO_2 from walking. The treadmill-based calibration produces calibration equations that tend to substantially overestimate both VO_2 and speed.

Keywords: Wearable devices, Energy expenditure, GPS, Physical activity, Exercise, Measurement

* Correspondence: Anthony.Barnett@acu.edu.au
[1]School of Exercise and Nutrition Sciences, Deakin University, 221 Burwood Highway, Burwood, VIC 3125, Australia
[2]Institute for Health & Ageing, Australian Catholic University, Melbourne, VIC 3000, Australia
Full list of author information is available at the end of the article

Background

Through its *Exercise is Medicine* initiative, the American College of Sports Medicine encourages regular assessment and inclusion of physical activity in treatment plans as a component of all medical care [1] and physical activity monitoring has become more common in clinical practice [2]. Clinical prescription and monitoring of post-diagnosis physical activity may benefit patients with specific disease states [3] and may be also used for morbidity prevention. Walking, a preferred and versatile form of physical activity, has been associated with decreased risks of cardiovascular disease and all-cause mortality [4, 5], decreased body fatness and resting diastolic blood pressure and increased aerobic fitness [6].

Due to between-individual variability in exercise capacity, health status and pre-intervention levels of physical activity, prescribed exercise intensity (e.g., walking speed) and duration should be determined on an individual basis. As self-reports can be influenced by poor recall and reporting bias, objective assessment is preferable when monitoring the patient during treatment [2]. Accelerometers are small, non-intrusive physical activity monitors appropriate for the clinical setting [2]. They are suited for objectively monitoring walking intensity, frequency and duration over many days. Actigraph is the most widely used brand of accelerometer [7].

Actigraph accelerometers have been extensively studied [8] and group calibration equations converting Actigraph outputs (counts per time unit) into energy expenditure (VO_2) and physical activity intensities have been derived [9]. However, substantial between-individual variations in the relationships between Actigraph outputs, walking speed and VO_2 have been reported [10–12]. This means that to accurately assess a patient's VO_2 and walking intensity, frequency and duration during treatment, determination of prescribed walking intensity should include establishment of individual specific accelerometer count, walking speed, VO_2 relationships [13]. This assessment can be undertaken using a graded intensity protocol on a treadmill or during overground walking. However, while equivalence was found between 3 % slope treadmill and horizontal overground walking counts using an RT3 accelerometer [14], Actigraph counts have been reported to be lower during horizontal treadmill than overground walking [12]. Conversely, VO_2 at a given walking speed has been found to be higher on a treadmill in comparison to overground walking [12, 15, 16]. Therefore, treadmill-based individual calibration may yield biased estimates of free-living level walking speed and VO_2.

A cost-effective, simple track-based calibration method to estimate free-living level walking speed and VO_2 using Actigraph counts has been proposed [10]. This method requires the participants to walk at four predetermined speeds controlled by a GPS monitor while wearing an Actigraph accelerometer and a mobile oxygen analyser. The calibration procedure is of similar duration to other calibration protocols [14, 17], but does not require a treadmill nor does it require a track. The protocol can be conducted on any flat, solid unobstructed pathway. Participants are asked to walk at four different speeds to allow the estimation of quadratic individual calibration equations, since the relationship between Actigraph output and energy expenditure from walking is curvilinear [18, 19]. This method has been shown to have good reliability and validity with respect to the estimation of free-living level walking speed [10]. However, its validity for the estimation of VO_2 from free-living level walking and how it compares to treadmill-based calibration is unknown.

The primary aim of this study was to compare the validity of the track- and treadmill-based calibration methods for estimating free-living level walking speed and VO_2 using the Actigraph monitor. The secondary aim was to explain between-method differences in accuracy of estimation of free-living walking speed and VO_2. To achieve the second aim, differences between calibration equations and relationships of calibration-trial walking speed with VO_2 and Actigraph counts obtained using the two methods were assessed.

Methods

Participants

Fifty healthy adults (32 women and 18 men), recruited either by word of mouth or by responding to local advertisements, participated in this study. The descriptive characteristics (mean (SD)) of the male participants were age 41 (14) years, height 182 (7) cm, and weight 81 (13) kg, and of the female participants age 40 (12) years, height 167 (7) cm, and weight 63 (9) kg. All participants provided written, informed consent and completed the Physical Activity Readiness Questionnaire. The Medical Research Ethics Committee at the University of Queensland approved the study.

Experimental protocol

Data were collected in 2006. Participants reported to the laboratory at the pre-arranged time (which varied across participants) and their height (stadiometer) and weight were measured. They then performed a treadmill walk, an outdoor track walk and a free-walk in randomized order on the same day. These walks were separated by a minimum of 10 min. For the duration of all walks VO_2 by indirect calorimetry (mobile oxygen analyser - Cosmed $K4b^2$, Cosmed, Rome, Italy) and accelerometer counts (Actigraph 7164) were recorded continuously. Clock times of the Cosmed, Actigraph and the GPS monitor (Forerunner 201, Garmin Ltd, Olathe, KS), used during the outdoor data collection, were synchronized to the time on the computer used to initialize the Actigraphs.

Treadmill walk (calibration trial)

Following a 5-min familiarization period and a 5-min recovery, participants walked on a calibrated treadmill (Bodyguard Cartier 312-C; Bodyguard Fitness, Quebec, Canada). The continuous protocol consisted of 5-min walks at 3.5, 4.5, 5.5 and 6.5 $km \cdot h^{-1}$. VO_2 ($ml \cdot kg^{-1} \cdot min^{-1}$) breath-by-breath data were collected over the last 2 min at each speed (allowing 3 min at each level to reach steady-state VO_2) and Actigraph count ($counts \cdot min^{-1}$) was taken as the mean of full minute counts at each speed.

Outdoor track walk (calibration trial)

The walk was carried out on a 400-m track with speed controlled by an investigator walking using a Forerunner GPS monitor and the subject instructed to maintain a distance of approximately 2 m behind. The Forerunner was set on lap speed function (400 m laps) as we have previously found this most appropriate for maintaining speed [10]. The walk was continuous and comprised of 400 m at 3.5, 4.5, and 5.5 $km \cdot h^{-1}$, and 800 m at 6.5 $km \cdot h^{-1}$. VO_2 and Actigraph count for each speed were determined in the same way as for the treadmill walk. The extra lap at 6.5 $km \cdot h^{-1}$ was undertaken to ensure time for adequate full-minute Actigraph counts. As each lap speed was determined separately and may vary from the protocol speed, VO_2 at this speed was determined for the last 2 min of each lap and the speeds and VO_2 values were then averaged.

Overground level walk (free-living walks)

A 3-km walk was undertaken on a flat, outdoor walking path. The walk comprised of 1-km walks at self-assessed slow, moderate and brisk pace in randomized order. To control distance and determine speed, participants wore a Forerunner with the lap function set to 1-km. At the end of each kilometer the Forerunner emitted an audible sound and the subject proceeded to the next walking pace (at 1 and 2 km) or the walk was terminated (at 3 km). Participants were asked to walk at a consistently maintained, self-paced speed without reference to the GPS display. For each 1-km walk, VO_2 ($ml \cdot kg^{-1} \cdot min^{-1}$) was estimated as the mean value from 3 min until the end point of the walk to ensure steady state values. Accelerometer counts during walking have some variation, even at a constant speed on a treadmill. To ensure the most representative count for that speed, Actigraph count was estimated as the mean of all full-minute counts during the 1 km. The minute counts at the transition from one speed to the next were excluded from the analysis.

Protocol without indirect calorimetry

To examine the possible effects of wearing a gas analyzer on the relationship between Actigraph counts and walking speed through alterations of walking patterns, a group of participants ($n = 15$) repeated the entire protocol without wearing the Cosmed.

Materials

GPS monitor

The Forerunner 201 GPS monitor was used to control calibration-trial walking speed and record distance and speed for the track walks. It was also used to control distance and record walking speed during the overground, free-living walks. GPS monitors determine speed by Doppler shift: the rate of change of satellite radio frequency signals resulting from movement of the receiver [20]. The Forerunner is designed to be worn on the wrist. We have previously found Forerunner and chronometer determined speeds during 400-m track walks ($n = 40$) to be virtually identical ($R^2 = 0.999$, slope = 1.001 and the intercept not significantly different from zero) [10]. Following each data collection period the Forerunner data were downloaded (Forerunner Logbook Version 2.5, Garmin Ltd, Olathe KS) to determine actual speeds for each trial component.

Actigraph accelerometer

The Actigraph 7164 is a uniaxial accelerometer and has been described in detail elsewhere [21]. Prior to each data collection session, the calibration of the Actigraph 7164 accelerometer was checked according to the manufacturer's instructions using the Actigraph Calibrator CAL71. All readings over the duration of the study were within the manufacturer's limits. The Actigraph was initialized using 1-min epochs. For the duration of each testing session, the Actigraph was worn against the skin at waist level on the right anterior-axillary line and held in place by a firmly-fitted elasticized belt. The Actigraph data were downloaded to a PC and the mean full-minute counts were determined for each speed in all trials.

Indirect calorimetry (VO_2)

Prior to each data collection session the mobile oxygen analyser was calibrated according to the manufacturer's instructions. A room air calibration and a reference calibration (15.1 % O_2 and 5.15 % CO_2) were undertaken to calibrate the oxygen and carbon dioxide analyzers. A 3-l syringe (Hans-Rudolf) was used to calibrate the flow turbine and a delay calibration was carried out to adjust for lag time between the expiratory flow and gas measurements. Ambient air calibrations were also undertaken prior to each trial. Breath-by-breath data were collected continuously during all trials and the mean VO_2 ($ml \cdot kg^{-1} \cdot min^{-1}$) for the relevant time period for each trial was determined. VO_2 data were adjusted for the mass of the equipment worn (1.2 kg).

Statistical analysis

Average full-minute Actigraph counts · min^{-1}, walking speed ($km \cdot h^{-1}$), and VO_2 ($ml \cdot kg^{-1} \cdot min^{-1}$) were computed for all walks, at all speeds in all participants.

Determination of individual calibration equations

To obtain individual calibration equations, ordinary-least-squares (OLS) linear regression models were used. Previous studies have found a linear relationship between calibration-trial walking speed and accelerometer counts [8, 10]. Consequently, to estimate individual calibration equations, calibration-trial walking speed (four walking speeds per calibration method per subject) was regressed onto Actigraph counts. This resulted in two walking speed-Actigraph counts individual calibration equations per subject, one for each calibration method. Each of these calibration equations yielded an intercept and a slope (regression coefficient) for each subject. The intercept value represented the estimated walking speed at 0 Actigraph counts · min^{-1}, while the slope represented the estimated increase in walking speed associated with a 1 unit increase in Actigraph counts · min^{-1} for a particular subject for a particular calibration method. As a curvilinear relationship between accelerometer counts and VO_2 has been reported [22], VO_2 was regressed onto Actigraph counts (linear) and their squared value (quadratic term). Two VO_2-Actigraph counts individual calibration equations per subject were obtained, one for each calibration method. Each of these calibration equations yielded an intercept and two slopes for each subject. The intercept value represented the estimated VO_2 at 0 Actigraph counts · min^{-1}, while the sum of the two slopes represented the estimated increase in VO_2 associated with a 1 unit increase in Actigraph counts · min^{-1} for a particular subject for a particular calibration method. The fit of linear and quadratic regression equations to the data were compared by examining their coefficients of determination (R^2).

Determination and comparison of validity of treadmill- and track-based calibration equations (primary study aim)

To examine and compare the validity of the two individual calibration methods for estimating free-living walking speed and VO_2 using Actigraph counts, differences between expected (estimated using the individual calibration equations) and actual (measured) values of speed and VO_2 collected during 1-km self-paced (free-living) walks were computed (here named prediction errors; Δ). The average prediction error for a calibration method represents its systematic bias of prediction. A value significantly greater than 0 indicates positive bias (overestimation of speed or VO_2), while a value significantly smaller than zero indicates negative bias (underestimation of speed or VO_2). Linear mixed models with random intercepts and slopes were then used to estimate: 1) the prediction errors for each calibration method for the 'average' subject walking at the 'average' speed (obtained by centering free-living walking speed around the group mean) on the free-living walks; 2) the between-participant (i.e., between-subject) variability in prediction errors; and 3) the extent to which the magnitude of the prediction errors (linearly or quadratically, based on an inspection of scatter plots with lowess smoother lines) depended on actual free-living walking speed.

Linear mixed models were used because the assumption of independency of observations was violated. Specifically, there were three sets of data points per subject, one for each free-living walk (participants undertook three 1-km self-paced walks). Thus, in order to obtain correct standard errors of regression coefficients, we needed to use models that take into account the existing correlation among data collected from the same participants. Linear mixed models with random intercepts and slopes were also considered appropriate in the context of this study because they fit the notion of person-specific effects implied by individual calibration by allowing intercept and slopes to vary across participants. They provide estimates of the values of the intercept and slopes for the average participant and also provide information on the variability of these across participants. Parameters were estimated using the residual maximum likelihood method (REML). The Aikake Information Criterion (AIC) and a modified likelihood ratio test [23] were used to test the significance of the between-subject variability in regression parameters. Additionally, standard errors of estimate (here called total error; TE) were computed using the formula: $TE = [\Sigma(Y - Y')^2/(N - 1)]^{0.5}$, where Y is the measured value of speed or VO_2 during a free walk, Y' is the estimated value of speed or VO_2 computed using the individual calibration equations and N is the number of observations. Total error represents the standard error of estimate obtained when an existing equation (e.g., an individual calibration equation) is cross-validated (i.e., its accuracy in predicting the newly collected data is evaluated) [24].

Differences between calibration methods (secondary study aim)

Between-method differences in individual calibration equations Paired t-tests were used to test the significance of the differences in OLS slopes and intercepts between the treadmill and track individual calibration equations described above for each outcome (speed and VO_2). Paired t-tests were used because estimates of two calibration equations obtained on the same participants were compared. While the relationship between Actigraph counts and speed was linear and quantified by one slope, the relationship between Actigraph counts and VO_2 was quadratic and quantified with two slopes (one for the linear and the other for quadratic term). Consequently, for VO_2, between-method differences were tested for the sum of the slopes of the linear and quadratic terms of Actigraph counts (representing the 'effect' of Actigraph counts). Also, *t*-tests were used to test the significance of the between-method difference in expected values of speed and VO_2 (as predicted by the respective individual calibration equations) at tertiles of Actigraph counts. The tertile values of Actipraph counts per minute were determined from data collected during the calibration trials.

Between-method differences in relationships of calibration-trial walking speed with Actigraph counts and VO_2 Linear mixed models with random intercepts and slopes were used to account for dependency in the observations (multiple data points per subject) and the fact that the relationships of interest vary across individuals. Actigraph counts $\cdot$ min^{-1} were modeled as a function of the linear term of calibration-trial walking speed centred at 3.5 $km \cdot h^{-1}$ (the lowest walking speed used), the calibration method (treadmill vs. track), and the interaction term of calibration-trial walking speed and calibration method, while VO_2 was modeled as a function of the linear and quadratic terms of speed, the calibration method, and the interaction terms of the calibration method and the linear and quadratic terms of speed. Between-participant variation in regression coefficients was tested using the modified likelihood ratio test and by comparing AIC values. Parameter estimation was performed using the REML method. However, to evaluate the significance of interaction terms, models with and without interaction terms were compared using AIC values estimated with the maximum likelihood method. Six additional sets of models as those described above but each with speed centered at one of the three remaining calibration-trial walking speeds (4.5, 5.5, and 6.5 $km \cdot h^{-1}$) and with different calibration-method reference categories (treadmill vs. track) were constructed. They were used to obtain estimates of the mean Actigraph counts and VO_2 (and associated standard errors and between-individual variability measures) at each calibration-trial walking speed and for each calibration method.

Differences in relationships between Actigraph counts and walking speed when wearing and not wearing the mobile oxygen analyser

Linear mixed models with random intercepts and slopes were used. A model for each component of the experimental protocol (i.e., treadmill-based calibration; track-based calibration; and free-living walks) was constructed to test the differences in calibration-trial and free-living walking speed-Actigraph counts relationship when wearing and not wearing the mobile oxygen analyser. Actigraph counts $\cdot$ min^{-1} were modeled as a function of the linear term of walking speed, the experimental condition (with or without the mobile oxygen analyser), and the interaction term of walking speed and experimental condition. Non-significant interaction terms were omitted from the models to re-estimate main effects. Speed was centered at 3.5 $km \cdot h^{-1}$. All slopes and intercepts were allowed to vary across participants. All analyses were conducted using Stata 9.0 (StataCorp) and MLwiN 2.02 (Multilevel Models Project).

Results

Determination of individual calibration equations

A linear relationship between Actigraph counts and speed of walking during the calibration trials was supported by individual scatter plots with superimposed fitted lines. Support was found for the hypothesis of a quadratic relationship between Actigraph counts and VO_2 from walking. The individual R^2 values from the quadratic regression models ranged from 0.91 to 1.00 (mean = 0.99). In contrast, the individual R^2 values from linear regression models ranged from 0.84 to 1.00 (mean = 0.95).

Determination and comparison of validity of treadmill- and track-based calibration equations (primary study aim)

Overall, the track-based individual calibration equations estimated free-living walking speed and VO_2 consumption from Actigraph counts more accurately than did the treadmill-based calibration equations (Table 1). The treadmill method tended to overestimate speed as well as VO_2 (see intercept values in Table 1). For example, for the 'average' subject walking at a speed of 5.7 $km \cdot h^{-}1$, which was the average speed of free-living walks across all individuals, the treadmill-based calibration equation overestimated actual speed by 0.7 $km \cdot h^{-1}$ (95 % CI: 0.56, 0.87 $km \cdot h^{-1}$). The average magnitude of the prediction error depended on the actual speed of walking (Fig. 1 and slopes for speed and $speed^2$ in Table 1). In contrast, the track-based calibration equation did not tend to yield biased estimates of speed for the average subject (Fig. 1) and the prediction error did not depend on actual free-living walking speed. Additionally, the between-individual variations in prediction error across values of actual free-living walking speed were smaller for the track-based than the treadmill-based method (smaller between-individual variability of intercept and slopes) (Table 1).

For the average subject walking at 5.7 $km \cdot h^{-1}$, the treadmill-based calibration equations overestimated VO_2 on average by 4.99 $ml \cdot kg^{-1} \cdot min^{-1}$ (95 % CI: 3.97,

Table 1 Regression models of prediction error for walking speed and VO_2 by calibration method

	Prediction error for speed of walking ($km \cdot h^{-1}$)		Prediction error for VO_2 ($ml \cdot kg^{-1} \cdot min^{-1}$)	
Regression parameter	Treadmill method	Track method	Treadmill method	Track method
	Coefficient (95 % CI) BPV	Coefficient (95 % CI) BPV	Coefficient (95 % CI) BPV	Coefficient (95 % CI) BPV
Intercept	0.71*** (0.56, 0.87) 0.54***	0.02 (−0.05, 0.08) 0.19***	4.99*** (3.96, 6.00) 3.26***	0.33 (−0.06, 0.73) 1.10***
Speed	0.15*** (0.06, 0.24) 0.26***	−0.04 (−0.09, 0.01) 0.08*	1.16*** (0.58, 1.75) 1.57***	−0.29** (−0.49, −0.08) –
(Speed)^2	−0.06* (−0.11, −0.01) 0.13*	−0.04 (−0.09, 0.01) 0.10**	– – –	−0.20* (−0.38, −0.02) –

These regression models report on average prediction error by calibration method (see intercept values) and if this error depends on walking speed (see regression coefficients for speed and speed^2). Coefficient = regression coefficient; 95 % CI = 95 % confidence interval; BPV = Between-participant variability in regression coefficients (expressed as standard deviations); – = not applicable (not significant regression term or between-participant variability based on a comparison of fixed and random slope models); *$p < .05$; **$p < .01$; ***$p < .001$. Speed ($km \cdot h^{-1}$) was centered at 5 · 7 km.h^{-1}

6.01 $ml \cdot kg^{-1} \cdot min^{-1}$; Table 1), which corresponds to ~ 1.43 METs (units of metabolic equivalent). The magnitude of the prediction error increased with an increase in actual free-living walking speed (Fig. 2 and slopes for speed and speed^2 in Table 1). No significant bias was observed for the track-based calibration method. The prediction error appeared to be curvilinearly related to actual speed of walking (slopes for speed and speed^2 in Table 1 and Fig. 2). However, when free-living walking speeds outside of the range of speeds used to derive the quadratic calibration equations for VO_2 (3.3 $km \cdot h^{-1}$ > speed > 6.7 $km \cdot h^{-1}$) were excluded from the model, the effect of speed on the prediction error for VO_2 was not significantly different from zero ($b_{speed} = -0.01$, 95 % CI; −0.36, 0.33; $b_{speed\wedge 2} = 0.05$, 95 % CI; −0.26, −0.40). The between-participant variability in prediction error for VO_2 was larger for the treadmill than the track calibration method (between-participant variability of intercepts: 3.28 vs. 1.10; see Table 1).

The total error (TE) for the estimation of free-living walking speed from Actigraph counts was 0.9 $km \cdot h^{-1}$ for the treadmill calibration method and 0.3 $km \cdot h^{-1}$ for the track method. The TE for the estimation of VO_2 from Actigraph counts was 6.11 $ml \cdot kg^{-1} \cdot min^{-1}$ for the treadmill and 1.50 $ml \cdot kg^{-1} \cdot min^{-1}$ for the track method. When limiting the computation to values of free-living walking speed that were within the ranges of values used for deriving the calibration trials the TE decreased to 5.49 $ml \cdot kg^{-1} \cdot min^{-1}$ and 1.45 $ml \cdot kg^{-1} \cdot min^{-1}$, respectively. These estimates need to be interpreted with care, especially those for the treadmill method, since the prediction error was dependent on free-living walking speed (Table 1).

Differences between calibration methods (secondary study aim)

Between-method difference in calibration equations

For given tertile values of Actigraph counts per minute (within the examined range of calibration-trial walking speeds), the treadmill method tended to give higher estimates of speed than the track method (Table 2). This

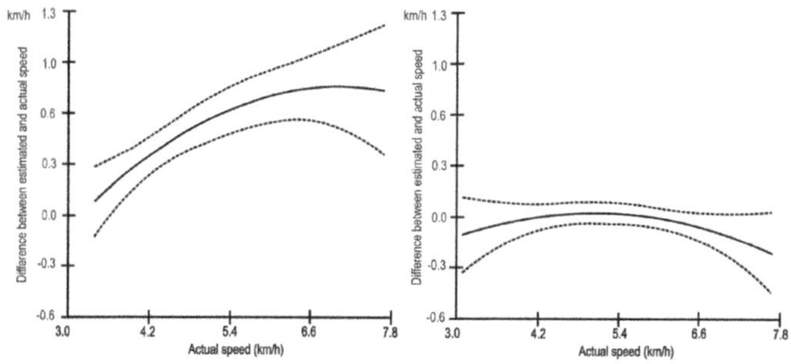

Fig. 1 Prediction error of walking speed on the free-living walks for treadmill- and track-based calibration methods. Figure 1 shows the relationship between mean prediction error for walking speed ($km \cdot h^{-1}$) and actual walking speed ($km \cdot h^{-1}$) on the free-living walks for the treadmill- (*left*) and track-based (*right*) calibration methods. *Dashed lines* are 95 % confidence intervals

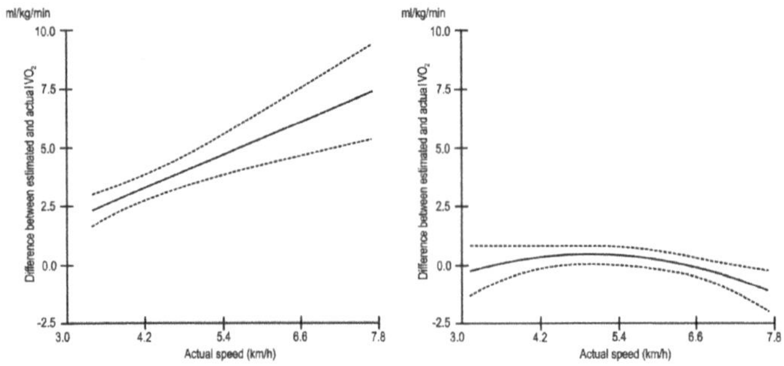

Fig. 2 Prediction error of VO_2 on the free-living walks for the treadmill- and track-based calibration methods. Figure 2 shows the relationship between mean prediction error for VO_2 (ml · kg^{-1} · min^{-1}) and actual walking speed (km · h^{-1}) on the free-living walks for the treadmill- (*left*) and track-based (*right*) calibration methods. *Dashed lines* are 95 % confidence intervals

was due to higher average slope values for the calibration equations based on the treadmill method (see slopes of Actigraph counts in Table 2). Significant between-method differences in intercepts were found for the calibration equations of VO_2 with the treadmill method yielding greater values of VO_2 than the track calibration method (Table 2). When examining the differences in estimated VO_2 at tertiles of Actigraph counts, it was found that the treadmill method was associated with higher estimates of VO_2. These differences ranged from 2.85 to 4.79 ml · kg^{-1} · min^{-1} of oxygen (see estimated speed or VO_2 at specific Actigraph counts in Table 2).

Between-method differences in relationships of calibration-trial walking speed with Actigraph counts and VO_2 Walking on a treadmill was associated with higher levels of VO_2 than walking on a track at a given speed (Tables 3 and 4). For the average subject walking at 3.5 km · h^{-1}, overground walking was associated with a 2.25 (95 % CI: −2.62, −1.89) ml · kg^{-1} · min^{-1} lower VO_2 as compared to walking on the treadmill (see regression coefficient for C. method in Table 3). This difference tended to remain stable across walking speeds (see regression coefficient for C. method by Speed in Table 3). Walking on a treadmill was associated with lower Actigraph counts than overground walking on a track. The average subject walking at 3.5 km · h^{-1} had 262 (95 % CI: 158, 366) more counts per minute when walking on a track than when walking on a treadmill (Table 4). This between-method difference tended to increase by 198 (95 % CI: 147, 249) counts · min^{-1} for each km · h^{-1} increase in speed. Between-participant variations in the between-method difference in VO_2 and Actigraph counts were observed (see BPV in Tables 3 and 4).

Differences in relationships between Actigraph counts and calibration-trial and free-living walking speeds when wearing and not wearing the mobile oxygen analyser No significant main effects of experimental condition (i.e., wearing and not wearing the mobile oxygen analyser) on Actigraph counts were found (all p-values > 0.13; in models without experimental condition by speed of walking interaction terms). Also, no significant interaction effects of experimental condition and speed of walking on

Table 2 Differences in speed and VO_2 calibration regression equation estimates between treadmill- and track-calibration methods

Regression estimates	Speed (km · h^{-1})	VO_2 (ml · kg^{-1} · min^{-1})
	Mean Δ treadmill – track (95 % CI)	Mean Δ treadmill – track (95 % CI)
Intercepts of calibration equations	−0.02 (−0.16, 0.12)	2.00 (1.18, 2.82)***
Slopes of Actigraph counts[a]	$1.5 \cdot 10^{-4}$ ($1.1 \cdot 10^{-4}$, $1.9 \cdot 10^{-4}$)***	$2.9 \cdot 10^{-4}$ ($4.1 \cdot 10^{-4}$, $9.8 \cdot 10^{-4}$)
Estimated speed or VO_2 at specific Actigraph counts		
... 2000 counts · min^{-1}	0.29 (0.19, 0.39)***	2.85 (0.42, 3.28)***
... 3300 counts · min^{-1}	0.49 (0.37, 0.61)***	3.71 (3.18, 4.24)***
... 4600 counts · min^{-1}	0.70 (0.54, 0.86)***	4.79 (3.87, 5.71)***

[a]While the relationship between Actigraph counts and speed was linear and quantified by one slope, the relationship between Actigraph counts and VO_2 was quadratic and quantified with two slopes (one for the linear and the other for quadratic term). Consequently, for VO_2, between-method differences were tested for the sum of the slopes of the linear and quadratic terms of Actigraph counts (representing the total 'effect' of Actigraph counts). Δ treadmill – track = difference between regression estimates of treadmill and track calibration equations; CI = confidence interval; ***$p < .001$

Table 3 Differences between calibration methods in regression models of Actigraph counts and VO_2 predicted by walking speed

Parameter	Outcome: Actigraph counts · min^{-1} Coef IPV	(95 % CI)	Outcome: VO_2 (ml · kg^{-1} · min^{-1}) Coef IPV	(95 % CI)
Intercept	1442*** 418***	(1319, 1565)	8.96*** 2.13***	(8.37, 9.55)
Speed (centred at 3.5km.h^{-1})	1134*** 247***	(1061, 1207)	1.56*** 0.61**	(1.28, 1.84)
(Speed)^2	– –	–	0.30*** 0.22***	(0.21, 0.40)
C. method	262*** 302***	(158, 366)	−2.25*** 1.10***	(−2.62, −1.89)
C. method × Speed	198*** 145***	(147, 249)	−0.33 0.37*	(−0.68, 0.02)
C. method × (Speed)^2	– –	–	0.08 0.12*	(−0.03, 0.19)

These regression models report on differences between calibration methods in Actigraph counts and VO_2 at 3.5 km.h^{-1}walking speed (see regression coefficients for C. method), and differences between calibration methods in associations of walking speed with Actigraph counts and VO_2 (see regression coefficients for C. method by Speed and C. method by (Speed^2)). Coef = regression coefficient; 95 % CI = 95 % confidence interval; BPV = between-participant variability in regression coefficients (expressed as standard deviations); – = not applicable; C. method = calibration method (treadmill is reference category); $^*p < .05$; $^{**}p < .01$; $^{***}p < .001$

Actigraph counts were observed (all p-values > 0.48). Finally, the data did not give sufficient support for the presence of between-individual variations in these effects.

Discussion

The primary aim of this study was to compare the validity of a new track-based and a traditional treadmill-based calibration method for estimating free-living level walking speed and VO_2 using the Actigraph monitor. The treadmill-based method tended to overestimate speed and, especially, VO_2 while the overground method did not. These differences were due to treadmill walking being associated with higher VO_2 and lower Actigraph counts than overground walking for a given walking speed. The average magnitude of overestimation of VO_2 (for the treadmill method) at the average free-living walking speed of 5.7 km · h^{-1} corresponded to approximately 1.4 METs. The average model prediction error increased at higher speeds of walking by ~ 0.33 METs per km · h^{-1}. The model prediction error for VO_2 varied across individuals and, for the average free-living walking speed, was (mean ± SD) 4.99 ± 3.28 ml · kg^{-1} · min^{-1}. This implies that the treadmill-based calibration method might overestimate energy expenditure from brisk level walking by more than 2 METs in 20 % of the population represented by the study sample. According to the data from this study, the average overestimation of energy expenditure for slow pace walking (up to 4 km · h^{-1}) would be approximately 0.86 METs and that for strolling (up to 3.2 km · h^{-1}) 0.60 METs. This is a substantial bias. The U.S. Department of Health and Human Services physical activity recommendations advocate at least 150 min of moderate-intensity physical activity per week [25], corresponding to activities of 3–5.9 METs [26]. While slow level walking is usually considered light-intensity activity (2.5 METs), with a positive bias of 0.86 METs, treadmill-based calibration equations would tend to classify it into moderate-intensity activities. Overestimation of energy expenditure by treadmill-based calibration equations has been also reported by Yngve and colleagues [12].

Table 4 Actigraph counts and VO_2 at given walking speeds by calibration method

	Actigraph counts · min^{-1}				VO_2 (ml · kg^{-1} · min^{-1})			
	Treadmill calibration		Track calibration		Treadmill calibration		Track calibration	
Speed (km · h^{-1})	mean (SE)	BPV	mean (SE)	BPV	mean (SE)	BPV	mean (SE)	BPV
3.5	1442 (63)	418	1704 (58)	454	8.96 (0.30)	2.32	6.86 (0.28)	2.38
4.5	2567 (78)	515	3036 (75)	556	10.62 (0.33)	2.73	8.47 (0.30)	2.73
5.5	3711 (199)	692	4368 (102)	741	13.44 (0.38)	3.80	10.86 (0.35)	3.80
6.5	4846 (136)	902	5700 (132)	963	16.53 (0.47)	5.75	14.02 (0.44)	6.35

Mean = estimated mean outcome value at specific walking speed; SE = standard error of the estimated mean; BPV = Between-participant variability around the mean (expressed as standard deviations). These estimates were obtained from models similar to those presented in Table 3 with speed centered at the various calibration-trial walking speeds (3.5, 4.5, 5.5, and 6.5 km.h^{-1}) and with a different calibration-method reference category

However, their study did not specifically focus on walking and they used pooled rather than individual calibration equations.

With regards to estimation of free-living walking speed, the average prediction error associated with the treadmill-based method ranged from 0.4 to 1.0 $km \cdot h^{-1}$ across the examined speeds. There was considerable between-individual variability in the prediction error as well as in the effect of actual free-living walking speed on the magnitude of prediction error. In contrast, the track-based method did not produce a significant bias at the average free-living walking speed (for the average subject), and the model prediction error was not significantly related to free-living walking speed. The results of this study, hence, give support for the hypothesis that treadmill walking is sufficiently different from overground walking in both biomechanical characteristics and energy economy to raise concerns about its utility for the estimation of free-living walking from accelerometer counts.

The secondary aim of this study was to explain differences in estimation of free-living walking speed and VO_2 between the two calibration methods. Lower Actigraph counts and higher VO_2 at a given speed during treadmill as compared to overground walking were found. These may be explained by reported differences in gait parameters during treadmill and overground walking. Most studies have found higher cadence and shorter stride length during treadmill walking [16, 27–30]. Reducing stride length at a given speed is associated with decreased vertical centre of mass displacement (flatter trajectory) and increased energy cost of walking [31, 32]. The flatter trajectory would be expected to result in lower accelerometer counts and a negative relationship between Actigraph counts and cadence has been reported [33].

In the present study, the total energy cost of walking on a treadmill was 33 % higher than that of walking on a track at 3.5 $km \cdot h^{-1}$. The proportional difference in energy cost between treadmill and overground walking decreased at higher walking speeds. This is in accordance with the finding that the economy of work production by muscles in flat-trajectory walking increased linearly with walking speed, while that of normal walking plateaus at a speed of around 4.5 $km \cdot h^{-1}$ [32].

Substantial between-individual variations were observed in intercepts and slopes of the calibration equations (Table 2). Additionally, between-individual differences were also found in the average prediction error of free-living level walking speed and VO_2. These between-individual differences were substantially greater for the treadmill- than the track-based calibration equations. This might be due to the fact that overground walking patterns are significantly more variable across individuals than are treadmill walking patterns. In this respect, Warabi and colleagues [28] observed greater between-individual variability in stance period, heel contact time and ratio of rear foot phase over stance period in overground, level walking than treadmill walking. This means that treadmill-based calibration equations cannot capture a significant portion of between-individual variability in walking patterns, while track-based calibration equations can. This explains why the between-individual variability in model prediction error from track-based equations were less than half those from the treadmill-based calibration equations.

Study limitations

The track-based calibration method validated in this study is limited in the sense that it can accurately work only for overground walking on flat ground. It is obvious that calibration equations obtained with this method will produce negatively biased estimates of VO_2 for graded walking or walking whilst carrying a weight. However, most walking appears to take place on flat ground [34]. Importantly, sedentary individuals, who are the principal target of public health initiatives, would seem more likely to adopt level than graded walking as a form of activity. Consequently, this calibration method has the potential to accurately estimate VO_2 from most daily ambulatory activities. However, future studies will need to verify this conjecture.

Disadvantages associated with overground calibration, such as lack of a suitable walking area and bad weather, are potential downsides to using overground rather than treadmill calibration. Therefore, despite the relative inaccuracy, the convenience of treadmill calibration may be preferred in some situations. Additionally, it would be more accurate, and therefore appropriate, for treadmill calibrations to be used when patients were to undertake their walking program on a treadmill.

There are several models of Actigraph accelerometers: the 7164 used in this study and new generation models such as the GT1M, GT3X and the GT3X+. Although this study was conducted using an old Actigraph model, there is correspondence between the output of the old and new models. A comparison between the 7164 and 3 versions of the GT1M found no statistically significant differences between outputs during walking and running [35] and, when using the low frequency extension range, the output of the GT3X+ has been shown to be comparable with the 7164 [8, 36]. Also, the mechanisms causing the differences in calibration equations across the treadmill and overground methods do not depend on the monitor and are likely to affect calibration equations obtained using different Actigraph models and other accelerometers in a similar way.

This study was based on a sample of 50 healthy adults. The literature recommends more than 100 participants to obtain reliable estimates of between-individual variability [37]. However, this study aimed at exploring whether the relationships of Actigraph counts with speed and VO_2 from walking varied across individuals rather than providing reliable estimates of between-individual variability in the population. Future larger-scale studies may want to find an answer to this issue as well as find predictors of between-individual differences in these relationships.

Conclusions

In conclusion, this study suggests that the proposed track-based individual calibration method can provide accurate and unbiased estimates of free-living walking speed and VO_2 from walking. It also suggests that treadmill-based calibration should be avoided as it produces calibration equations that tend to substantially overestimate both VO_2 and speed. Apart from being more valid, the proposed track-based calibration can be undertaken at a lower cost than its treadmill counterpart and may be more acceptable to individuals, especially to those who are not accustomed to walking on a treadmill.

Competing interests

The authors declare that they have no competing interests.

Authors' contributions

AB conceptualized the track-based calibration method. AB and EC designed the study and led the writing of the manuscript. CV, AM and DJ coordinated the study, collected the data and critically commented on versions of the manuscript. All authors read and approved the final manuscript.

Acknowledgements

This study was funded by the University of Queensland New Staff Research Start-Up Fund, Ref 20040001471 (Australia). Ester Cerin is supported by an Australian Research Council Future Fellowship (FT3), #FT140100085. The authors thank Mr. Gary Wilson for his technical advice and assistance.

Author details

[1]School of Exercise and Nutrition Sciences, Deakin University, 221 Burwood Highway, Burwood, VIC 3125, Australia. [2]Institute for Health & Ageing, Australian Catholic University, Melbourne, VIC 3000, Australia. [3]School of Public Health, The University of Hong Kong, Pokfulam, Hong Kong SAR. [4]Centre for Physical Activity Studies, Central Queensland University, Rockhampton, QLD 4702, Australia. [5]Baker IDI Heart and Diabetes Institute, 75 Commercial Road, Melbourne, VIC 3004, Australia. [6]School of Human Movement and Nutrition Sciences, The University of Queensland, Brisbane, QLD 4072, Australia.

References

1. American College of Sports Medicine. Exercise is medicine. 2014. http://exerciseismedicine.org/index.php. Accessed 2 Jan 2015.
2. Trost SG, O'Neil M. Clinical use of objective measures of physical activity. Br J Sports Med. 2014;48:178–81.
3. Bao PP, Zheng Y, Nechuta S, Gu K, Cai H, Peng P, et al. Exercise after diagnosis and metabolic syndrome among breast cancer survivors: a report from the Shanghai Breast Cancer Survival Study. Cancer Causes Control. 2013;24:1747–56.
4. Hamer M, Chida Y. Walking and primary prevention: a meta-analysis of prospective cohort studies. Br J Sports Med. 2008;42:238–43.
5. Kelly P, Kahlmeier S, Götschi T, Orsini N, Richards J, Roberts N, et al. Systematic review and meta-analysis of reduction in all-cause mortality from walking and cycling and shape of dose response relationship. Int J Behav Nutr Phys Act. 2014;11:132.
6. Murphy MH, Nevill AM, Murtagh EM, Holder RL. The effect of walking on fitness, fatness and resting blood pressure: a meta-analysis of randomised, controlled trials. Prev Med. 2007;44:377–85.
7. Bassett DR, Troiano RP, McClain JJ, Wolff DL. Accelerometer-based physical activity: total volume per day and standardized measures. Med Sci Sports Exerc. 2015;47:883–8.
8. Cain KL, Conway TL, Adams MA, Husak LE, Sallis JF. Comparison of older and newer generations of ActiGraph accelerometers with the normal filter and the low frequency extension. Int J Behav Nutr Phys Act. 2013;10:51.
9. Crouter SE, DellaValle DM, Haas JD, Frongillo EA, Bassett DR. Validity of ActiGraph 2-regression model, Matthews cut-points, and NHANES cut-points for assessing free-living physical activity. J Phys Act Health. 2013;10:504–14.
10. Barnett A, Cerin E. Individual calibration for estimating free-living walking speed using the MTI monitor. Med Sci Sports Exerc. 2006;38:761–7.
11. Schutz Y, Weinsier S, Terrier P, Durrer D. A new accelerometric method to assess the daily walking practice. Int J Obes. 2002;26:111–8.
12. Yngve A, Nilsson A, Sjönström M, Ekelund U. Effect of monitor placement and of activity setting on the MTI accelerometer output. Med Sci Sports Exerc. 2003;35:320–6.
13. Aadland E, Steene-Johannessen J. The use of individual cut points from treadmill walking to assess free-living moderate to vigorous physical activity in obese subjects by accelerometry: is it useful? BMC Med Res Methodol. 2012;12:172.
14. Vanhelst J, Béghin L, Rasoamanana P, Theunynck D, Meskini T, Iliescu C, et al. Calibration of the RT3 accelerometer for various patterns of physical activity in children and adolescents. J Sports Sci. 2010;28:375–9.
15. Berryman N, Gayda M, Nigam A, Juneau M, Bherer L, Bosquet L. Comparison of the metabolic energy cost of overground and treadmill walking in older adults. Eur J Appl Physiol. 2012;112:1613–20.
16. Stolze H, Kuhtz-Buschbeck JP, Mondwurf C, Boczek-Funcke A, Jöhnk K, Deuschl G, et al. Gait analysis during treadmill and overground locomotion in children and adults. Electroencephalogr Clin Neurophysiol. 1997;105:490–7.
17. Ozemek C, Cochran HL, Strath SJ, Byun W, Kaminsky LA. Estimating relative intensity using individualized accelerometer cutpoints: the importance of fitness level. BMC Med Res Methodol. 2013;13:53.
18. Browning RC, Baker EA, Herron JA, Kram R. Effects of obesity and sex on the energetic cost and preferred speed of walking. J Appl Physiol. 2006;100:390–8.
19. Schmitz KH, Treuth M, Hannan P, McMurray R, Ring KB, Catellier D, et al. Predicting energy expenditure from accelerometry counts in adolescent girls. Med Sci Sports Exerc. 2005;37:155–61.
20. Schutz Y, Herren R. Assessment of speed of human locomotion using a differential satellite global positioning system. Med Sci Sports Exerc. 2000;32:642–6.
21. Tyron WW, Williams R. Fully proportional actigraphy: a new instrument. Behav Res Methods Instrum Comput. 1996;28:393–403.
22. Crouter SE, Clowers KG, Bassett Jr DR. A novel method for using accelerometer data to predict energy expenditure. J Appl Physiol. 2006;100:1324–31.
23. Snijders TAB, Bosker RJ. Multilevel analysis. London: Sage Publications; 1999.
24. Mahar MT, Rowe DA. Construct validity in physical activity research. In: Welk GJ, editor. Physical activity assessments for health-related research. Champaign: Human Kinetics; 2002. p. 51–72.
25. U.S. Department of Health and Human Services. 2008 Physical activity guidelines for Americans. Washington, DC: U.S. Department of Health and Human Services; 2008. Office of Disease Prevention and Health Promotion Publication No. U0036. http://www.health.gov/paguidelines. Accessed 2 Jan 2015.
26. Ainsworth BE, Haskell WL, Herrmann SD, Meckes N, Bassett Jr DR, Tudor-Locke C, et al. 2011 Compendium of Physical Activities: a second update of codes and MET values. Med Sci Sports Exerc. 2011;43:1575–81.
27. Alton F, Baldey L, Caplan S, Morrissey MC. A kinematic comparison of overground and treadmill walking. Clin Biomech (Bristol, Avon). 1998;13:434–40.
28. Warabi T, Kato M, Kiriyama K, Yoshida T, Kobayashi N. Treadmill walking and overground walking of human subjects compared by recording sole-floor reaction force. Neurosci Res. 2005;53:343–8.
29. Watt JR, Franz JR, Jackson K, Dicharry J, Riley PO, Kerrigan DC. A three-dimensional kinematic and kinetic comparison of overground and treadmill walking in healthy elderly subjects. Clin Biomech (Bristol, Avon). 2010;25:444–9.

30. Wearing SC, Reed LF, Urry SR. Agreement between temporal and spatial gait parameters from an instrumented walkway and treadmill system at matched walking speed. Gait Posture. 2013;38:380–4.
31. Gordon KE, Ferris DP, Kuo AD. Metabolic and mechanical energy costs of reducing vertical center of mass movement during gait. Arch Phys Med Rehabil. 2009;90:136–44.
32. Massaad F, Lejeune TM, Detrembleur C. The up and down bobbing of human walking: a compromise between muscle work and efficiency. J Physiol. 2007;582:789–99.
33. Brage S, Wedderkopp N, Franks PW, Andersen LB, Froberg K. Reexamination of validity and reliability of the CSA monitor in walking and running. Med Sci Sports Exerc. 2003;35:1447–54.
34. Levine JA, Baukol PA, Westerterp KR. Validation of the Tracmor triaxial accelerometer system for walking. Med Sci Sports Exerc. 2000;33:1593–7.
35. John D, Tyo B, Bassett DR. Comparison of four ActiGraph accelerometers during walking and running. Med Sci Sports Exerc. 2010;42:368–74.
36. Ried-Larsen M, Brønd JC, Brage S, Hansen BH, Grydeland M, Andersen LB, et al. Mechanical and free living comparisons of four generations of the Actigraph activity monitor. Int J Behav Nutr Phys Act. 2012;9:113.
37. Hox J. Multilevel analysis: techniques and applications. Mahwah, NJ: Lawrence Erlbaum Associates; 2002. p. 304.

3

Do non-elite older runners slow down more than younger runners in a 100 km ultra-marathon?

Christoph A Rüst[1], Thomas Rosemann[1], Matthias A Zingg[1] and Beat Knechtle[1,2*]

Abstract

Background: This study investigated changes in normalised running speed as a proxy for effort distribution over segments in male elite and age group 100 km ultra-marathoners with the assumption that older runners would slow down more than younger runners.

Methods: The annual ten fastest finishers (*i.e.* elite and age group runners) competing between 2000 and 2009 in the '100 km Lauf Biel' were identified. Normalised average running speed (*i.e.* relative to segment 1 of the race corrected for gradient) was analysed as a proxy for pacing in elite and age group finishers. For each year, the ratio of the running speed from the final to the first segment for each age cohort was determined. These ratios were combined across years with the assumption that there were no 'extreme' wind events etc. which may have impacted the final relative to the first segment across years. The ratios between the age cohorts were compared using one-way ANOVA and Tukey's post-hoc test. The ratios between elite and age group runners were investigated using one-way ANOVA with Dunnett's multiple comparison post-hoc tests. The trend across age groups was investigated using simple regression analysis with age as the dependent variable.

Results: Normalised average running speed was different between age group 18–24 years and age groups 25–29, 30–34, 35–39, 40–44, 45–49, 50–54, 55–59 and 65–69 years. Regression analysis showed no trend across age groups ($r^2 = 0.003$, $p > 0.05$).

Conclusion: To summarize, (*i*) athletes in age group 18–24 years were slower than athletes in most other age groups and (*ii*) there was no trend of slowing down for older athletes.

Keywords: Running, Men, Long-distance, Master athlete

Background

Ultra-marathon running involves any race distance longer than the classical marathon distance of 42.195 km [1]. Among the different race distances, the 100 km ultra-marathon distance is highly popular where the number of female and male finishes increased exponentially in the last 50 years [2].

For 100 km ultra-marathon running, age [3] and the origin [2] of the fastest finishers are known. For elite 100 km ultra-marathoners, the pacing strategy has also been investigated [4]. Faster runners started at a faster running speed, finished the race within 15% of their starting speed, and maintained their starting speed for ~50 km before slowing down [4]. Slower runners showed a greater percent decrease in running speed and were unable to maintain their initial pace for as long [4]. Apart from elite 100 km ultra-marathoners, the pacing strategy has recently been investigated for elite 161 km ultra-marathoners [5]. Winners in 161 km ultra-marathons remained relatively close behind the leading runners before taking the lead in the middle half of the race, and then avoided slowing down as much as the other top runners in the latter stages of the race [5].

Age seems to be an important predictor variable in running performance in marathoners [6] and ultra-marathoners [7,8]. Running performance in male 100 km ultra-marathoners was fastest at the age of ~35 years [3] and decreased after the age of ~45 years [9]. Since running performance in 100 km ultra-marathon running decreased with increasing age, we may assume that older runners (*i.e.* older than ~35-45 years) will slow

* Correspondence: beat.knechtle@hispeed.ch
[1]Institute of Primary Care, University of Zurich, Zurich, Switzerland
[2]Gesundheitszentrum St. Gallen, Vadianstrasse 26, 9001 St. Gallen, Switzerland

down faster during a 100 km than younger runners (*i.e.* younger than ~35-45 years). This study investigated changes in normalised running speed (as a proxy for effort distribution) over segments in male elite and age group 100 km ultra-marathoners in the '100 km Lauf Biel' held in Switzerland [10] with the assumption that older runners would slow down more than younger runners [11].

Methods

Ethics

The present study was approved by the Institutional Review Board of St. Gallen, Switzerland, with a waiver of the requirement for informed consent given that the study involved the analysis of publicly available data.

The race

The '100 km Lauf Biel' held in Biel, Switzerland, is one of the most traditional and largest 100 km ultra-marathons in Europe [10]. The race takes place during the night of the first weekend in June. All runners start the race at 10:00 p.m. The race held is held as one large loop of 100 km with a total change in altitude of ~645 m. The organizer provides a total of 17 aid stations offering an abundant variety of food and beverages such as hypotonic sports drinks, tea, soup, caffeinated drinks, water, bananas, oranges, energy bars and bread. The athletes are allowed to be supported by a cyclist for additional food and clothing, if necessary. The fastest finishers complete the race within ~7 h and arrive early in the morning at around sunrise of the following day.

Data sampling and data analysis

The data set for this study was obtained from the race website of the '100 km Lauf Biel' [10]. In this race, split times at three time stations (TS) at TS1 'Oberramsern' (38 km), TS2 'Kirchberg' (56.1 km) and TS3 'Bibern' (76.7 km) were taken using an electronic chip during the 2000–2009 period. In earlier and later years, split times were taken differently. For each edition, we extracted the ten fastest men overall and the ten fastest male age group finishers for 5-year age groups (*i.e.* 18–24 yrs, 25–29 yrs, 30–34 yrs, 35–39 yrs, 40–44 yrs, 45–49 yrs, 50–54 yrs, 55–59 yrs, 60–64 yrs, and 65–69 yrs). Since too few women competed in this race, we had to limit to male competitors. Normalised average running speed (*i.e.* relative to segment 1 of the race corrected for gradient) was analysed as a proxy for pacing in elite (*i.e.* the annual fastest) and age group finishers. Elite runners (*i.e.* the annual ten fastest) were considered as a kind of 'gold standard' of pacing from start to end since we may assume that they have got their pacing right. We obtained for each year the ratio of the running speed from the final to the first segment for elite athletes and each age cohort. We combined these ratios across years with the assumption that there were no 'extreme' wind events etc. that may have impacted the final segment relative to the first across years. We plotted then the mean and standard deviations of these ratios on a graphic with age cohort on the X-axis.

Statistical analysis

The ratios between the age cohorts were compared using measures one-way analysis of variance (ANOVA) and Tukey's post-hoc test. The ratios between elite runners and age group runners were investigated using one-way ANOVA with Dunnett's multiple comparison post-hoc tests. The trend across age groups (*i.e.* from elite runners to runners in age group 65–69 years) seemed linear and we conducted a simple regression analysis with age as the dependent variable. Statistical analyses were performed using IBM SPSS Statistics (Version 22, IBM SPSS, Chicago, IL, USA) and GraphPad Prism (Version 6.01, GraphPad Software, La Jolla, CA, USA). Significance was accepted at $p < 0.05$ (two-tailed for *t*-tests). Data are given as mean ± standard deviation (SD).

Results

Normalised average running speed was different between athletes ranked in age group 18–24 years and athletes ranked in age groups 25–29 years, 30–34 years, 35–39 years, 40–44 years, 45–49 years, 50–54 years, 55–59 years and 65–69 years (Table 1 and Figure 1). Regression analysis showed no trend across age groups ($r^2 = 0.003$, $p > 0.05$).

Discussion

We investigated changes in normalised running speed over segments in male elite and age group 100 km ultra-marathoners in the '100 km Lauf Biel' held in Switzerland and hypothesized that older runners would slow down more than younger runners. The most important findings were (*i*) athletes in age group 18–24 years were slower than athletes in most other age groups and (*ii*) older runners were not slowing down compared to younger runners.

Athletes in age group 18–24 years were slower than athletes in older age groups

A rather surprising finding was that athletes in age group 18–24 years were slower than athletes in most other age groups. Age has been reported as a major predictor variable in 100 km apart from running speed during training and weekly running kilometers [7]. The age of 18–24 years is not the typical age of successful ultra-marathoners [8]. Ultra-marathoners are typically ~45 years old and male ultra-marathoners achieve their fastest running times at the age of ~ 30–49 years [3,8]. Cejka et al. [3] investigated the change in 100 km running performance and in the age

Table 1 Results of the Tukey's multiple comparisons test

	Mean 1	Mean 2	Mean diff.	95% CI of diff.	Significance
18-24 *versus* 25-29	90.69	92.65	−1.96	−3.90 to −0.02	*
18-24 *versus* 30-34	90.69	94.03	−3.34	−5.28 to −1.40	****
18-24 *versus* 35-39	90.69	93.67	−2.98	−4.92 to −1.04	****
18-24 *versus* 40-44	90.69	94.20	−3.51	−5.45 to −1.57	****
18-24 *versus* 45-49	90.69	94.03	−3.34	−5.28 to −1.40	****
18-24 *versus* 50-54	90.69	93.46	−2.77	−4.71 to −0.83	***
18-24 *versus* 55-59	90.69	93.57	−2.88	−4.82 to −0.94	***
18-24 *versus* 60-64	90.69	92.19	−1.50	−3.44 to 0.43	ns
18-24 *versus* 65-69	90.69	93.06	−2.37	−4.31 to −0.43	**
25-29 *versus* 30-34	92.65	94.03	−1.37	−3.31 to 0.56	ns
25-29 *versus* 35-39	92.65	93.67	−1.01	−2.95 to 0.92	ns
25-29 *versus* 40-44	92.65	94.20	−1.55	−3.49 to 0.38	ns
25-29 *versus* 45-49	92.65	94.03	−1.37	−3.31 to 0.56	ns
25-29 *versus* 50-54	92.65	93.46	−0.80	−2.74 to 1.13	ns
25-29 *versus* 55-59	92.65	93.57	−0.91	−2.85 to 1.02	ns
25-29 *versus* 60-64	92.65	92.19	0.46	−1.47 to 2.40	ns
25-29 *versus* 65-69	92.65	93.06	−0.40	−2.34 to 1.53	ns
30-34 *versus* 35-39	94.03	93.67	0.35	−1.58 to 2.29	ns
30-34 *versus* 40-44	94.03	94.20	−0.17	−2.11 to 1.76	ns
30-34 *versus* 45-49	94.03	94.03	−0.00	−1.94 to 1.93	ns
30-34 *versus* 50-54	94.03	93.46	0.56	−1.37 to 2.50	ns
30-34 *versus* 55-59	94.03	93.57	0.45	−1.48 to 2.39	ns
30-34 *versus* 60-64	94.03	92.19	1.83	−0.10 to 3.77	ns
30-34 *versus* 65-69	94.03	93.06	0.96	−0.97 to 2.90	ns
35-39 *versus* 40-44	93.67	94.20	−0.53	−2.47 to 1.40	ns
35-39 *versus* 45-49	93.67	94.03	−0.35	−2.29 to 1.58	ns
35-39 *versus* 50-54	93.67	93.46	0.21	−1.73 to 2.15	ns
35-39 *versus* 55-59	93.67	93.57	0.09	−1.84 to 2.03	ns
35-39 *versus* 60-64	93.67	92.19	1.48	−0.45 to 3.42	ns
35-39 *versus* 65-69	93.67	93.06	0.60	−1.33 to 2.54	ns
40-44 *versus* 45-49	94.20	94.03	0.17	−1.76 to 2.11	ns
40-44 *versus* 50-54	94.20	93.46	0.74	−1.19 to 2.68	ns
40-44 *versus* 55-59	94.20	93.57	0.63	−1.30 to 2.57	ns
40-44 *versus* 60-64	94.20	92.19	2.01	0.07 to 3.95	*
40-44 *versus* 65-69	94.20	93.06	1.14	−0.79 to 3.08	ns
45-49 *versus* 50-54	94.03	93.46	0.56	−1.37 to 2.50	ns
45-49 *versus* 55-59	94.03	93.57	0.45	−1.48 to 2.39	ns
45-49 *versus* 60-64	94.03	92.19	1.84	−0.10 to 3.78	ns
45-49 *versus* 65-69	94.03	93.06	0.96	−0.97 to 2.90	ns
50-54 *versus* 55-59	93.46	93.57	−0.11	−2.05 to 1.82	ns
50-54 *versus* 60-64	93.46	92.19	1.27	−0.66 to 3.21	ns

Table 1 Results of the Tukey's multiple comparisons test *(Continued)*

50-54 *versus* 65-69	93.46	93.06	0.39	−1.54 to 2.33	ns
55-59 *versus* 60-64	93.57	92.19	1.38	−0.55 to 3.32	ns
55-59 *versus* 65-69	93.57	93.06	0.51	−1.42 to 2.45	ns
60-64 *versus* 65-69	92.19	93.06	−0.87	−2.81 to 1.06	ns

* = $p < 0.05$, ** = $p < 0.01$, *** = $p < 0.001$, **** = $p < 0.0001$, ns = non significant.

of peak performance for 100 km ultra-marathoners competing worldwide between 1960 and 2012. Considering the world-wide trend in 100 km ultra-running, the fastest race times are achieved by athletes at the age of ~40 years. Running speed of the top ten athletes increased across calendar years from 8.67 km/h to 15.65 km/h and the age of the top ten athletes increased across calendar years from 29 years to 40 years [3]. The age of the best ultra-marathon performance is also higher in the longest race distances. When athletes competing from 6 hours to 10 days were investigated, the age of the best ultra-marathon performance increased with increasing race duration [12].

Athletes at the age of ~20 years may also have too little experience in ultra-marathon running. Younger ultra-marathoners have not finished as many ultra-marathoners as older ultra-marathoners have [8]. Hoffman and Krishnan [13] investigated the past-year and lifetime exercise patterns of 1,345 current and former ultra-marathoners. Median age at the first ultra-marathon was 36 years, and the median number of years of regular running before the first ultra-marathon was 7 years [13]. Active ultra marathoners had a previous year median running distance of 3,347 km, which was minimally related to age but mostly related to their longest ultra-marathon competition of the year. A recent study investigating ultra-marathoners competing from 6 hours to 10 days showed that the age of peak ultra-marathon performance increased with increasing number of finishes [12].

Older runners were not slowing down compared to younger runners

We hypothesized that older runners would slow down more than younger runners. However, older runners were not slowing down compared to elite and younger age group runners. Apart from the aspect of experience discussed above, also psychological reasons for decision taking in pacing strategy should also be considered [14-16]. The performance level of the athletes seems the most important reason. Renfree and St Clair Gibson [14] investigated the influence of different performance standards on pacing strategy in elite female marathoners competing in the IAAF Women's Marathon Championship in 2009. Athletes finishing in the first 25% of all finishers ran the first two 5-km segments at a relatively lower speed than athletes in the second to fourth 25% of all finishers but at a relatively higher sped after km 35. The authors concluded that psychological factors influenced decision

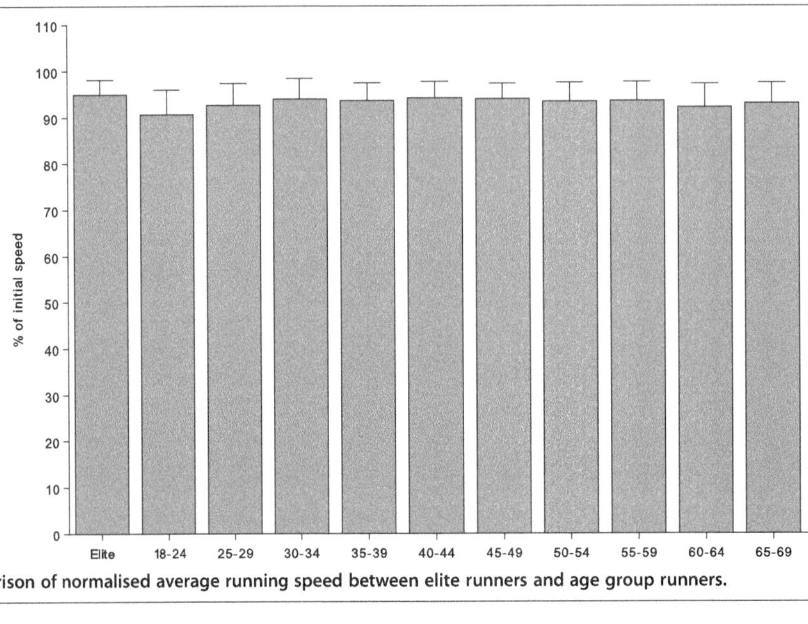

Figure 1 **Comparison of normalised average running speed between elite runners and age group runners.**

making in a major competitive event. Similarly, top runners in the 'New York City Marathon' tried to maintain an even pacing profile by avoiding an excessively fast start which might result in a decrease in running speed in the second half of the race [15]. Esteve-Lanao et al. [16] investigated the pacing strategy in World Cross Country Championships between 2007 and 2013. They showed that top ten finishers displayed a more even pacing compared to the other finishers who showed a more positive pacing.

Limitations

This study is limited since the aspect of environmental factors such as wind has not been included. An actual study reported that headwind was significant factor in running speed variability in the world record marathon runs in 2008 and 2011 [17].

Practical applications

This analysis shows that athletes in age group 18–24 years were slower than athletes in most other age groups. Younger athletes intending to compete in a 100 km should be very cautious about pacing and are recommended to complete many shorter races in advance.

Conclusions

In summary, the comparison of normalized average running speed between elite runners and age group runners showed that athletes in age group 18–24 years were slower than athletes in most other age groups. Across age groups, there was no trend of slowing down for older athletes compared to younger athletes.

Competing interests

The authors declare that they have no competing interests.

Authors' contributions

All authors have been involved in collecting data, writing, drafting and revising the manuscript. CR performed the statistical analyses and drafted the manuscript. BK and MZ collected the data. TR participated in the design of the study and revised the manuscript critically for important intellectual content. All authors read and approved the final manuscript.

References

1. Ultramarathon Running Resource. website www.ultramarathonrunning.com.
2. Cejka N, Rüst CA, Lepers R, Onywera V, Rosemann T, Knechtle B. Participation and performance trends in 100-km ultra-marathons worldwide. J Sports Sci. 2014;32:354–66.
3. Cejka N, Knechtle B, Rüst CA, Rosemann T, Lepers R. Performance and age of the fastest female and male 100-km ultra-marathoners worldwide from 1960 to 2012. J Strength Cond Res. [Epub ahead of print].
4. Lambert MI, Dugas JP, Kirkman MC, Mokone GG, Waldeck MR. Changes in running speeds in a 100 km ultra-marathon race. J Sports Sci Med. 2004;3:167–73.
5. Hoffman MD. Pacing by winners of a 161-km mountain ultramarathon. Int J Sports Physiol Perform. 2014;9:1054–6.
6. March DS, Vanderburgh PM, Titlebaum PJ, Hoops ML. Age, sex, and finish time as determinants of pacing in the marathon. J Strength Cond Res. 2011;25:386–91.
7. Knechtle B, Knechtle P, Rosemann T, Lepers R. Predictor variables for a 100-km race time in male ultra-marathoners. Percept Mot Skills. 2010;111:681–93.
8. Knechtle B. Ultramarathon runners: nature or nurture? Int J Sports Physiol Perform. 2012;7:310–2.
9. Knechtle B, Rüst CA, Rosemann T, Lepers R. Age-related changes in 100-km ultra-marathon running performance. Age (Dordr). 2012;34:1033–45.
10. 100 km Lauf Biel. website www.100km.ch.
11. Abbiss CR, Laursen PB. Describing and understanding pacing strategies during athletic competition. Sports Med. 2008;38:239–52.
12. Knechtle B, Valeri F, Zingg MA, Rosemann T, Rüst CA. What is the age for the fastest ultra-marathon performance in time-limited races from 6 h to 10 days? Age (Dordr). 2014;36:9715.
13. Hoffman MD, Krishnan E. Exercise behavior of ultramarathon runners: baseline findings from the ULTRA study. J Strength Cond Res. 2013;27:2939–45.
14. Renfree A, St Clair Gibson A. Influence of different performance levels on pacing strategy during the Women's World Championship marathon race. Int J Sports Physiol Perform. 2013;8:279–85.
15. Santos-Lozano A, Collado PS, Foster C, Lucia A, Garatachea N. Influence of sex and level on marathon pacing strategy: insights from the New York City race. Int J Sports Med. 2014;35:933–8.
16. Esteve-Lanao J, Larumbe-Zabala E, Dabab A, Alcocer-Gamboa A, Ahumada F. Running World Cross Country Championships: a unique model for pacing study. Int J Sports Physiol Perform. 2014;9:1000–5.
17. Angus SD. Did recent world record marathon runners employ optimal pacing strategies? J Sports Sci. 2014;32:31–45.

4

Sporting programs for inactive population groups: factors influencing implementation in the organized sports setting

Linda Ooms[1*], Cindy Veenhof[2], Nicolette Schipper-van Veldhoven[3] and Dinny H. de Bakker[1,4]

Abstract

Background: The organized sports sector has received increased attention as a setting to promote health-enhancing physical activity (HEPA) to the general population. For significant public health impact, it is important that successful HEPA programs are widely adopted, implemented and continued as ongoing practice. The importance of evaluating the context in which programs are implemented has been identified as critical. However, little research has focused on understanding the organized sports implementation context, including factors facilitating and impeding implementation. In this study, the main factors influencing implementation of HEPA programs in the organized sports setting were studied.

Methods: Fourteen sporting programs in the Netherlands aimed at increasing participation in sports by inactive population groups and funded within the National Action Plan for Sport and Exercise (NAPSE) were investigated. The programs were developed by ten Dutch National Sports Federations (NSFs) and implemented by different sports clubs in the Netherlands over a 3-year implementation period (June 2008–June 2011). The qualitative research component involved yearly face-to-face interviews (i.e. fourteen interviews each year, $n = 12$ program coordinators) and a group meeting with the program coordinators of the NSFs ($n = 8$). Cross-case comparisons and thematic analyses were performed to identify and categorize important facilitating and impeding factors respectively. The quantitative research component, used to identify the most important facilitating and impeding factors across all sporting programs, consisted of ranking of factors according to importance by the program coordinators ($n = 12$).

Results: Different factors act during six identified (implementation) phases. When comparing factors across phases, several key learnings were evident. Successful implementation relied, for example, on program design and enthusiastic individuals within sporting organizations. On the other hand, inactive people were hard to reach and participation of sports clubs was not self-evident. The findings were discussed in a broader context.

Conclusions: This study adds to the knowledge base concerning the implementation of sporting programs, aimed at inactive people, in the organized sports setting. The main factors facilitating and impeding implementation were identified. The results of this study can be used by sports practitioners and policy makers when developing and implementing HEPA programs in this setting.

Keywords: Organized sports setting, Sporting program, Implementation, Health-enhancing physical activity promotion

* Correspondence: l.ooms@nivel.nl
[1]Netherlands Institute for Health Services Research (NIVEL), PO Box 1568, 3500 BN Utrecht, The Netherlands
Full list of author information is available at the end of the article

Background

Participation in regular physical activity impacts positively on physical and mental health [1–3]. However, an alarming number of people are not sufficiently active to receive these benefits. In the Netherlands, this comprises 34 % of adults and 51 % of children and youth [4]. Worldwide, 31 % of adults do not engage in enough physical activity. According to the World Health Organization, insufficient physical activity is the fourth leading risk factor for mortality causing an estimated 3.2 million deaths globally each year [5]. The greatest improvements in health are obtained by increasing physical activity levels of the most inactive people, rather than getting those already active to do a little more [3].

Given the low levels of physical activity, many countries are investing resources in strategies to increase population-wide levels of health-enhancing physical activity (HEPA) [6]. Recognizing the complexity of physical activity behavior and the multiple factors influencing this behavior, more attention is paid to holistic and multi-disciplinary approaches to physical activity promotion. One such approach commonly used in health promotion is the settings-based approach, which is based on the idea that changes in people's health and health behavior are easier to achieve if health promoters focus on settings instead of individuals [7]. This approach builds on the Ottawa Charter of 1986 that stated: "Health is created and lived by people within the settings of their everyday life; where they learn, work, play and love [8]." The settings-based approach has an ecological perspective and acknowledges the multiple levels of influence on behavior, i.e. personal, organizational, environmental and policy. It, therefore, takes into account the complexity of systems and societies in which people make their health choices [9–12]. The settings-based approach has been applied to different settings, like schools and workplaces [7, 9, 10]. A setting that has received increased attention in promoting health, including HEPA, is the organized sports sector [13–23].

There is large potential for the organized sports sector as a setting in which to promote HEPA to the general population, given the large numbers of participants, the extent of community reach and the availability of many different sports. The Dutch sports system, for example, consists of 76 National Sports Federations, approximately 25,000 sports clubs and 4.8 million sports club members [24]. Another positive aspect of participation in organized sports is that those people who are involved in organized sports are significantly more likely to meet levels of HEPA than those who are not [4]. Moreover, it has been suggested that participation in sports clubs is associated with improved psychosocial health in addition to improvements (in health) attributable to participation in physical activity [25]. Also, the social and informal nature of the sports setting has been argued to be advantageous for promoting HEPA [22, 26]. Therefore, further increasing physical activity levels of sports participants who do not meet levels of HEPA and increasing participation in sports by inactive population groups seems to be a promising strategy to enhance public health.

Different countries have already been investing resources in the organized sports sector for promoting health. Good examples of strategies can be derived from Australia. Early Australian efforts, for example, focused on delivering health promotion messages at sponsored sporting events [21]. More recently, the focus is on the creation of healthy (e.g. smoke-free settings, healthy food choices) and welcoming sporting environments as a means to increase participation in sport for health benefits [14–16, 19]. In Finland, guidelines have been developed for youth sports clubs to develop, implement and assess health promotion within their activities [23]. Another example is the "11 for Health" program, a football-based health education program, which was developed by the Fédération Internationale de Football Association (FIFA) Medical Assessment and Research Center for children in Africa. The program combined learning football skills with health education messages and was implemented in different countries in Africa [27]. Furthermore, in the Netherlands, the Dutch Ministry of Health, Welfare and Sport initiated the National Action Plan for Sport and Exercise (NAPSE). This program was aimed at increasing the number of Dutch people meeting levels of HEPA [18]. Within the NAPSE, National Sports Federations (NSFs) were asked to develop sporting programs aimed at increasing participation in sports by inactive population groups. Seventeen NSFs developed twenty-four programs which were pilot tested by a dozen local sports clubs. Based on results of a process evaluation and monitoring study [28], fourteen programs of ten NSFs were funded to be implemented more broadly by sports clubs in the Netherlands over a 3-year implementation period. Examples include a 6-week training program for adult novice runners and an adjusted form of weekly hockey for seniors played with soft balls and soft sticks.

For significant public health impact, it is important that successful HEPA programs are widely adopted, implemented and continued as ongoing practice. In this regard, the importance of evaluating the context in which programs are implemented has been identified as critical [29–33]. The primary provider of sport in the Netherlands and in many other countries (e.g. Australia, Finland, Norway) is the sports club. Any HEPA sporting program to be implemented must be interpreted and implemented by the representatives of the sports club, which are mainly volunteers and whose main focus is on providing sports activities and organizing sports competitions [32, 33]. Nonetheless, sports clubs are aware of the healthy outcomes of sport and sometimes use this as legitimacy for their activities [33].

To date, little research has focused on understanding the organized sports implementation context, including factors facilitating and impeding implementation of health programs or activities [29–31]. A few studies have been conducted in Australia concerning the development of healthy and welcoming environments (HWEs) in sports clubs [14–16, 19]. Important factors facilitating the implementation of HWEs, both for the funded State Sporting Associations and implementing sports clubs, were the availability of funding; guidance and support (e.g. training, advice, materials); understanding of benefits (i.e. increased participation at sports clubs); a positive attitude towards the HWE concept; and support of key individuals within the organization. The barriers to implementation were mainly the inverse of the facilitators. Other important barriers were State Sporting Associations' limited capacity and power to influence activities at the club level; limited capacity of volunteer-based sports clubs; no clear outlining of expectations and responsibilities; unrealistic timeframes for implementation; and structural impediments (e.g. a lack of facilities, costs). Furthermore, the Finnish "Health Promoting Sports Club" guidelines provide fourteen consecutive steps for local youth sports clubs to enhance health promotion as part of their activities [23]. The guidelines are divided into policy development actions and activities a club needs to perform before the club actors (e.g. coaches) can implement health promotion as part of their daily practice, like "prioritize the most relevant health promotion aims" (policy development) and "educate coaches and other club officials" (practice development). For each guideline, the rationale and practical examples are provided.

The aforementioned studies have a relatively broad focus when it comes to health promotion. Less is known about the implementation of HEPA programs per se. The promotion of HEPA is more closely related to the core business of sporting organizations (i.e. the provision of sports activities) than other health promotion actions and may, therefore, result in different implementation successes or challenges. There is one Australian study that focused on partnership and capacity-building strategies associated with successful implementation of cross-sectoral (e.g. sports, recreation, health) sports and recreation programs [13]. The investigated programs had a strong emphasis on participation in physical activity that would benefit people who were not currently active and on low incomes. The findings showed that engagement of key stakeholders, formalization of the partnership agreement and capacity (diversity of skills and resources within the partnership) to develop and implement sports and recreation programs facilitated program implementation. In addition, addressing the development of partnerships, implementing a phased approach to program development and implementation was suggested to assist the sports and recreation sector build capacity to participate in partnership approaches to health promotion. The researchers focused on cross-sectoral HEPA programs and addressed only a particular aspect of the implementation process (i.e. partnership and capacity-building strategies). Therefore, to gain a broader understanding of the implementation of HEPA programs in the organized sports setting, this study focused on HEPA programs initiated by sporting organizations and the implementation process as a whole. Specifically, the main factors influencing implementation of the fourteen NAPSE sporting programs, initiated by NSFs and implemented by sports clubs in the Netherlands, were studied. The study results will support sports practitioners and policy makers with developing and implementing HEPA programs in this setting. The findings of this study are of international interest, particularly in countries where the organized sports sector is used as a setting to promote HEPA.

Methods

Sample

This study focused on the fourteen NAPSE sporting programs and the ten funded NSFs, i.e. the program coordinators who were designated to facilitate implementation of these programs in local sports clubs in the Netherlands. The programs varied with regard to targeted age group, content and duration. A description of the programs can be found in Table 1. The NAPSE sporting programs were implemented by different sports clubs over a 3-year implementation period (June 2008–June 2011). Sizes of the NSFs, as well as program aims and the extent to which NSFs were successful in achieving these aims, varied widely. The actual reach of the programs ranged from 9 (45 % of aim reached) to 680 (159 %) participating locations (a sports club could implement the program in different locations) and 85 (43 %) to 273,896 (304 %) participants (see Table 2).

Design

This research was part of a larger study in which both a process and effectiveness evaluation of the programs were conducted [34]. It consisted of a qualitative component to explore factors facilitating and impeding implementation of the individual sporting programs followed by a quantitative component to identify a generic set of factors (i.e. the most important factors across all sporting programs) influencing implementation. The qualitative component results informed the quantitative component. When performing the study, ethical guidelines were followed (i.e. with regard to

Table 1 Description Dutch NAPSE sporting programs

NSF	Sporting program	Target group	Description
Athletics	Start to Run	Adults	Six-week training program for novice runners aimed at running 3 km continuously. The program is offered by athletics clubs and running stores.
Judo	Judo in school	Children, adolescents	During a few weeks judo lessons in school provided by a qualified judo trainer.
Walking	Through 4 days Marches	Adults	Six-month training program for the Four Days Marches of Nijmegen. Participants can take part in the program individually or at a walking club.
Walking	Working by Walking	Adults	Walking program of at least 16 weeks aimed at improving health parameters. The program is provided by qualified walking trainers.
Gymnastics	Trendy Weeks for Masters	Older adults (45+)	During 8–12 weeks gymnastic classes with a specific theme (e.g. Move on music) at a gymnastics club.
Hockey	Fit Hockey	Older adults (50+)	Hockey played in a team with soft sticks and soft balls; training opportunities are provided continuously at the hockey club.
Swimming	My Swimming Coach	Adults	A membership of the NSF, including access to an online swimming coach and opportunities to participate in swim clinics and events.
Bridge	Thinking and Doing	Older adults (55+)	A project of two years in which bridge is used to create communities of older people. After a year physical activities are offered.
Sportive cycling	Cycle-Fit	Adults	Six-week training program for novice cyclers (speed cycling, mountain biking). The program is offered by (sportive) cycling clubs and cycling stores.
Sportive cycling	Cycle & Enjoy Nature	Older adults (45+)	Regular recreational cycling activities with a focus on relaxing and enjoying nature at a cycling club; or and individual introduction package including a cycling magazine, a training manual, a map with cycling routes and a calendar with cycling events.
Triathlon	Trio-Triathlon	Adults	Organization of Trio-Triathlon (the three sports of a triathlon are performed by three different individuals) events.
Volleyball	Beach volleyball	Children, adolescents, adults	Organization of different beach volleyball activities (e.g. clinics, tournaments, workshops) at schools, (beach) volleyball clubs, companies and (beach) volleyball events.
Volleyball	Cool Moves Volley	Children	A volleyball approach adapted to the abilities and needs of kids. Training opportunities are provided continuously at volleyball clubs; clinics are provided in schools.
Volleyball	Ultimate Volley Xperience	Adolescents	A volleyball event in a Caribbean atmosphere. The event is held at a special location and includes music and spectacular side-events.

avoiding undue intrusion, avoiding adverse consequences, confidentiality, enabling participation, informed consent and data protection) [35]. Before the start of the implementation phase, a group meeting was held with the program coordinators of the NSFs to explain in plain language the purpose of the research, the methods, demands, potential risks and possible outcomes of the research. In addition, it was explained that monitoring implementation progress was part of the NAPSE funding agreement, but that NSFs were not judged on the basis of the program or research results (i.e. the NSFs had a best-efforts obligation with regard to implementing the programs). Written informed consent for participation in the study was obtained from the NSFs when they applied for the funding. According to Dutch legislation, approval by a medical ethics committee was not obligatory, as participants were not subjected to procedures, nor were they required to follow rules of behavior. The privacy regulations of the study were approved by the Dutch Data Protection Authority. For reporting of results, the RATS guidelines were used as a guidance [36].

Procedures

Qualitative part

Face-to-face interviews

Face-to-face interviews were conducted with the program coordinators of the NSFs ($n = 12$; one program coordinator per NAPSE sporting program; two program coordinators were responsible for two programs). Overall, fourteen (i.e. one interview per program) semi-structured interviews of 60–90 min duration were conducted yearly (in 2009, 2010 and 2011) during the 3-year implementation period by the primary researcher (LO). The same program coordinators participated in the interviews, except for five sporting programs. For these programs, there was a change in program coordinator during the implementation period. The interview questions focused on implementation progress in the past year and factors that respondents believed have facilitated and/or hindered implementation. Also, other topics were considered, like the number of participants, obtained results, developed products, collaboration with other parties, the follow-up activities offered and continuation of the program after cessation of funding. The latter topics,

Table 2 Size NSFs and reach programs in relation to aims

NSF	Size NSF[a]	Sporting program	Locations*: aim (N)[b]	Locations*: result (N, % of aim)	Participants: aim (N)[c]	Participants: result (N, % of aim)
Athletics	Large	Start to Run	150	120 (80 %)	26.000	25.777 (99 %)
Judo	Medium	Judo in school	No aim	474 (NA)	10.000	53.804 (538 %)
Walking	Medium	Through 4 days Marches	NA	NA	3.500	4.650 (133 %)
Walking	Medium	Working by Walking	20	9 (45 %)	200	85 (43 %)
Gymnastics	Large	Trendy Weeks for Masters	220	218 (99 %)	7.500	3.110 (41 %)
Hockey	Large	Fit Hockey	20	15 (75 %)	1.000	989 (99 %)
Swimming	Large	My Swimming Coach	130	70 (54 %)	19.000	11.350 (60 %)
Bridge	Large	Thinking and Doing	38	71 (187 %)	2.925	4.055 (139 %)
Sportive cycling	Medium	Cycle-Fit	420	228 (54 %)	8.000	3.057 (38 %)
Sportive cycling	Medium	Cycle & Enjoy Nature	No aim	47 (NA)	1.000	446 (45 %)
Triathlon	Small	Trio-Triathlon	40	66 (165 %)	9.600	13.014 (136 %)
Volleyball	Large	Beach volleyball	52	104 (200 %)	90.000	273.896 (304 %)
Volleyball	Large	Cool Moves Volley	428	680 (159 %)	14.000	49.883 (356 %)
Volleyball	Large	Ultimate Volley Xperience	220	164 (75 %)	56.750	34.658 (61 %)

*A sports club could implement the program in different locations
[a]Large > 100,000 club members, medium 25,000–100,000 club members, small < 25,000 club members
[b]Aimed number of locations in which the sporting program will be implemented
[c]Aimed number of participants of sporting program
NA = not applicable

however, were asked in light of the general process evaluation. In this research, they were only used as background information. The interview questions were partly based on interview questions used during the pilot study [28] and further developed by an expert panel consisting of the two researchers (LO and CV) and representatives of the Netherlands Olympic Committee and Netherlands Sports Federation (NOC*NSF), the Dutch Ministry of Health, Welfare and Sport, the Netherlands Institute for Sport and Physical Activity and four NSFs. The interviews were recorded with a digital voice recorder and transcribed later on. A transcript summarizing the main findings was sent for review and revision to the interviewees.

Extraction and categorizing of factors

For each sporting program, facilitating and impeding factors were extracted from the interview transcripts and summarized. Subsequently, a list of facilitating and impeding factors for all sporting programs was created. For this purpose, cross case analyses [37] were performed with the individual sporting programs representing the cases. Factors were compared between sporting programs to investigate commonalities: Comparable factors between sporting programs were summarized and added as a single factor. For instance, multiple program coordinators indicated that it was important to visit sports clubs personally when asking for participation. This was summarized as the facilitating factor: "approaching sports clubs personally". Unique factors were added as a single factor to the list. Finally, thematic analyses [38] were performed to categorize the factors according to themes. Extraction of factors, cross-case and thematic analyses were performed manually by the primary researcher (LO) using Microsoft Word 2010 (Microsoft Corporation, Redmond, United States). To enhance rigor, all analyses were checked by a second researcher (CV). Differences between researchers were discussed. This resulted in only minor adjustments.

Meeting with program coordinators

To verify the obtained factors and categorizing according to themes or, in this case, phases, the results were presented and discussed at a meeting with the program coordinators ($n = 8$, the others were unable to attend). In a general discussion which was led by the primary researcher (LO), consensus was reached about the phases. In addition, the program coordinators were asked whether they agreed on the identified factors and whether any important factors were missing. For this purpose, they circulated along paper boards. On each board, a phase with its accompanying factors was presented. Program coordinators could add or remove factors. This led to the addition of 16 new facilitating factors and three new impeding factors. These factors are presented in bold in Additional file 1 [See Additional file 1 - Overview of all factors and their ranking scores]. No factors were removed. Subsequently, a final overview of factors categorized by phases was made by the researcher (LO).

Quantitative part

Ranking of factors

To identify the most important facilitating and impeding factors across all sporting programs, the final overview was sent to the program coordinators ($n = 12$) by email. The program coordinators were asked to rank the factors in an attached ranking form, whereby ranking was done by phase and for facilitating and impeding factors separately. The most important (facilitating or impeding) factor was assigned ranking 1, the second most important factor was assigned ranking 2, etc. As the number of factors varied by phase, the number of assigned rankings also varied. Completed ranking forms ($n = 12$) were returned by email.

Calculating mean ranking scores and composing the top three of factors

The mean ranking score for each factor was calculated (i.e. sum of ranks divided by number of program coordinators ($n = 12$)) by the researcher (LO) using Stata statistical software version 10.1 (Stata Corporation, College Station, Texas). Then, the factors were placed in order of importance, with the lower mean ranking scores corresponding to more important factors. Subsequently, the top three facilitating and impeding factors were composed per phase. In case there were three or less than three factors, all factors are presented.

Results

Phases and final overview of factors

Based on thematic analyses and the meeting with the program coordinators of the NSFs, factors were categorized according to six phases through which all programs proceeded in a consecutive manner:

1) Program development: factors that influenced implementation, but had to be dealt with during program development, i.e. the phase proceeding implementation;
2) Organizational (pre)conditions: factors that influenced implementation at the level of the NSF;
3) Recruiting local sports clubs: factors that affected the recruitment of local sports clubs;
4) Recruiting participants: factors that facilitated or impeded recruitment of participants for the program;
5) Local implementation: factors that were important during local implementation, i.e. at the level of the sports club;
6) Securing continuation of the program: factors that had to be considered during implementation and influenced continuation of the program after implementation, both at the level of the NSF and sports clubs.

The final overview of factors, comprising the six phases, contained a total of 56 facilitating and 29 impeding factors [See Additional file 1 - Overview of all factors and their ranking scores]. The number of facilitating factors varied by phase from 7 to 12, the number of impeding factors varied by implementation phase from 2 to 7. In each phase, there were more facilitating than impeding factors.

Ranking results

Based on the ranking of factors according to importance, the top three facilitating and impeding factors per phase were identified. These results are presented in Tables 3 and 4 for facilitating and impeding factors respectively. Comparing both tables, it is apparent that the impeding factors were mainly the inverse of the facilitating factors. Furthermore, the range of rankings shows that there were some differences in ranking by the program coordinators. Under the headings of the six phases, the factors will be explained in more detail and illustrated with examples provided by the program coordinators in the interviews. Since the impeding factors were often the inverse of the facilitators, they are not always explained separately. In the additional file, all factors and their ranking scores are presented [See Additional file 1 - Overview of all factors and their ranking scores].

Program development

It was reported that, when developing a program, it is important to consider the needs, wishes and possibilities of the target group. Both the content of the program (e.g. sport, intensity of activity) as well as organizational aspects (e.g. day and time of activities) have to be tailored to the target group.

The NAPSE sporting programs were aimed at inactive people. For this particular target group, the threshold for participation had to be low. This meant that people with no previous training experiences or specific sport skills could participate and sports activities were offered in a non-threatening manner to non-sport participants. The NSFs lowered barriers for participation by using graded training programs (i.e. starting with small amounts of physical activity and gradually increasing intensity over time), simplified sport techniques and/or rules and easy to use (soft and non-threatening) sport materials.

Furthermore, it was important to consider the needs, wishes and possibilities of local sports clubs, because they were the ones actually implementing the programs. The main focus of sports clubs was to provide sports competition and they generally relied on volunteers. Implementation was facilitated when the program was easy to implement locally, i.e. the program required little in terms of materials, manpower and time. In contrast, high implementation costs (i.e. a costly program) were perceived as a barrier to local implementation. For

Table 3 The top three facilitating factors per phase based on ranking by NAPSE program coordinators ($n = 12$)

Phase (total number of factors in phase)	Top three factors	Mean ranking score[a]	Range assigned rankings[b]
1. Program development ($n = 12$)	• The program matches the target group's needs, wishes and possibilities	1.1	1–2
	• The program is easy to implement locally	3.8	2–7
	• Low threshold for participation of inactive people	3.9	1–7
2. Organizational (pre)conditions ($n = 10$)	• Having a "dedicated" program coordinator	2.9	1–8
	• Sufficient time (in man-hours) to coordinate the program	3.1	1–6
	• Internal support for the program	3.9	1–9
3. Recruiting local sports clubs ($n = 10$)	• Providing a complete (readily usable) package to sports clubs	3.8	1–7
	• Approaching sports clubs personally	4.3	1–10
	• Support for the program by sports clubs	4.7	1–10
4. Recruiting participants ($n = 9$)	• Support for the program by the target group	3.3	1–6
	• A good promotion/marketing strategy nationally and locally	3.4	1–8
	• The sports activities are organized in close proximity to the target group	3.6	1–6
5. Local implementation ($n = 8$)	• Enthusiastic people within sports clubs delivering (high-)quality performances	2.9	1–7
	• Sports clubs are (personally) supported by the NSF when implementing the program locally	3.8	1–7
	• Availability of follow-up sports activities locally that match participants' needs, wishes and possibilities	3.8	1–8
6. Securing continuation of the program ($n = 7$)	• The program is part of the NSF's long-term policy	2.6	1–5
	• The NSF has sufficient financial resources available to continue the program/ secure the program for the future	2.7	1–6
	• The program is part of the sports club's long-term policy	3.0	1–6

[a]For each factor: Sum of rankings divided by the number of program coordinators ($n = 12$)
[b]Lowest and highest ranking of factor

example, intensive personal guidance of participants, expensive program materials, (regular) transportation of sports equipment and the need to rent a specific (sports) accommodation contributed to high implementation costs.

Organizational (pre)conditions

A major facilitator of implementation at the level of the NSF was having a "dedicated" program coordinator, i.e. someone who was committed to the program and believed in it. Additionally, it was important that this person had sufficient time to coordinate the program. Preferably, he or she was only working on the program and was not being distracted by other projects or activities.

Another key factor to successful implementation at the level of the NSF was having support for the program within the NSF's organization of both individuals that were involved in the program as well as individuals that were not directly involved (e.g. staff members and other NSF departments). High level management and administrative commitment and support was especially needed in cases where the program required large organizational or structural changes. For example, for one sporting program a new type of membership was introduced, whereby individual sports participants became a direct member of the NSF. In absence of support, it took longer to get programs running and, in some cases, this led to delayed implementation.

Other main factors at the level of the NSF impeding implementation were insufficient finances for coordination/ implementation and internal organizational changes. The NAPSE programs were all funded programs. For the implementation of two programs additional co-financing of municipalities was taken into account, so that the programs could be implemented in more locations than was possible with the NAPSE funding alone. Many municipalities have a budget to stimulate sports participation. However, municipalities were not always willing or able (i.e. there was no budget or the budget was already spent) to provide financial resources, which hindered the implementation of the programs in certain locations. Next to that, the NSFs agreed that, in general, insufficient finances are an important barrier to implementation of these kind of sporting programs. Examples of (unfavorable) organizational changes that took place were staff turnover, policy changes and a reorganization of the NSF. Particularly, a change of program coordinator resulted in slowed

Table 4 The top three impeding factors per phase based on ranking by NAPSE program coordinators ($n = 12$)

Phase (total number of factors in phase)	Top three factors	Mean ranking score[a]	Range assigned rankings[b]
1. Program development ($n = 6$)	• The program does not match the target group's needs, wishes and/or possibilities	1.8	1–6
	• The (implementation of the) program (locally) is costly	3.2	1–5
	• The program does not match the needs, wishes and/or possibilities of sports clubs	3.3	1–5
2. Organizational (pre)conditions ($n = 3$)	• Insufficient finances to coordinate and implement the program	1.4	1-2
	• No or insufficient support for the program internally	1.9	1–3
	• Internal organizational changes	2.7	1–3
3. Recruiting local sports clubs ($n = 6$)	• No or insufficient qualified trainers locally	2.2	1–4
	• No or insufficient support for the program by sports clubs	2.4	1–6
	• Unavailability of additional (local) funding possibilities	3.6	1–6
4. Recruiting participants ($n = 7$)	• The target group is unfamiliar with the program or the sport	3.0	1–5
	• No or insufficient support for the program by the target group	3.3	1–7
	• The program does not reach/engage inactive people	3.4	1–5
5. Local implementation ($n = 5$)	• No enthusiastic and/or incompetent people within sports clubs	1.5	1–4
	• No clear division of roles, tasks and responsibilities between the NSF and sports clubs	3.0	1–5
	• No (appropriate) follow-up sports activities for participants locally	3.2	1–5
6. Securing continuation of the program ($n = 2$)	• The NSF has insufficient financial resources available to continue the program/secure the program for the future	1.4	1–2
	• Sports clubs have insufficient financial resources available to continue the program locally/secure the program for the future	1.6	1–2

[a]For each factor: Sum of rankings divided by the number of program coordinators ($n = 12$)
[b]Lowest and highest ranking of factor

implementation of planned activities within the programs. This was due to the time required for the NSF to employ a new program coordinator and for the new program coordinator to become oriented with the program and sports clubs.

Recruiting local sports clubs

Local sports clubs were more willing to participate when they valued the program and supported it. The opposite, was a great barrier to recruiting sports clubs. Most NSFs experienced (some) resistance from their sports clubs, especially when the programs were first introduced. The NSFs described the sports clubs as being traditional: Their primary focus was on running their sports competitions and regular training programs. Providing physical activity opportunities for inactive people was something else and beyond their core business. However, during the 3-year implementation period, resistance often ceased because sports clubs became familiar with the program and/or were positively affected by other sports clubs implementing the program. Sports clubs were introduced to the successes of other sports clubs through the NSF website, the NSF (online) newsletter, adverts in local newspapers and (meetings with) trainers of other sports clubs. Also, different sports clubs provided demonstrations of the sporting programs (e.g. during large sports events) and implementation successes were spread by partner organizations of the NSF and implementing sports clubs.

Nonetheless, to convince sports clubs to participate a more personal approach was required. Preferably, the NSF visited the club personally to explain the program and ask for participation. Furthermore, a complete (readily usable) package with all necessary materials (e.g. trainer manual, sport materials, promotional materials) enhanced participation of sports clubs, because this saved them a lot of time during local implementation.

A main factor impeding participation of sports clubs was having no or insufficient qualified trainers. Finding volunteers with the appropriate skills (i.e. volunteers that were able to work with non-sport participants) was an issue for many sports clubs. Most NSFs developed and organized special trainer courses to grow their trainer database.

For implementation of the programs, it was sometimes required that sports clubs invested their own financial resources (e.g. to produce promotional materials, pay trainers or buy sports equipment). However, sports clubs did not always have enough internal financial resources and they depended on external financial resources to participate. Unavailability of (local) funding possibilities, therefore, impeded the recruitment of sports clubs as well.

Recruiting participants

As with the recruitment of sports clubs, recruitment of participants was facilitated when (potential) participants valued the program and supported it. In addition, a good promotion and marketing strategy, both nationally and locally, was needed. According to the NSFs, promoting the program at a national level was necessary to get people familiar with the program. For the actual recruitment of participants, however, local marketing was more important. The NSFs marketed their programs via national press, the internet, television and partner organizations. Local marketing was done by sports clubs through the distribution of posters, flyers and leaflets. Also, adverts were placed in local newspapers, demonstrations were given and participants were recruited by word of mouth. On the other hand, when the target group was unfamiliar with the program or the sport in general, recruitment was impeded. Some sports, for example, had the image of being tough (e.g. hockey, sports of a triathlon) or only to be played by certain (sub)groups (e.g. hockey).

Organizing the sports activities in close proximity to the target group was another factor facilitating recruitment. In this way, travel distance was no barrier to participation. Providing the program in many different locations in the Netherlands was one way that some NSFs dealt with this. Others organized the sports activities in places where the target group gathered; for example, activities for children were organized in elementary schools.

Finally, the NAPSE sporting programs were all aimed at increasing physical activity levels of inactive people. However, some NSFs stated that it was very difficult to attract large numbers of inactive people to their sports activities. Most participants were already a little or very physically active. A NSF summarized this as not having the right people and channels to reach this target group.

Local implementation

For the program to be successfully implemented by a local sports club, it was important to have people (e.g. a trainer) within the club who were enthusiastic about the program and skilled in running the program. The NSFs stated that, when the program was of high-quality (i.e. participants had good experiences due to trainer capabilities), participants gladly came back to the club to participate in (additional) sports activities.

(Personal) support of sports clubs by the NSF was another factor positively influencing local implementation. During the implementation period, the NSFs supported sports clubs in different ways, for example, by providing them with personal guidance, financial resources, advice and (promotional) materials. In this way, local barriers were overcome and sports clubs spent less time on decision making and developing new products.

A main factor hindering implementation locally was an unclear division of roles, tasks and responsibilities between the NSF and sports clubs. For the NSF, this resulted in doing more supportive work than initially planned; and for the sport club, this led to a slowing down of planned activities.

Finally, to stimulate continuous participation in physical activity and to recruit new members for the sports club, it was important to have follow-up activities at the sports club that matched participants' needs, wishes and possibilities. Follow-up activities consisted, for example, of a few additional introductory training sessions for free or at low costs at the club. Sports clubs also offered membership options at a reduced rate with continuation of activities in an appropriate beginners' group. In cases where there were no suitable follow-up activities at the sports club, it was difficult to capture participants' interest for the sport and they were often lost to club membership.

Securing continuation of the program

Including the program in both the NSF's and sports club's long-term policy was reported to enhance continuation of the program. This ensured integration of the program in the organization and available time and resources to run the program. With regard to resources, having sufficient financial resources was reported as a separate facilitating factor. At the same time, a lack of financial resources was seen as a great barrier to sustaining a program, both for the NSF as well as the sports clubs. Of the fourteen NAPSE sporting programs, ten were reported to be continued after the funding period. Programs that were self-sustaining after the implementation period spent funds to develop the program infrastructure, such as educating trainers and providing equipment and resources. These programs could be financed from internal financial resources and/or membership/participation fees. Other programs still relied on external financial resources following cessation of funding. In these cases, the program infrastructure was not fully developed and program costs (e.g. costs related to use of accommodations or facilities, sports equipment, payment of trainers, promotion and recruitment strategies) could not be covered by internal financial resources or membership/participation fees. At the time of the last interview, some NSFs were still struggling with finding sponsors or funding opportunities. Others already found a sponsor for their programs for the next year, like a health insurance company and an international bank.

Summary of results

Given the ecological perspective of the settings-based approach [9–12], an ecological model is used to summarize the results (see Fig. 1). The organized sports setting and the different levels of influence - policy, NSF and sports clubs (organizational and environmental level) and non-sport participants (personal level) - are presented on the left. The factors are presented on the right in the form of a checklist, which can be used as guidance when developing and implementing HEPA programs in the organized sports setting. The arrows indicate the influence of the different ecological levels on the implementation process. Behind each factor, the exact level of influence is indicated (NSF, SC, P). For instance, at the non-sport participants and sports club level, program development must consider how the program can be tailored to the target group (inactive people) and sports clubs; and at the non-sport participants level, recruitment must consider both national and local promotion strategies. Furthermore, the results show that the major factors influencing implementation of HEPA programs by the organized sports setting do not act on the policy level (e.g. regulations for facilities, safety laws). Therefore, the arrow representing this influence is dashed.

Discussion

A new setting of interest in the promotion of health, including health-enhancing physical activity (HEPA), is the organized sports sector [13–23]. In this study, the main factors facilitating and impeding implementation of sporting programs, aimed at inactive population groups, were identified (see Tables 3, 4 and Fig. 1). The results showed that different factors acted during the different phases of the implementation process. When comparing factors across phases, several key learnings are evident. These will be discussed here in a broader context.

First, program design is an important influencer of implementation. HEPA sporting programs must be tailored to the needs, wishes and possibilities of both inactive populations groups as well as the implementing sports clubs. This could be achieved by engaging and actively involving these parties in the program development and

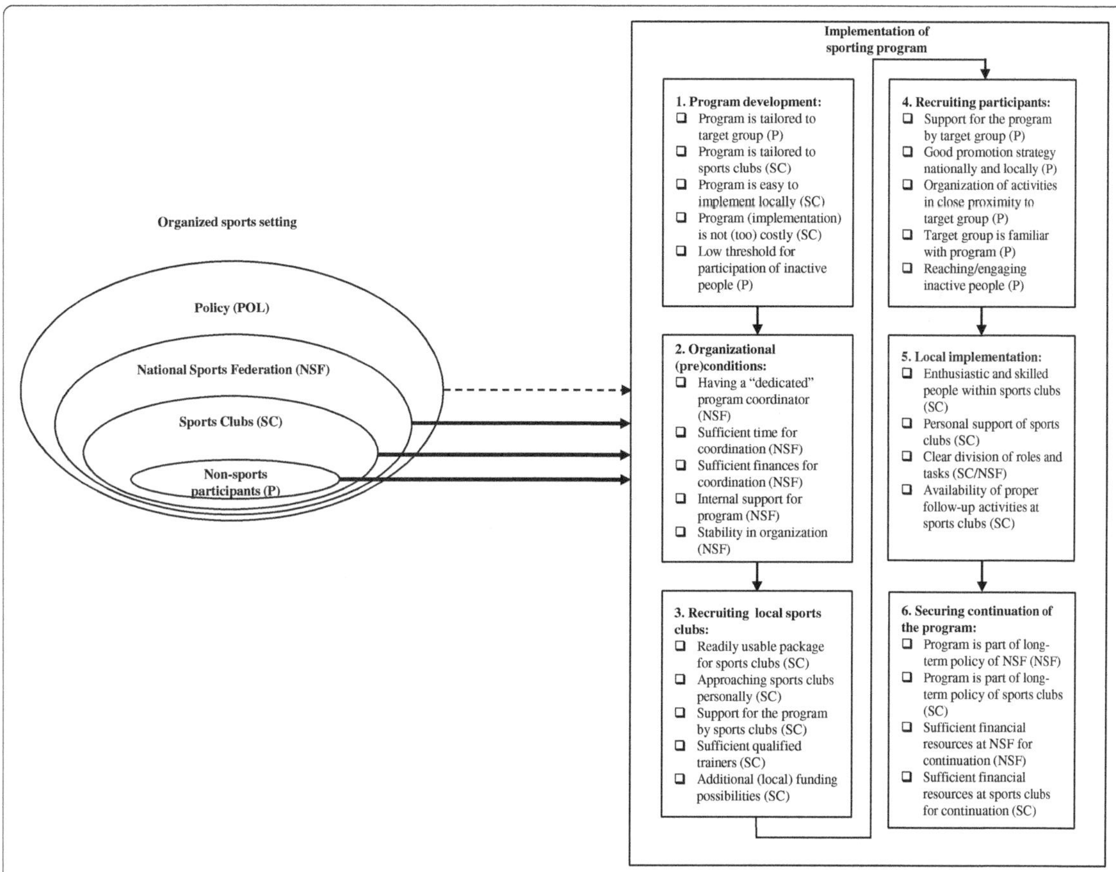

Fig. 1 Summary of results in an ecological model

implementation process [39]. Consequently, support for and implementation of the program will be enhanced. In addition, there are different formative research strategies (e.g. interviews, observations, focus groups) that can be used before a program is developed or implemented to obtain detailed information about the target group and implementers of the program [40]. In this study, the focus was on implementation and not on program development. Therefore, it is not known how the programs were developed and whether non-sport participants and sports clubs were involved in program design. However, all programs were pilot tested before advancing to broader implementation [28], which suggests that needs of both participants and sports clubs have been addressed. Satisfaction of participants with the programs was measured during the effectiveness evaluation of the programs [34]. The results showed that a majority (87–99 %) of participants of the sporting programs enjoyed participation and liked the sports activities offered. The average rating of the programs varied between 7.6 and 8.4 (scale 0–10; 0 being very poor and 10 being excellent), which indicates that the sporting programs were suitable for their participants.

However, the actual target group, i.e. inactive people, was not always reached, at least not in great numbers. It seems that the organized sports sector is not yet "a setting of everyday life" for this target group. The results of the effectiveness evaluation confirm this [34]. The percentage of inactive people varied from 0 to 15 % per sporting program. In addition, for seven sporting programs enough data were available to assess effectiveness on increasing levels of HEPA. Three sporting programs showed significant increases in physical activity levels of participants six months after the start of the programs and in comparison with a control group. For two of these programs, this was accompanied by a significant increase in the percentage of participants meeting levels of HEPA (+26 and +12 % compared to baseline). For the remaining four sporting programs, no significant changes in levels of physical activity of participants were observed. Therefore, to engage more inactive people into organized sports activities, sporting organizations should focus on proper recruitment methods and channels to reach this target group. In this regard, they may consider engaging in partnerships with primary health care, community health or other relevant organizations to get closer to this target group [41].

Another important finding was that successful implementation was largely dependent upon enthusiastic people within sporting organizations (e.g. program coordinator, trainer at a sports club) that were willing to invest time in coordinating/running the program. These people needed to possess the right skills, especially the local trainers, to provide high-quality training programs. This ensured participants returned to the club for (additional) sports activities.

For continued participation in sport of (initially) inactive people, however, suitable follow-up activities were required at the sports club. This was also advocated in a study which investigated structural links between sports participation programs conducted in schools and participation in community-based sports clubs [42]. The school-based sporting programs were seen as ineffective in promoting sustained sports participation and club membership due to a lack of formal strategies linking program participants with sports clubs. Repeated or additional experiences in the sport at the sports club was one of the strategies suggested to encourage engagement of participants in a local sports club. In addition, it was recommended that sporting organizations tailor their school-based programs using recognized health promotion planning principles (including taking into account the needs of participants and sports clubs) rather than continuing their current "one-size-fits-all" approach.

Furthermore, within the NAPSE, the NSFs received the funding, but the sports clubs were the ones actually implementing the HEPA programs. (Financial) resources of the mainly voluntary-based sports clubs were often limited. In addition, their primary focus was on running their sports competitions and regular training programs. Therefore, it was not self-evident that sports clubs implemented the HEPA programs in addition to their regular sports activities. Similar conclusions were drawn in a study which investigated the work of sports clubs as seen by representatives of sports clubs [33]. Sports clubs do what is familiar to them and respond to their local environment [32]. In the current study, it was also seen that sports clubs' support for the programs increased when they became familiar with the programs and were introduced to successes of other sports clubs implementing the programs. These latter sports clubs can be seen as the "early adopters" in the diffusion of innovations theory [43] and can thus be used to recruit other sports clubs. Nonetheless, to convince sports clubs to actually participate a more personal approach was required. Moreover, the support that NSFs offered to sports clubs (i.e. providing sports clubs with personal guidance, financial resources, advice and (promotional) materials) was essential and facilitated implementation at the sports club level. At the same time, this highlights the need to allocate (financial) resources directly to the implementing sports club and it should be considered in funding arrangements in which the implementing sports club is not the receiver of the funding.

Finally, for population health gains, all programs for promoting HEPA through sport will need to be sustained over a long period of time [17]. Of the fourteen NAPSE programs, ten were reported to be continued after the funding period. A lack of financial resources was seen as a great barrier to sustaining a program, both for the NSFs as well as the sports clubs. The sustainability of health promotion programs within sport and recreation organizations also relied heavily on continued funding [44]. Hence, it is important that program funds are spent to develop the program infrastructure so that the program is self-sustaining and can be financed from internal financial resources and/or membership/participation fees. It should be noted that it is unknown whether the NAPSE programs will actually be sustained in the absence of ongoing funding. This was also a limitation of the study concerning the sustainability of health promotion programs within sport and recreation organizations [44]. Thus, further research is required to examine factors influencing the long-term sustainability of HEPA programs in the organized sports setting.

The findings of this study add to those found in the study regarding partnership and capacity-building strategies associated with successful implementation of cross-sectoral sport and recreation programs [13]. In addition, the identified factors are comparable to those found in the studies concerning the implementation of HWEs [14–16, 19] and the factors acting on the sports club level support the "Health Promoting Sports Club" guidelines [23]. For instance, the guideline "determine the current state of will to practice health promotion in your club" is a prerequisite for the identified facilitating factor "support for the program by sports clubs" and the guideline "educate coaches and other club officials" is the solution to the impeding factor "no or insufficient qualified trainers locally". This implies there are generic factors, independent of the health program or activity being implemented, influencing implementation in the organized sports setting. Nonetheless, some factors are specific to the implementation of HEPA programs, such as the factor "low threshold for participation of inactive people (program development)".

In contrast to the organized sports setting, a lot of research is available concerning the implementation of promotion and prevention programs in other settings, like schools and the health care setting (e.g. [45, 46]). Surprisingly, the identified factors in this study reflect some of the major facilitators (and barriers) to program implementation in these settings, such as the availability of funding, skill proficiency (of providers) (vs. trainers with the appropriate skills), compatibility of the innovation (vs. a program that matches the needs, wishes and possibilities of sports clubs), the existence of a program champion (vs. enthusiastic people within sporting organizations) and provision of training and technical assistance (vs. providing (personal) support to sports clubs) [45]. Nevertheless, some caution in interpreting this findings is needed. The practical realization of factors may, for example, be quite different between programs or settings (e.g. training volunteers in sports clubs to provide HEPA programs vs. training health professionals in providing substance abuse prevention programs). Therefore, the context in which programs are implemented remains important [29–31].

Overall, the findings of this study can assist sports practitioners and policy makers with developing and implementing HEPA programs in the organized sports setting. Figure 1, in which the results are summarized, can be used as guidance to tailor programs and implementation strategies to this setting. Also, the practical examples provided in the results section may be of value for realization of factors. Moreover, the results can be used to guide funding guidelines (e.g. allocating (a part of the) financial resources directly to implementing sports clubs and using funds for developing program infrastructure). Considering the main facilitating and impeding factors during the development and implementation process will concurrently facilitate successful implementation [29–31].

This study was designed to contribute to the understanding of the implementation of HEPA programs in the organized sports setting. A strength of the study was that the implementation process was studied longitudinally. Interviews were conducted yearly during the 3-year implementation period. In this way, the (time-)specific features of the implementation process were better captured and recall bias was reduced. Moreover, the (partly) qualitative nature of the study (i.e. semi-structured interviews, meeting) revealed detailed information about the implementation process. A disadvantage of self-report might be the introduction of social desirability biases. However, given the fact that the program coordinators of the NSFs reported both the facilitators and barriers to implementation, it appears there was limited social desirability bias. In addition, it is believed that the different evaluation rounds ensured the reliability of this study.

With regard to quantitative ranking of factors, the mean ranking score was calculated from an ordinal ranking scale. It is not certain whether the difference in ranking between one and two is the same as that, for example, between three and four on a ordinal ranking scale. Moreover, when the mean ranking score of factor A is two and four of factor B, this does not necessarily mean that factor A was twice as important as factor B. In addition, there were some differences in ranking of factors between program coordinators. This could be due to differences in programs (e.g. content, size) and/or NSFs (e.g. size, organizational structure), making some factors more or less relevant. However, the sum of ranks and the mode of ranks (results not presented in this article) did not yield a different ordering of factors. Therefore, it is believed that the mean ranking score was appropriate to identify the top three facilitating and impeding factors in this study.

Furthermore, in this study, the focus was on the perceptions of the program coordinators of the NSFs, because they were the ones designated to facilitate implementation of the programs in local sports clubs. Information was not directly obtained from representatives of the sports clubs, i.e. the actual implementers of the programs. This could be seen as a limitation of the study. However, the program coordinators worked in close collaboration with the sports clubs and were, therefore, well-informed about the implementation process locally. Nonetheless, in future research it would be interesting to evaluate directly at the sports club level.

Conclusions

Considering both the strengths and limitations, this study does add to knowledge base concerning the implementation of sporting programs, aimed at inactive people, in the organized sports setting. The main factors facilitating and impeding implementation were identified. The results of this study can be used by sports practitioners and policy makers when developing and implementing HEPA programs in this setting. Moreover, the results can be used to guide funding guidelines. In future research, it would be interesting to evaluate implementation directly at the sports club level and to study factors influencing the long-term sustainability of HEPA programs. This will further contribute to the understanding of the implementation context of the organized sports setting, and will, consequently, improve the implementation and sustainability of HEPA programs in this setting.

Additional file

Additional file 1: Overview of all factors and their ranking scores. In the additional file, an overview of all facilitating and impeding factors per (implementation) phase can be found, including their ranking scores (i.e. mean ranking score and range assigned rankings).

Abbreviations

HEPA: Health-enhancing physical activity; HWEs: Healthy and welcoming sporting environments; FIFA: Fédération Internationale de Football Association; NAPSE: National Action Plan for Sport and Exercise; NOC*NSF: Netherlands Olympic Committee and Netherlands Sports Federation; NSF: National Sports Federation; P: Non-sport participants; POL: Policy; SC: Sports Clubs.

Competing interests

The authors declare that they have no competing interests.

Authors' contributions

LO contributed to the design of the study, participated in the data collection process, performed data analysis and drafted the manuscript. CV verified data analyses as second researcher. Both CV and DHB contributed to the design of the study, advised on the analytical approach and reviewed and commented on the manuscript. NS contributed to the design of the study and reviewed and commented on the manuscript. All authors read and approved the final manuscript.

Acknowledgements

The authors gratefully acknowledge the contribution of the NSFs. This study was funded by NOC*NSF. NOC*NSF had no role in data collection and analysis and interpretation of data.

Author details

[1]Netherlands Institute for Health Services Research (NIVEL), PO Box 1568, 3500 BN Utrecht, The Netherlands. [2]Physical Therapy Research, Program in Clinical Health Sciences & Department of Rehabilitation, Nursing Science and Sport, Brain Center Rudolf Magnus, University Medical Center Utrecht, PO Box 85500, 3508 GA Utrecht, The Netherlands. [3]Netherlands Olympic Committee and Netherlands Sports Federation (NOC*NSF), PO Box 302, 6800 AH Arnhem, The Netherlands. [4]Scientific Center for Transformation in Care and Welfare (Tranzo), Tilburg University, PO Box 90153, 5000 LE Tilburg, The Netherlands.

References

1. Haskell WL, Lee IM, Pate RR, Powell KE, Blair SN, Franklin BA, et al. Physical activity and public health: updated recommendation for adults from the American College of Sports Medicine and the American Heart Association. Med Sci Sports Exerc. 2007;39:1423–34.
2. Ströhle A. Physical activity, exercise, depression and anxiety disorders. J Neural Transm. 2009;116:777–84.
3. Warburton DE, Nicol CW, Bredin SS. Health benefits of physical activity: the evidence. CMAJ. 2006;174:801–9.
4. Bernaards C. TNO monitor physical activity and health - Physical activity in the Netherlands 2000–2010. Leiden, the Netherlands: TNO Healthy Living; 2011.
5. World Health Organization (WHO). Global status report on noncommunicable diseases 2010. Geneva, Switzerland: WHO; 2011.
6. World Health Organization (WHO). Review of physical activity promotion policy development and legislation in European Union Member States. Copenhagen, Denmark: WHO; 2010.
7. Whitelaw S, Baxendale A, Bryce C, MacHardy L, Young I, Witney E. 'Settings' based health promotion: a review. Health Promot Int. 2001;16:339–53.
8. World Health Organization (WHO). Ottawa charter for health promotion. Geneva, Switzerland: WHO; 1986.
9. Dooris M. Healthy settings: challenges to generating evidence of effectiveness. Health Promot Int. 2006;21:55–65.
10. Dooris M. Holistic and sustainable health improvement: the contribution of the settings-based approach to health promotion. Perspect Public Health. 2009;129:29–36.
11. McLeroy KR, Bibeau D, Steckler A, Glanz K. An ecological perspective on health promotion programs. Health Educ Q. 1988;15:351–77.
12. Sallis JF, Owen N, Fisher EB. Ecological models of health behavior. In: Glanz K, Rimer BK, Viswanath K, editors. Health behavior and health education: theory, research and practice. San Francisco, USA: Jossey-Bass; 2008. p. 465–85.
13. Casey MM, Payne WR, Eime RM. Partnership and capacity-building strategies in community sports and recreation programs. Managing Leisure. 2009;14:167–76.
14. Casey MM, Payne WR, Eime RM. Organisational readiness and capacity building strategies of sporting organisations to promote health. Sport Manage Rev. 2012;15:109–24.
15. Crisp BR, Swerissen H. Critical processes for creating health-promoting sporting environments in Australia. Health Promot Int. 2003;18:145–52.
16. Dobbinson SJ, Hayman JA, Livingston PM. Prevalence of health promotion policies in sports clubs in Victoria, Australia. Health Promot Int. 2006;21:121–9.
17. Donaldson A, Finch CF. Sport as a setting for promoting health. Br J Sports Med. 2012;46:4–5.
18. Dutch Ministry of Health, Welfare and Sport. Time for sport: exercise, participate, perform. The Hague, the Netherlands: Dutch Ministry of Health, Welfare and Sport; 2005.
19. Eime RM, Payne WR, Harvey JT. Making sporting clubs healthy and welcoming environments: a strategy to increase participation. J Sci Med Sport. 2008;11:146–54.
20. European Commission. Communication from the commission to the European parliament, the council, the European economic and social committee and the committee of the regions - Developing the European Dimension in Sport. Brussels, Belgium: European Commission; 2011.

21. Holman CD, Donovan RJ, Corti B, Jalleh G, Frizzell SK, Carroll AM. Banning tobacco sponsorship: replacing tobacco with health messages and creating health-promoting environments. Tob Control. 1997;6:115–21.
22. Kokko S, Kannas L, Villberg J. The health promoting sports club in Finland - a challenge for the settings-based approach. Health Promot Int. 2006;21:219–29.
23. Kokko S. Guidelines for youth sports clubs to develop, implement, and assess health promotion within its activities. Health Promot Pract. 2014;15:373–82.
24. NOC*NSF. Membership NOC*NSF 2010. Arnhem, the Netherlands: NOC*NSF; 2011.
25. Eime RM, Young JA, Harvey JT, Charity MJ, Payne WR. A systematic review of the psychological and social benefits of participation in sport for adults: informing development of a conceptual model of health through sport. Int J Behav Nutr Phys Act. 2013;10:135.
26. Eime RM, Harvey JT, Brown WJ, Payne WR. Does sports club participation contribute to health-related quality of life? Med Sci Sports Exerc. 2010;42:1022–8.
27. Fuller CW, Junge A, Dorasami C, DeCelles J, Dvorak J. '11 for Health', a football-based health education programme for children: a two-cohort study in Mauritius and Zimbabwe. Br J Sports Med. 2011;45:612–8.
28. Pisters MF, Veenhof C. Evaluation of the pilot phase of the National Action Plan for Sport and Exercise: the sports setting. Utrecht, the Netherlands: NIVEL; 2008.
29. Finch C. A new framework for research leading to sports injury prevention. J Sci Med Sport. 2006;9:3–9.
30. Finch CF, Donaldson A. A sports setting matrix for understanding the implementation context for community sport. Br J Sports Med. 2010;44:973–8.
31. Finch CF. No longer lost in translation: the art and science of sports injury prevention implementation research. Br J Sports Med. 2011;45:1253–7.
32. Skille EA. Understanding sport clubs as sport policy implementers - a theoretical framework for the analysis of the implementation of central sport policy through local and voluntary sport organizations. Int Rev Sociol Sport. 2008;43:181–200.
33. Skille EA. Competitiveness and health: the work of sport clubs as seen by sport clubs representatives - a Norwegian case study. Int Rev Sociol Sport. 2010;45:73–85.
34. Ooms L, Veenhof C. Evaluation of the implementation phase of the National Action Plan for Sport and Exercise, the sports setting: results process and effectiveness evaluation. Utrecht, the Netherlands: NIVEL; 2011.
35. Webster S, Lewis J, Brown A. Ethical considerations in qualitative research. In: Ritchie J, Lewis J, McNaughton Nicholls C, Ormston R, editors. Qualitative research practice - a guide for social science students and researchers. London, England: SAGE Publications, Ltd; 2014. p. 77–110.
36. Clark JP. How to peer review a qualitative manuscript. In: Godlee F, Jefferson T, editors. Peer review in health sciences. 2nd ed. London, England: BMJ Books; 2003. p. 219–35.
37. Patton MQ. Qualitative analysis and interpretation. In: Qualitative research & evaluation methods. Thousand Oaks, California: SAGE Publications, Inc; 2015. p. 520–651.
38. Boyatzis RE. Transforming qualitative information: thematic analysis and code development. Thousand Oaks, California: SAGE Publications, Inc; 1998.
39. Donaldson A, Finch CF. Planning for implementation and translation: seek first to understand the end-users' perspectives. Br J Sports Med. 2012;46:306–7.
40. Gittelsohn J, Steckler A, Johnson CC, Pratt C, Grieser M, Pickrel J, et al. Formative research in school and community-based health programs and studies: "state of the art" and the TAAG approach. Health Educ Behav. 2006;33:25–39.
41. Casey MM, Payne WR, Brown SJ, Eime RM. Engaging community sport and recreation organisations in population health interventions: Factors affecting the formation, implementation, and institutionalisation of partnership efforts. Ann Leisure Res. 2009;12:129–47.
42. Eime RM, Payne WR. Linking participants in school-based sport programs to community clubs. J Sci Med Sport. 2009;12:293–9.
43. Haider M, Kreps GL. Forty years of diffusion of innovations: utility and value in public health. J Health Commun. 2004;9(S1):3–11.
44. Casey MM, Payne WR, Eime RM, Brown SJ. Sustaining health promotion programs within sport and recreation organisations. J Sci Med Sport. 2009;12:113–8.
45. Durlak JA, DuPre EP. Implementation matters: a review of research on the influence of implementation on program outcomes and the factors affecting implementation. Am J Community Psychol. 2008;41:327–50.
46. Meyers DC, Durlak JA, Wandersman A. The quality implementation framework: a synthesis of critical steps in the implementation process. Am J Community Psychol. 2012;50:462–80.

5

Sport-2-Stay-Fit study: Health effects of after-school sport participation in children and adolescents with a chronic disease or physical disability

Maremka Zwinkels[1,2], Olaf Verschuren[1,2], Kristel Lankhorst[2,3], Karin van der Ende-Kastelijn[2,3], Janke de Groot[2,3], Frank Backx[4], Anne Visser-Meily[1,4], Tim Takken[2,5*] and on behalf of the Sport-2-Stay-Fit study group

Abstract

Background: Children and adolescents with a chronic disease or physical disability have lower fitness levels compared to their non-disabled peers. Low physical fitness is associated with reduced physical activity, increased cardiovascular diseases, and lower levels of both cognitive and psychosocial functioning. Moreover, children and adolescents with a chronic disease or physical disability participate less in both recreational and competitive sports. A variety of intervention studies have shown positive, but only temporary, effects of training programs. Next to issues related to the chronic condition itself, various personal and environmental factors play a key role in determining the extent to which they participate in sports or physical activities. Due to these barriers, sport participation in the immediate after-school hours seems to be a feasible solution to get these children and adolescents physical active structurally. To investigate if an after school sport program can sustain the positive effects of an intervention, a standardized interval training will be given to improve physical fitness levels. High-intensity Interval Training (HIT) is superior to moderate-intensity continuous training in improving physical fitness in patients with chronic diseases. Therefore, the Sport-2-Stay-Fit study will investigate whether after school sport participation can increase the sustainability of a HIT program in children and adolescents with a chronic disease or physical disability.

Methods: The Sport-2-Stay-Fit study is a clinical controlled trial. A total of 74 children and adolescents in the age of 6–19 years with a chronic disease or physical disability will be included. This could be either a cardiovascular, pulmonary, metabolic, musculoskeletal or neuromuscular disorder. Both children and adolescents who are ambulatory or propelling a manual wheelchair will be included. All participants will follow a HIT program of eight weeks to improve their physical fitness level. Thereafter, the intervention group will participate in sport after school for six months, while the control group receives assessment only. Measurements will take place before the HIT, directly after, as well as, six months later. The primary objective is anaerobic fitness. Secondary objectives are agility, aerobic fitness, strength, physical activity, cardiovascular health, cognitive functioning, and psychosocial functioning.
(Continued on next page)

* Correspondence: t.takken@umcutrecht.nl
[2]Partner of Shared Utrecht Pediatric Exercise Research (SUPER) Lab, Utrecht, the Netherlands
[5]Child Development and Exercise Center, University Medical Center Utrecht, Wilhelmina Children's Hospital, P.O. Box 850903508AB, Utrecht, the Netherlands
Full list of author information is available at the end of the article

(Continued from previous page)

Discussion: If effective, after school sport participation following a standardized interval training could be implemented on schools for special education to get children and adolescents with a chronic disease or physical disability active on a structural basis.

Trial registration: This trial is registered at the Dutch Trial Register #NTR4698.

Keywords: Children, Adolescents, Physical fitness, Health, Chronic disease, Physical disability, Interval training, Exercise, Sport participation

Background

Children and adolescents with a chronic disease or physical disability have lower fitness levels compared to their non-disabled peers [1–6]. Low physical fitness is highly associated with reduced physical activity, increased cardiovascular diseases and overall mortality in healthy populations [7–10]. Additionally, cardiovascular risk factors such as dyslipidemia, hypertension, hyperinsulinemia or insulin resistance, and obesity often exist in children and young adults [11, 12]. To be healthy later in life, it is assumed that children and adolescents should be physically active on a structural basis.

At the same time, children and adolescents who are healthy [13] or physical active [14, 15] perform better at school. Moreover, childhood physical fitness is associated with higher levels of cognition [15–17]. Physical fitness level is a strong predictor in children and adolescents of school performance and level of cognition one year later [18, 19]. School performance has improved in children and adolescents who are typically developing by intervention programs stimulating physical activity and sports [20, 21]. However, this relationship between physical fitness and cognition level is still unknown in children and adolescents with a chronic disease or physical disability.

Another positive effect related to participation in sports is improving quality of life. This relation has been found in children and adolescents with cerebral palsy [22, 23]. In addition, children with lower motor skills have a lower global self-perception than their well-coordinated peers [24]. Perceptions of physical competence are strong predictors of self-perception among children with motor coordination difficulties [24, 25]. Successful performance experiences are the strongest means of changing self-perception; sport participation [26, 27]. Short-term sport interventions, however, did not significantly improve the self-perception of children with a physical disability although motor skills did improve [28, 29]. The long-term effect of sport participation on self-perception in children and adolescents with a chronic disease or physical disability still has to be established.

It can be assumed that the benefits of participating in sports are universal for all children, including those with a chronic disease or physical disability. However, they participate less in competitive and recreational sports compared to their non-disabled peers [30, 31]. A variety of interventions have shown that training programs improved physical fitness levels and participation in physical activities or sports. However, the positive effects following the training program did never sustain [23, 32, 33]. Therefore, more recently a shift in focus has moved from interventions to improve fitness to interventions to increase physical activity [30, 34].

For children and adolescents with a chronic disease or physical disability it is difficult to participate in sports or physical activities. Next to issues related to the chronic condition itself, various personal and environmental factors play a key role [35–37]. The most important barriers are: physical ability of the child, decreased motivation, lack of awareness of sports possibilities and lack of access to transportation. Most of these barriers can possibly be eliminated when an adapted sports program is provided at school. Interventions to promote sports in healthy young people conducted in the hours after school are effective in improving physical fitness, physical activities and health [38, 39]. A few special schools in the Netherlands are experienced in organizing and facilitating an after-school sports program. Although they anecdotally notice a lot of progress in these children, they have never measured the effect accurately in a scientific and systematic way.

To investigate if an after school sport program can sustain physical fitness level, health, and both cognitive and psychosocial functioning, a baseline fitness level is needed. Standardized exercise training with prescribed work-rest ratios, intensity, volume and time are more effective in improving physical fitness, especially short term [23, 32, 33]. In this regard, high-intensity Interval Training (HIT) is superior to moderate-intensity continuous training in improving physical fitness in patients with chronic diseases [40–42]. Furthermore, HIT is feasible for these children and adolescents [23]. Therefore, prior to the after-school sport program, a HIT program will be given to improve physical fitness level.

The current study, denoted as the Sport-2-Stay-Fit study, will investigate whether an after school sports program can increase the sustainability of a HIT program in children and adolescents with a chronic disease or physical disability. In addition, sport participation in these children may have positive effects on cardiovascular health, and both cognitive and psychosocial functioning. While these positive relationships have been reported in children and adolescents who are typically developing, the benefits are not established in those with a chronic disease or physical disability.

Methods

Design

The Sport-2-Stay-Fit study is a controlled clinical trial. All children and adolescents will participate in an eight week HIT program to improve their physical fitness level. Thereafter, the intervention group will participate in an after-school sports program for six months, while the control group will receive assessments only. Outcome measures will be assessed at baseline (T0), immediately after eight weeks of HIT (T1), and at completion of six months intervention (T2) (Fig. 1). Similar outcome measures will be evaluated at T0, T1 and T2 except for physical activity at T1, because no effect or changed difference between groups was expected [43, 44]. The current study is part of a larger project in which children and adolescents with a chronic disease or physical disability who are active in sports will be compared to their non-sporting peers [45].

Setting

In total 74 participants will be recruited from four schools for special education in the Netherlands: Ariane de Ranitz|De Hoogstraat Rehabilitation in Utrecht, Lichtenbeek in Arnhem, Mariendael in Arnhem, and Heliomare in Wijk aan Zee. Schools experienced in organizing and facilitating an after school sports program, will be included in the intervention group. To prevent bias, the control group will only be included at schools where no after school sport is provided. In this way, the research design is close to reality and participants are not unethically prohibited to sport at school. Both ethics approval and administrative site approvals were granted by the Medical Ethical Committee of UMC Utrecht in the Netherlands (#14–118). Additionally, all parents, and participants from 12 years of age, have to provide informed consent prior to study initiation.

Participants

Children and adolescents between the age of 6 and 19 with a chronic disease or physical disability will be included. This could be either cardiovascular, pulmonary, musculoskeletal, metabolic or neuromuscular disorders. Both children and adolescents who are ambulatory or propelling a manual wheelchair are asked to participate. They may participate in sports at most once a week during leisure time in the preceding three months or have a treatment goal on fitness level prescribed by their physician. Participants have to understand simple commands and are able to perform the physical fitness tests. Children and adolescents using electric wheelchair or having progressive diseases will be excluded. In addition, during the length of the study, children and adolescents are not allowed to participate in other research projects which might influence current study results.

Intervention

All participants will follow a training program of eight weeks to increase their physical fitness level. A HIT program will be given twice a week at school by a physical educator and/or a physical therapist. Every training session will consist of a prescribed intensity, volume and time (Table 1). According to the review of Baquet et al. the 30 seconds all out approach for interval training is recommended in youth [46]. An active recovery has been suggested in order to effectively aid the process of lactate removal [47]. Sitting will therefore be forbidden during the interval training and children will be encouraged to motivate and support the others while exercising. After eight weeks of HIT, the

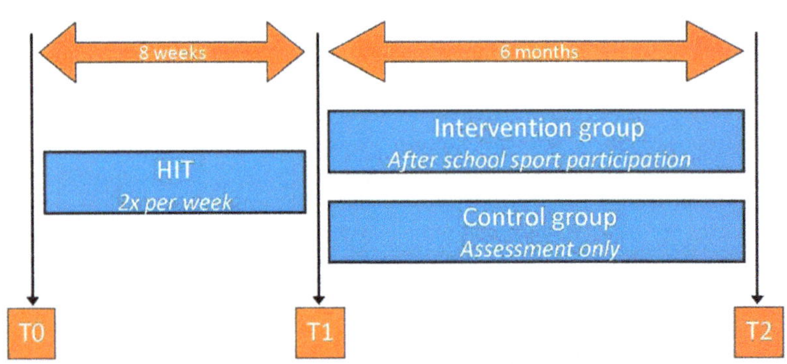

Fig. 1 Schematic research design of the Sport-2-Stay-Fit study. HIT: High-intensity interval training

Table 1 Schematic design of the HIT program. HIT: High-intensity interval training

	Week 1	Week 2	Week 3	Week 4	Week 5	Week 6	Week 7	Week 8
Frequency (p/w)	2	2	2	2	2	2	2	2
Duration	30 sec	30 sec	30 sec	30 sec	30 sec	30 sec	30 sec	30 sec
Intensity	max	max	max	max	max	max	max	max
Work:rest ratio	1:4	1:4	1:4	1:4	1:3	1:3	1:3	1:3
Repetitions	8	8	10	10	12	12	12	12
Total time	20 min	20 min	25 min	25 min	24 min	24 min	24 min	24 min

experimental group will participate in an after school sport program for six months. This is an extra sport lesson additional to the regular physical education schedule. During regular physical education half of the time is spend on skill practice, physical education knowledge and management in children with a physical disability [48]. In contrast, sport is about being physical active, playing the game, and being competitive.

Outcome measures

A general screening questionnaire will be used to inquire about possible factors influencing the outcomes: age, sex, physical activities, health status, injuries. The following outcome measures can be divided: physical fitness, cardiovascular health, physical activity, cognitive functioning, and psychosocial functioning (Table 2).

Primary outcomes

Anaerobic fitness is the primary outcome measure in the current study, because daily physical activity in children most often consists of brief, intermittent bouts of intense movement [49, 50]. Consequently, the anaerobic fitness of healthy individuals involved in recreational sport programs is significantly better than that of those individuals who are not involved in any activities [51]. The Muscle Power Sprint Test (MPST) will be used to evaluate anaerobic fitness. This test is suitable and validated for both children and adolescents who are typically developing, and with cerebral palsy who are ambulant or self-propel a manual wheelchair [6, 52–54]. Subjects have to complete six 15-meter runs at a maximum pace. The MPST is an intermittent sprint test, in which the child starts and stops at standardized intervals. Power output will be calculated for each of the six sprints. Peak power will be defined as the highest calculated power, while mean power will be defined as average power over the six sprints.

Secondary outcomes

Agility

The 10x5 meter sprint test will be performed to asses agility, either while running or propelling a wheelchair. This is a reliable field test to measure agility in children with cerebral palsy [52, 53]. During this test, the child has to sprint as fast as possible for 10 times in between two lines that are five meters apart. Since there is no resting period, the participant has to turn as fast as possible.

Table 2 Overview of the outcome measures of the Sport-2-Stay-Fit

Outcome measure	Parameter	Measurement
Physical Fitness	Anaerobic fitness	Muscle Power Sprint Test (MPST)
	Agility	10x5 meter sprint
	Aerobic fitness	Shuttle run/ride test (SRT)
	Strength	Grip strength
		Reverse curl
		Seated push up
		Standing broad jump/One stroke push
	Flexibility	Modified Apley test
		Modified Thomas test
Cardiovascular Health	Morphologic	Length, weight, BMI
		Bioelectrical impedance analysis
	Metabolic	Sphygmomanometer
		Arteriograph
		Finger puncture
Physical Activity	Modality	Activ8
		Activity diary
Cognitive functioning	School performance	Type of education
		Educational achievement test
	Attention	Bourdon-Vos
		Cancellation task
		Capture task
Psychosocial functioning	Self-perception	Self-Perception Profile for Children (SPPC)
	Quality of life	Disabkids
	Self-efficacy	Exercise Self-efficacy Scale (ESES)

Aerobic fitness

Aerobic fitness, generally expressed as peak oxygen uptake (VO_2peak), is a good predictor of cardiovascular risk [55, 56]. VO_2peak will be measured with a field test. Shuttle run/ride test (SRT) is a field test in which a participant runs, walks or rides between two markers. The SRT starts at 1.5 km/h, 2 km/h or 5 km/h and has shown to be a valid and reliable test in children with cerebral palsy measuring aerobic fitness [57, 58]. The children have to adjust their running, walking or wheelchair propulsion pace to the beep-signals, until they fail to reach the line two times in a row, despite encouragements. Subsequently, a participants mode of locomotion will be identified in order to apply a proper testing protocol (Table 3). Based on clinical observations, participants will be divided into four groups: subjects who are able to run, subjects who walk independently but are not able to run, subjects using walking devices, and wheelchair users. Running is defined in the ICF as moving with quick steps so that both feet may be simultaneously off the ground [59].

Each test will last until volitional exhaustion and protocols will be chosen with the aim to achieve a total exercise time between 6 and 15 min [60, 61]. The shuttle tests will be evaluated with the Cortex Metamax 3X (Samcon bvba, Melle, Belgium), a valid and reliable cardio-pulmonary exercise testing system [62–64]. The Cortex Metamax 3X consists of a facemask, transmitting unit attached to a harness containing oxygen and carbon dioxide analysers, and a receiving unit. Metabolic stress test software (Metasoft Studio) will be used to measure minute ventilation, oxygen uptake (VO_2), carbon dioxide production (VCO_2), heart rate, and respiratory exchange ratio ($RER = VCO_2/VO_2$) every 10 seconds.

Strength

To assess explosive functional strength, the standing broad jump and one stroke push will be performed in children who are ambulatory and propel a manual wheelchair, respectively. Lower limbs strength will be measured by the distance jumped with two legs together from standing position [65] and upper limbs strength by measuring the distance covered in a wheelchair by one push [66]. The following tests are chosen from the Brockport Physical Fitness Test, which was designed to test fitness of youths with various disabilities and is both health related and criterion referenced. Grip strength represents the general strength in healthy children [67]. The grip strength of the dominant hand will be tested through the use of a hand held dynamometer, as described by Beenakker et al. [68] The reverse curl is designed as a measure of hand, wrist, and arm strength [69]. In this test, the participant attempts to pick up a 0.5-kg dumbbell with the preferred arm while seated in a chair or wheelchair. The seated push up is designed to measure upper-body strength and endurance [69]. The participant attempts to perform a seated push-up and holds it for up to 20 seconds.

Flexibility

To test flexibility, the Modified Apley Test and the Modified Thomas Test were chosen from the Brockport Physical Fitness Test. To measure upper-body flexibility with the Modified Apley test, participants attempt to reach back and touch the superior medial angle of the opposite scapula with one hand [69]. The Modified Thomas Test is designed to assess the length of participant's hip flexor muscles: iliopsoas and rectus femoris muscles [69].

Cardiovascular health

BMI, body mass index, will be calculated as weight (kg)/ length $(m)^2$. Height will be measured in standing position in case of ambulant subjects and supine in case of wheelchair bound persons. When a person has spastic legs, arm span width will be measured and corrected as described by Dosa et al. 2009 [70]. Fat free mass will be determined with bioelectrical impedance analysis (BIA), using the Bodystat Quadscan 4000 (Euromedix, Leuven, Belgium). BIA is a non-invasive test comparing conductivity and resistance in the body to distinguish lean body mass and fat [71].

Increased arterial stiffness is associated with a higher likelihood of cardiovascular disease [72]. Arterial stiffness exists of two independent values. The Pulse Wave Velocity (PWV) is measured as the speed at which an aortic pulse travels; increased speed will indicate stiffer arteries. The Augmentation Index (AIX) provides information on the peripheral resistance of the endothelial vessels. Blood pressure and arterial stiffness measurements will be performed using arteriography. The arteriograph (Litra, Amsterdam, the Netherlands) will measure blood pressure, as well as arterial stiffness, using oscillometric tonometry. This method is valid

Table 3 Overview of different SRT protocols. SRT: shuttle run/ride test

Participants	Protocol	Distance	Starting pace	Increasement per min
Able to run	SRT I	10-meter line	5.0 km/h	0.25 km/h
Walk independently (not able to run)	SRT II	10-meter line	2.0 km/h	0.25 km/h
Using walking devices	SRT II	7.5-meter square	1.5 km/h	0.19 km/h
Wheelchair users	SRT II	10-meter line	2.0 km/h	0.25 km/h

compared with the golden standard: invasive measurement during cardiac catheterization [73]. Each subject will rest for at least 10 min prior to the recording. The measurement will be executed using an inflatable cuff at the right upper arm. The participants may not move or talk during the measurement.

To determine metabolic parameters, a finger puncture will be performed to measure cholesterol, low density lipoprotein, high density lipoprotein, glucose and triglyceride. The finger puncture will be performed using a Cholestech LDX analyzer (Mediphos Medical Supplies BV, Renkum, the Netherlands). Participants may not eat or drink for three hours prior to this procedure.

Physical activity

An Activ8 (2M Engineering, Valkenswaard, the Netherlands) accelerometer will be used to measure the type, duration, frequency and intensity of physical activity in daily life. The system is valid and reliable to detect the type, duration, frequency and intensity of physical activity in persons able to walk [74]. Both children who are ambulatory and wheelchair dependent wear the Activ8 on their upper leg for five consecutive days: three weekdays and two weekend days. Wearing the activity monitor will be no burden for the participants; all activities in daily life and during sport activities can be performed. The general activity pattern, incidence and type of injury during the last 3 months will be measured by a questionnaire.

Cognitive functioning

Childhood physical fitness is associated with higher levels of cognition; attention and school performance [15, 16, 75]. For quantifying school performance, a Dutch educational achievement test will be used, which should be administered at school annually. All scores can be converted to a didactic age equivalent. In addition, a more sensitive outcome measure has been chosen to detect changes longitudinally. Cognition was operationalized into three components: sustained attention, search efficiency and distractibility. All tasks will be performed on a tablet (Asus Eee Slate Tablet, with a 12.1 inch display and clock speed of 1.33 GHz) overcoming coordination problems and guaranteeing detection of subtle improvements in performance. Sustained attention will be measured using an adapted digitalized version of the Bourdon-Vos task [76, 77]. The Bourdon-Vos Test is a cancellation test requiring high-speed visual selectivity and a repetitive motor response [76]. Given the length and duration of the test, sustained attention will be assessed [78, 79]. Children are instructed to cross out the target items, i.e., the dot patterns with four dots on a tablet covered in three, four, and five dot patterns. Dependent variables are performance and accuracy over time indicating fluctuations in attention. To assess search efficiency an object cancellation task was used. The presented screen contained 130 stimuli: red and green apples, green and brown pears, letters, and strings of letters. Children had to cancel all apples, while ignoring all other stimuli. Search efficiency will be measured including consistency of search direction, distance between two clicks, and number of intersections. The original capture task used in van der Stigchel & Nijboer was adapted to measure distractibility [80]. Each trial starts with the presentation of central fixation cross. When the cross disappeared, the target, represented as an apple, appeared in one of the corners. In 50 % of the trials, a distractor will appear as well. Reaction time will be measured for both conditions to calculate distractibility.

Psychosocial functioning

In children who are typical developing several studies proved a positive correlation between sports participation and self-perception [81]. To evaluate self-perception, the self-perception profile for children will be used [82]. This is a self-report scale that measures five specific domains of self-concept and the sense of general self-worth.

Children with physical disabilities who participate in sports had significantly higher health related quality of life satisfaction scores compared to their non-sporting peers [83]. The Disabkids questionnaire will be used to assess health related quality of life of children with chronic health conditions [84]. The questionnaire consists of 37 Likert-scaled items and is associated with three domains: mental, social and physical. Additionally, the three domains can be subdivided to six dimensions: independence, emotion, social inclusion, social exclusion, limitation, and treatment. The Disabkids has been developed and validated for children of age 4–16 years [85–87]. Older kids probably have not been included before, because some questions are related to school situations. Since all participants are still attending school, the questionnaire is considered to be applicable for all participants.

To establish the extent of participation in and adherence to a program of regular exercise or physical activity, the Exercise Self-Efficacy questionnaire scale (ESES) will be conducted [88]. A persons self-efficacy is largely influenced by past performances and accomplishments, or mastery experiences.

Sample size

According to a study of Verschuren et al. an average decline of 10 ± 27 % in anaerobic fitness was calculated 3–4 months following a training program [23]. It has been hypothesized that participants following the sports program will show a difference of 20 % compared to the control group. The effect of 20 % seems realistic, since we previously found a 24 % increase in anaerobic fitness in children with cerebral palsy after a training program [23]. With an alpha of 0.05 and bèta of 0.20 (power of 0.80) a sample size of 32 subjects per group will be required. When taking a failure rate of 15 % into account, 74 subjects should be included in total in the Sport-2-Stay-Fit study.

Statistical analyses

The effect of the HIT program and six months after-school sports program will be analysed using a multivariate repeated measures ANOVA. The possible differences between and within T0, T1 and T2 for the intervention group and control group will be calculated with a statistical significance level of $P = 0.01$. If there is a significant difference, a post-hoc test (a Bonferroni or LSD) will be executed to further investigate group differences. Quantitative descriptive statistics will be used to present demographics of the primary and secondary study parameters. All statistical analyses will be performed using SPSS for Windows (version 21.0, SPSS Inc, Chicago, Ill.) with a statistical significance level of $P = 0.05$.

Discussion

The Sport-2-Stay-Fit study will provide insight in the effectiveness of an eight weeks HIT program in children and adolescents with a chronic disease or physical disability. Furthermore, the current study gives answer to the important question whether an after school sports program can increase the sustainability of the effectiveness of a HIT program. To our knowledge, this is the first study investigating the sustainability of a standardized training with a sport program in a group of children and adolescents with a chronic disease or physical disability.

In addition, sport participation in these children may have positive effects on cardiovascular health, injuries, and both cognitive and psychosocial functioning. While these positive relationships have been reported in healthy children, the benefits are not yet established in children with a chronic disease or physical disability.

The Sport-2-Stay-Fit study provide insight and understanding in both the effectiveness and feasibility of an after-school sport program following a standardized interval training. Changing physical activity during leisure time is complicated. Especially in children and adolescents with a chronic disease or physical disability who experience a lot of barriers in joining sport clubs. In this perspective, after-school sport participation may be a feasible solution to get those children and adolescents structurally active. The results are expected to be available in 2017.

Abbreviations

HIT: high-intensity interval training; MPST: muscle power sprint test; SRT: shuttle run/ride test; VO_2peak: peak oxygen uptake; VCO_2: carbon dioxide production; RER: respiratory exchange ratio; BIA: bioelectrical impedance analysis; BMI: body mass index; PWV: pulse wave velocity; AIX: augmentation index.

Competing interests

The authors declare that they have no competing interests.

Authors' contribution

MZ, KL, and KvdEK participated in the design of the study, collection of data and helped to draft the manuscript. TT, OV, JdG, FB, AVM and TT conceived of the study, and participated in its design and coordination and helped to draft the manuscript. All authors read and approved the final manuscript.

Authors' information

Not applicable.

Acknowledgments

The study was funded by an unconditional grant of the Dutch Organization of Health Research (ZONMW) grant number: 525001005.

Sport-2-Stay-Fit study group

FJG Backx (Department of Rehabilitation, Nursing Science and Sports, and Brain Center Rudolf Magnus, University Medical Center Utrecht, Utrecht, the Netherlands), JF de Groot (University of Applied Sciences, Utrecht, the Netherlands), T Takken (Child Development and Exercise Center, University Medical Center Utrecht, Utrecht, the Netherlands), DW Smits (Department of Rehabilitation, Nursing Science and Sports, and Brain Center Rudolf Magnus, University Medical Center Utrecht, Utrecht, the Netherlands), O Verschuren (Center of Excellence for Rehabilitation Medicine and Brain Center Rudolf Magnus and, De Hoogstraat Rehabilitation and University Medical Center Utrecht, Utrecht, the Netherlands), JMA Visser-Meily (Department of Rehabilitation, Nursing Science and Sports, and Center of Excellence for Rehabilitation Medicine and Brain Center Rudolf Magnus, De Hoogstraat Rehabilitation and University Medical Center Utrecht, Utrecht, the Netherlands), MJ Volman (Faculty of Social Sciences, Department of General and Special Education, Utrecht University, Utrecht, the Netherlands), HW Wittink (University of Applied Sciences, Utrecht, the Netherlands), M Zwinkels (Center of Excellence for Rehabilitation Medicine and Brain Center Rudolf Magnus and, De Hoogstraat Rehabilitation and University Medical Center Utrecht, Utrecht, the Netherlands), T Nijboer (Department of Rehabilitation, Nursing Science and Sports, and Center of Excellence for Rehabilitation Medicine and Brain Center Rudolf Magnus, De Hoogstraat Rehabilitation and University Medical Center Utrecht, Utrecht, the Netherlands), G Steenweg (University of Applied Sciences, Arnhem and Nijmegen, the Netherlands).

Author details

[1]Center of Excellence for Rehabilitation Medicine and Brain Center Rudolf Magnus, De Hoogstraat Rehabilitation and University Medical Center Utrecht, Utrecht, the Netherlands. [2]Partner of Shared Utrecht Pediatric Exercise Research (SUPER) Lab, Utrecht, the Netherlands. [3]Research Group Lifestyle and Health, Institute of Human Movement Studies, University of Applied Sciences, Utrecht, the Netherlands. [4]Department of Rehabilitation, Nursing Science and Sports, University Medical Center Utrecht, Utrecht, the Netherlands. [5]Child Development and Exercise Center, University Medical Center Utrecht, Wilhelmina Children's Hospital, P.O. Box 850903508AB, Utrecht, the Netherlands.

References

1. van Brussel M, Lelieveld OTHM, van der Net J, Engelbert RHH, Helders PJM, Takken T. Aerobic and anaerobic exercise capacity in children with juvenile idiopathic arthritis. Arthritis Care Res. 2007;57(6):891–7.
2. Takken T, Van den Beuken C, Wulffraat NM, Helders PJM, van der Net J. Exercise tolerance in children with juvenile idiopathic arthritis after autologous SCT. Bone Marrow Transplant. 2008;42(5):351–6.

3. Takken T, van der Net J, Helders PJM. Anaerobic exercise capacity in patients with juvenile-onset idiopathic inflammatory myopathies. Arthritis Care Res. 2005;53(2):173–7.
4. Takken T, Van Bergen MWM, Sakkers RJB, Helders PJM, Engelbert RHH. Cardiopulmonary exercise capacity, muscle strength, and physical activity in children and adolescents with achondroplasia. J Pediatr. 2007;150(1):26–30.
5. Takken T, Terlingen HC, Helders PJM, Pruijs H, Van Der Ent CK, Engelbert RHH. Cardiopulmonary fitness and muscle strength in patients with osteogenesis imperfecta type I. J Pediatr. 2004;145(6):813–8.
6. Verschuren O, Takken T. Aerobic capacity in children and adolescents with cerebral palsy. Res Dev Disabil. 2010;31(6):1352–7.
7. Erikssen G. Physical fitness and changes in mortality. Sports Med. 2001;31(8):571–6.
8. Arraiz GA, Wigle DT, Mao Y. Risk assessment of physical activity and physical fitness in the Canada Health Survey mortality follow-up study. J Clin Epidemiol. 1992;45(4):419–28.
9. Blair SN, Kohl HW, Paffenbarger RS, Clark DG, Cooper KH, Gibbons LW. Physical fitness and all-cause mortality: A prospective study of healthy men and women. JAMA. 1989;262(17):2395–401.
10. Colditz GA, Samplin-Salgado M, Ryan CT, Dart H, Fisher L, Tokuda A, et al. Harvard Report on Cancer Prevention, Volume 5 Fulfilling the potential for cancer prevention: policy approaches. Cancer Causes Control. 2002;13(3):199–212.
11. Bao W, Srinivasan SR, Wattigney WA, Berenson GS. Persistence of multiple cardiovascular risk clustering related to syndrome X from childhood to young adulthood: the Bogalusa Heart Study. Arch Intern Med. 1994;154(16):1842–7.
12. Smoak CG, Burke GL, Webber LS, Harsha DW, Srinivasan SR, Berenson GS. Relation of obesity to clustering of cardiovascular disease risk factors in children and young adults. The Bogalusa Heart Study. Am J Epidemiol. 1987;125(3):364–72.
13. Basch C. Healthier students are better learners: high-quality, strategically planned, and effectively coordinated school health programs must be a fundamental mission of schools to help close the achievement gap. J Sch Health. 2011;81(10):650–62.
14. Singh A, Uijtdewilligen L, Twisk JWR, van Mechelen W, Chinapaw MJM. Physical activity and performance at school: a systematic review of the literature including a methodological quality assessment. Arch Pediatr Adolesc Med. 2012;166(1):49–55.
15. Chaddock L, Pontifex M, Hillman C, Kramer A. A review of the relation of aerobic fitness and physical activity to brain structure and function in children. J Int Neuropsychol Soc. 2011;17(6):975–85.
16. Tomporowski P, Davis C, Miller P, Naglieri J. Exercise and Children's Intelligence, Cognition, and Academic Achievement. Educ Psychol Rev. 2008;20(2):111–31.
17. Pontifex MB, Scudder MR, Drollette ES, Hillman CH. Fit and vigilant: the relationship between poorer aerobic fitness and failures in sustained attention during preadolescence. Neuropsychology. 2012;26(4):407.
18. Chaddock L, Hillman C, Pontifex M, Johnson C, Raine L, Kramer A. Childhood aerobic fitness predicts cognitive performance one year later. J Sports Sci. 2012;30(5):421–30.
19. London R, Castrechini S. A longitudinal examination of the link between youth physical fitness and academic achievement. J Sch Health. 2011;81(7):400–8.
20. Donnelly J, Greene J, Gibson C, Smith B, Washburn R, Sullivan D, et al. Physical Activity Across the Curriculum (PAAC): a randomized controlled trial to promote physical activity and diminish overweight and obesity in elementary school children. Prev Med. 2009;49(4):336–41.
21. Sallis JF, McKenzie TL, Kolody B, Lewis M, Marshall S, Rosengard P. Effects of health-related physical education on academic achievement: project SPARK. Res Q Exerc Sport. 1999;70(2):127–34.
22. Groff DG, Lundberg NR, Zabriskie RB. Influence of adapted sport on quality of life: Perceptions of athletes with cerebral palsy. Disabil Rehabil. 2009;31(4):318–26.
23. Verschuren O, Ketelaar M, Gorter J, Helders PJM, Uiterwaal CSPM, Takken T. Exercise training program in children and adolescents with cerebral palsy: a randomized controlled trial. Arch Pediatr Adolesc Med. 2007;161(11):1075–81.
24. Rose B, Larkin D, Berger BG. Coordination and gender influences on the perceived competence of children. Adapt Phys Activ Q. 1997;14(3):210–21.
25. Piek JP, Dworcan M, Barrett NC, Coleman R. Determinants of self-worth in children with and without developmental coordination disorder. Int J Disability Dev Educ. 2000;47(3):259–72.
26. Feltz DL, Landers DM, Raeder U. Enhancing self-efficacy in high-avoidance motor tasks: A comparison of modeling techniques. J Sport Psychol. 1979;1(2):112–22.
27. Bandura A, Adams NE, Beyer J. Cognitive processes mediating behavioral change. J Pers Soc Psychol. 1977;35(3):125–39.
28. Hedrick BN. The effect of wheelchair tennis participation and mainstreaming upon the perception of competence of physically disabled adolescents. Ther Recreation J. 1985;19(2):34–46.
29. Mazzoni ER, Purves PL, Southward J, Rhodes RE, Temple VA. Effect of indoor wall climbing on self-efficacy and self-perceptions of children with special needs. Adapt Phys Activ Q. 2009;26(3):259–73.
30. Van Brussel M, van der Net J, Hulzebos E, Helders PJM, Takken T. The Utrecht approach to exercise in chronic childhood conditions: the decade in review. Pediatr Phys Ther. 2011;23(1):2–14.
31. Murphy N, Carbone P. Promoting the participation of children with disabilities in sports, recreation, and physical activities. Pediatrics. 2008;121(5):1057–61.
32. Van Brussel M, Takken T, Uiterwaal CSPM, Pruijs H, Van der Net J, Helders PJM, et al. Physical training in children with osteogenesis imperfecta. J Pediatr. 2008;152(1):111–6.
33. de Groot J, Takken T, van Brussel M, Gooskens R, Schoenmakers M, Versteeg C, et al. Randomized controlled study of home-based treadmill training for ambulatory children with spina bifida. Neurorehabil Neural Repair. 2011;25(7):597–606.
34. World Health Organization. Global recommendations on physical activity for health. 2010.
35. Verschuren O, Wiart L, Hermans D, Ketelaar M. Identification of facilitators and barriers to physical activity in children and adolescents with cerebral palsy. J Pediatr. 2012;161(3):488–94.
36. Lindert C. Sport voor mensen met een handicap in Nederland: op weg naar Olympisch niveau? 2012.
37. Bloemen M, Verschuren O, van Mechelen C, Borst H, de Leeuw A, van der Hoef M, et al. Personal and environmental factors to consider when aiming to improve participation in physical activity in children with Spina Bifida: a qualitative study. BMC Neurol. 2015;15:11.
38. Atkin A, Gorely TB, Stuart JH, Cavill N, Foster C. Interventions to promote physical activity in young people conducted in the hours immediately after school: a systematic review. Int J Behav Med. 2011;18(3):176–87.
39. Heath G, Parra D, Sarmiento O, Andersen L, Owen N, Goenka S, et al. Evidence-based intervention in physical activity: lessons from around the world. Lancet (London, England). 2012;380(9838):272–81.
40. Weston K, Wisløff U, Coombes J. High-intensity interval training in patients with lifestyle-induced cardiometabolic disease: a systematic review and meta-analysis. Br J Sports Med. 2014;48(16):1227-34.
41. Haykowsky M, Timmons M, Kruger C, McNeely M, Taylor D, Clark A. Meta-analysis of aerobic interval training on exercise capacity and systolic function in patients with heart failure and reduced ejection fractions. Am J Cardiol. 2013;111(10):1466–9.
42. Gibala M, Little J, Macdonald M, Hawley J. Physiological adaptations to low-volume, high-intensity interval training in health and disease. J Physiol (Lond). 2012;590(5):1077–84.
43. Slaman J, Roebroeck M, Dallmijer A, Twisk J, Stam H, Van Den Berg-Emons R. Can a lifestyle intervention programme improve physical behaviour among adolescents and young adults with spastic cerebral palsy? A randomized controlled trial. Dev Med Child Neurol. 2015;57(2):159–66.
44. Van Wely L, Balemans A, Becher J, Dallmeijer A. Physical activity stimulation program for children with cerebral palsy did not improve physical activity: a randomised trial. J Physiother. 2014;60(1):40–9.
45. Lankhorst K, van der Ende-Kastelijn, Zwinkels M, Muselaers E, Verschuren O, Takken T, et al. Sport participation reduces sedentary time, but does it improve physical fitness in youth with a physical disability or chronic disease? Pediatric Exercise Science, 2015;27(SupplAugust):50.
46. Baquet G, van Praagh E, Berthoin S. Endurance training and aerobic fitness in young people. Sports Med. 2003;33(15):1127–43.
47. Billat LV. Interval training for performance: a scientific and empirical practice. Special recommendations for middle- and long-distance running. Part I: aerobic interval training. Sports Med. 2001;31(1):13–31.
48. Sit CHP, McManus A, McKenzie TL, Lian J. Physical activity levels of children in special schools. Prev Med. 2007;45(6):424–31.
49. Bailey RC, Olson J, Pepper SL, Porszasz J, Barstow TJ, Cooper DM. The level and tempo of children's physical activities: an observational study. Med Sci Sports Exerc. 1995;27(7):1033–41.

50. Verschuren O, Ketelaar M, Gorter J, Helders PJM, Takken T. Relation between physical fitness and gross motor capacity in children and adolescents with cerebral palsy. Dev Med Child Neurol. 2009;51(11):866–71.
51. Hoffman JR, Kang J, Faigenbaum AD, Ratamess NA. Recreational sports participation is associated with enhanced physical fitness in children. Res Sports Med. 2005;13(2):149–61.
52. Verschuren O, Zwinkels M, Obeid J, Kerkhof N, Ketelaar M, Takken T. Reliability and validity of short-term performance tests for wheelchair-using children and adolescents with cerebral palsy. Dev Med Child Neurol. 2013;55(12):1129–35.
53. Verschuren O, Takken T, Ketelaar M, Gorter JW, Helders PJ. Reliability for running tests for measuring agility and anaerobic muscle power in children and adolescents with cerebral palsy. Pediatr Phys Ther. 2007;19(2):108–15.
54. Bongers BC, Werkman MS, Blokland D, Eijsermans MJ, Van der Torre P, Bartels B, et al. Validity of the Pediatric Running-Based Anaerobic Sprint Test to Determine Anaerobic Performance in Healthy Children. Pediatr Exerc Sci. 2015;27(2):268–76.
55. Shephard R, Benade A, Benade A, Davies C, Di Prampero P, Hedman R, et al. The maximum oxygen intake. An international reference standard of cardiorespiratory fitness. Bull World Health Organ. 1968;38(5):757–64.
56. Aspenes ST, Nilsen TI, Skaug EA, Bertheussen GF, Ellingsen O, Vatten L, et al. Peak oxygen uptake and cardiovascular risk factors in 4631 healthy women and men. Med Sci Sports Exerc. 2011;43(8):1465–73.
57. Verschuren O, Zwinkels M, Ketelaar M, Reijnders-van Son F, Takken T. Reproducibility and validity of the 10-meter shuttle ride test in wheelchair-using children and adolescents with cerebral palsy. Phys Ther. 2013;93(7):967–74.
58. Verschuren O, Takken T, Ketelaar M, Gorter JW, Helders PJM. Reliability and validity of data for 2 newly developed shuttle run tests in children with cerebral palsy. Phys Ther. 2006;86(8):1107–17.
59. World Health Organization. Chapter 4 Mobility. International Classification of Functioning, Disability, and Health: Children & Youth Version: ICF-CY. Geneva, Switzerland: World Health Organization; 2007. p. 157.
60. Buchfuhrer M, Hansen J, Robinson T, Sue D, Wasserman K, Whipp B. Optimizing the exercise protocol for cardiopulmonary assessment. J Appl Physiol Respir Environ Exerc Physiol. 1983;55(5):1558–64.
61. Hebestreit H. Exercise testing in children – what works, what doesn't, and where to go? Paediatr Respir Rev. 2004;5(Suppl A):S11–4.
62. Meyer T, Georg T, Becker C, Kindermann W. Reliability of gas exchange measurements from two different spiroergometry systems. Int J Sports Med. 2001;22(8):593–7.
63. Medbø JI, Mamen A, Welde B, Von Heimburg E, Stokke R. Examination of the Metamax I and II oxygen analysers during exercise studies in the laboratory. Scand J Clin Lab Invest. 2002;62(8):585–98.
64. Brehm MA, Harlaar J, Groepenhof H. Validation of the portable VmaxST system for oxygen-uptake measurement. Gait Posture. 2004;20(1):67–73.
65. Deitz JC, Kartin D, Kopp K. Review of the Bruininks-Oseretsky test of motor proficiency, (BOT-2). Phys Occup Ther Pediatr. 2007;27(4):87–102.
66. Verschuren O, Ketelaar M, De Groot J, Vila Nova F, Takken T. Reproducibility of two functional field exercise tests for children with cerebral palsy who self-propel a manual wheelchair. Dev Med Child Neurol. 2013;55(2):185–90.
67. Wind AE, Takken T, Helders PJ, Engelbert RH. Is grip strength a predictor for total muscle strength in healthy children, adolescents, and young adults? Eur J Pediatr. 2010;169(3):281–7.
68. Beenakker EA, van der Hoeven JH, Fock JM, Maurits NM. Reference values of maximum isometric muscle force obtained in 270 children aged 4–16 years by hand-held dynamometry. Neuromuscul Disord. 2001;11(5):441–6.
69. Winnick JP, Short FX. The Brockport physical fitness training guide. Champaign, Illinois: Human Kinetics Publishers; 1999.
70. Dosa NP, Foley JT, Eckrich M, Woodall-Ruff D, Liptak GS. Obesity across the lifespan among persons with spina bifida. Disabil Rehabil. 2009;31(11):914–20.
71. Mok E, Letellier G, Cuisset JM, Denjean A, Gottrand F, Hankard R. Assessing change in body composition in children with Duchenne muscular dystrophy: anthropometry and bioelectrical impedance analysis versus dual-energy X-ray absorptiometry. Clin Nutr. 2010;29(5):633–8.
72. Mattace-Raso FU, van der Cammen TJ, Hofman A, van Popele NM, Bos ML, Schalekamp MA, et al. Arterial stiffness and risk of coronary heart disease and stroke: the Rotterdam Study. Circulation. 2006;113(5):657–63.
73. Horváth IG, Németh A, Lenkey Z, Alessandri N, Tufano F, Kis P, et al. Invasive validation of a new oscillometric device (Arteriograph) for measuring augmentation index, central blood pressure and aortic pulse wave velocity. J Hypertens. 2010;28(10):2068–75.
74. Erasmus MC University Medical Center Rotterdam. Validation of the Activ8 Activity Monitor: detection of body postures and movements. 2013.
75. Westendorp M, Houwen S, Hartman E, Visscher C. Are gross motor skills and sports participation related in children with intellectual disabilities? Res Dev Disabil. 2011;32(3):1147–53.
76. Vos P. De Bourdon concentratietest voor kinderen.[The Bourdon concentration test for children]. 1992.
77. De Sonneville L. Amsterdam Neuropsychological Tasks: A computer-aided assessment program. Comput Psychol. 1999;6:187–203.
78. Bloemers F, Collard D, Paw MC, Van Mechelen W, Twisk J, Verhagen E. Physical inactivity is a risk factor for physical activity-related injuries in children. Br J Sports Med. 2012;46(9):669–74.
79. Lezak M. Neuropsychological assessment. Oxford, UK: Oxford University Press; 2004.
80. Van der Stigchel S, Nijboer TCW. The imbalance of oculomotor capture in unilateral visual neglect. Conscious Cogn. 2010;19(1):186–97.
81. Eime RM, Young JA, Harvey JT, Charity MJ, Payne WR. A systematic review of the psychological and social benefits of participation in sport for children and adolescents: informing development of a conceptual model of health through sport. Int J Behav Nutr Phys Act. 2013;10(1):98.
82. Harter S. Manual for the self-perception profile for children. Denver, Colorado: University of Denver; 1985.
83. Yazicioglu K, Yavuz F, Goktepe AS, Tan AK. Influence of adapted sports on quality of life and life satisfaction in sport participants and non-sport participants with physical disabilities. Disabil Health J. 2012;5:249–53.
84. Baars RM, Atherton CI, Koopman HM, Bullinger M, Power M. The European DISABKIDS project: development of seven condition-specific modules to measure health related quality of life in children and adolescents. Health Qual Life Outcomes. 2005;3:70.
85. Panepinto J, O'Mahar K, DeBaun M, Rennie K, Scott JP. Validity of the child health questionnaire for use in children with sickle cell disease. J Pediatr Hematol Oncol. 2004;26(9):574–8.
86. Simeoni MC, Schmidt S, Muehlan H, Debensason D, Bullinger M. Field testing of a European quality of life instrument for children and adolescents with chronic conditions: the 37-item DISABKIDS Chronic Generic Module. Qual Life Res. 2007;16(5):881–93.
87. Janssens L, Gorter JW, Ketelaar M, Kramer WLM, Holtslag H. Health-related quality-of-life measures for long-term follow-up in children after major trauma. Qual Life Res. 2008;17(5):701–13.
88. Nooijen CFJ, Post MWM, Spijkerman DCM, Bergen M, Stam H, van den Berg-Emons RJG. Exercise self-efficacy in persons with spinal cord injury: psychometric properties of the Dutch translation of the Exercise Self-Efficacy Scale. J Rehabil Med. 2013;45(4):347–50.

6

Gender differences in myocardial function and arterio-ventricular coupling in response to maximal exercise in adolescent floor-ball players

Åsa Fomin[1†], Cristina Da Silva[2,3†], Mattias Ahlstrand[1], Anders Sahlén[2], Lars Lund[2], Marcus Stahlberg[2], Anders Gabrielsen[1†] and Aristomenis Manouras[2,3,4*†]

Abstract

Background: The hemodynamic and cardiac responses to exercise have been widely investigated in adults. However, little is known regarding myocardial performance in response to a short bout of maximal exercise in adolescents. We therefore sought to study alterations in myocardial function and investigate sex-influences in young athletes after maximal cardiopulmonary testing.

Methods: 51 adolescent (13-19 years old) floor-ball players (24 females) were recruited. All subjects underwent a maximal exercise test to determine maximal oxygen uptake (VO2max) and cardiac output. Cardiac performance was investigated using conventional and tissue velocity imaging, as well as 2D strain echocardiography before and 30 minutes following exercise. Arterio-ventricular coupling was evaluated by means of single beat ventricular elastance and arterial elastance.

Results: Compared to baseline the early diastolic myocardial velocity (E'LV) at the basal left ventricular (LV) segments declined significantly (females: E'LV: 14.7 +/- 2.6 to 13.6 +/- 2.9 cm/s; males: 15.2 +/- 2.2 to 13.9 +/- 2.3 cm/s, $p < 0.001$ for both). Similarly, 2D strain decreased significantly following exercise (2D strain LV: from 21.5 +/- 2.4 to 20.2 +/- 2.7% in females, and from 20 +/- 1 to 17.9 +/- 1.5% in males, $p < 0.05$ for both). However, there were no significant changes in LV contractility estimated by elastance in either sex following exercise ($p > 0.05$). Arterial elastance) Ea) at baseline was identified as the only predictor of VO2max in males ($r = 0.76$, $p < 0.001$) but not in females ($p > 0.05$).

Conclusions: The present study demonstrates that vigorous exercise of short duration results in a significant decrease of longitudinal myocardial motion in both sexes. However, in view of unaltered end systolic LV elastance (Ees), these reductions most probably reflect changes in the loading conditions and not an attenuation of myocardial function per se. Importantly, we show that arterial load at rest acts as a strong predictor of VO2max in males but not in female subjects.

Keywords: Exercise, Echocardiography, Elastance, Tissue Doppler Imaging, Adolescent, Sex, Exercise stress test, Contractility, Peak VO2

* Correspondence: aristomenis.manouras@karolinska.se
†Equal contributors
[2]Department of Cardiology, Karolinska University Hospital, Stockholm, Sweden
[3]School of Technology and Health, Royal Institute of Technology, Stockholm, Sweden
Full list of author information is available at the end of the article

Background

Numerous studies have documented the beneficial effects of moderate physical activity on cardiovascular health [1-3]. However, there is a substantial body of evidence supporting the notion that prolonged exercise might be less favorable regarding its immediate effects on cardiac function. Indeed, it has been demonstrated that ventricular performance is attenuated following strenuous exercise, a phenomenon that has been designated "exercise-induced cardiac fatigue" (EICF) [4]. Conversely, there is a paucity of data on EICF after a short bout of maximal exercise and the evidence available indicates that ventricular function is either unaltered or even improved during recovery [5]. While the physiological explanation of EICF is as yet not clear, some investigators support the notion that the observed alterations in cardiac function may be the result of preload reduction following exercise [6], whereas others advocate that a reduction of the intrinsic myocardial function might also contribute to the development of EICF.

Echocardiography is the method most frequently employed in studies of EICF due to its non-invasive nature and its broad availability. Moreover, the rapid development of instrumentation during the last decades has significantly enriched the arsenal of echocardiographic cardiac assessment with modalities such as tissue Doppler imaging (TDI) and 2D strain contributing substantially in the diagnostics of myocardial function. Although, the aforementioned echocardiographic modalities have been shown to provide robust quantification of the heart function, it is established today, that these techniques are susceptible to changes in hemodynamic loading. Conversely, ventricular elastance (E_{es}) has been shown to be less load-dependent and the development of non-invasive algorithms for measuring E_{es} has provided novel possibilities for a more precise and robust quantification of the cardiac function.

To date, the studies investigating the EICF have mainly interrogated the cardiac alterations either in children or in adult population and a number of investigations have demonstrated significant sexual dimorphism in metabolic responses during exercise [7]. Despite the increasing number of teenagers participating in competitive sports during past decades [8,9], there is a lack of studies regarding the hemodynamic responses following short bouts of exercise in adolescent athletes. Furthermore, although significant sex-related differences after acute bout of exercise have been demonstrated [7,10], detailed knowledge is limited regarding this issue in adolescent exercise physiology. The lack of knowledge regarding EICF in adolescents impedes ones interpretation of the cardiovascular and respiratory responses to exercise and limits the guidance available for adolescents in competitive in exercise programs.

In light of the aforementioned and based on previously demonstrated sexual disparities in neuroendocrine responses during exercise we hypothesized that adolescents may behave in a different hemodynamic manner following a short bout of exercise. Thus, we undertook the present study on adolescent floor-ball players to investigate: 1. the myocardial and hemodynamic responses following maximal exercise testing and to assess whether intense exercise of short duration impacts on the myocardial function; 2. possible differences in heart function following exercise between the two sexes.

Methods

Study population

51 adolescent floor-ball players (24 female and 27 male), aged between 13 and 19 years old were recruited from a local floor-ball club. Floor-ball is a well known sport with its origin in Sweden and a significant number of participants of both genders. It is classified as a sport activity with a high aerobic and a low to moderate anaerobic component [11]. Informed consent was given from the participants and their parents following an oral and written explanation of the study objectives and protocol. The subjects reported initially to the study room and underwent a health and a physical examination. All subjects were healthy, had no history of cardiovascular disease and were not taking any medication. The investigation was approved by the ethical committee of Northern Stockholm (Young athlete Heart study, 2009/1246-31/1).

Study protocol

Blood samples

Blood samples were collected from an indwelling catheter placed in the ante-cubital vein. Total hemoglobin, creatinine and N-terminal pro B-type natriuretic peptide (NT-proBNP) concentration were analyzed. Baseline venous blood gas samples were obtained (ABL 700, Radiometer, Copenhagen, Denmark) for analyses of blood lactate concentration and for metabolic assessment (base-excess, HCO_3^-, pH). Ten minutes post exercise, new blood samples were collected and analyzed.

Blood pressure recording

For the purposes of the echocardiographic measurements, systolic (SBP) and diastolic (DBP) blood pressure were recorded using a semi-automatic blood pressure (BP) measure device (Omron 7051 T, Omron Healthcare) directly after the termination of each echocardiographic examination with the patient supine. Additional BP recordings were obtained during the exercise test using a BP cuff and a Doppler flow measuring probe positioned over the radial artery.

Exercise test

A baseline supine resting 12-lead ECG was recorded and the subjects were subsequently placed on the exercise bicycle. One female participant was diagnosed with a

Wolf-Parkinson-White type pre-excitation but was included in the study as she was completely asymptomatic. Following the study she was referred for cardiac electrophysiological evaluation. Her other exams and test results, beside the ECG, were completely normal. The exercise test was performed on a Rodby Ergometer Bike RE990 stress bicycle using a standard protocol (60 watt initial load applying load increments of 20 watt per minute). A 12 lead ECG was recorded at rest and during the whole exercise period.

Ventilation, gas exchange, pulmonary blood flow and cardiac output acquisition

During the exercise test, ventilation, O_2 and CO_2 were measured on a breath-by-breath basis using an Innocor® device (Innovision, Odense, Denmark) connected through a breathing mouth piece to the subject with a continuous inspiratory and expiratory sampling for the flow analysis. VO_2max was derived as the average VO_2 obtained during the last 30 seconds of exercise and normalized to the total body weight. Using the inert gas re-breathing technique, the Innocor® device provided measurements of the pulmonary flow at baseline and at peak exercise with the patient seated on the bicycle ergometer. To measure the pulmonary blood flow the subject performed a 30 seconds of closed re-breathing circle from a bag containing a gas mixture of 50% oxygen (O_2), 0,5% Nitric Oxide (N_2O) (soluble gas) and 0,1% sulphur hexafluoride (SF_6) (insoluble gas) in nitrogen (N_2) diluted with ambient room air. The re-breathing bag volume was set 30% higher than the expected tidal volume in each case. Pulmonary blood flow was calculated using standard validated formulas incorporated in the Innocor® software [12,13]. Pulmonary blood flow was assumed to equal cardiac output as there were no signs of pulmonary blood shunting. Subsequently cardiac index (CI) was calculated according to the standard formula.

Echocardiography

All subjects underwent transthoracic echocardiography (TTE) at two occasions i.e., prior the exercise and 30 minutes following the exercise termination, using a commercially available equipment (Vivid *i*, GE Vingmed, Horten, Norway) equipped with a standard phased array 2.5 MHz multi-frequency transducer. TTE was performed according to the current recommendations of the European Society of echocardiography [14] with the patient lying at the left lateral recumbent position. All measurements were performed offline by the same investigator (CDS) using commercially dedicated software (EchoPAC PC, version 11.0.0.0 GE Ultrasound, Waukesha, Wisconsin). Measurements were performed in three cardiac cycles and the values obtained averaged.

Measurements of the left ventricular (LV) end-diastolic diameter (LVEDD), septal and posterior wall thickness were assessed from the parasternal long-axis view using 2D. The LV mass was obtained according to the formula proposed by the American society of echocardiography [15]. From the apical window the LV end-diastolic (LVEDV), end-systolic (LVESV) volumes and ejection fraction (EF) were assessed employing the Simpson's formula in 4- and 2 chamber apical view while ensuring that any apical foreshortening was avoided. Left atrial area (LA-area) was measured from the apical 4-chamber view. All volumetric measurements were indexed to Body Surface Area (BSA). BSA was calculated using the DuBois formula: $BSA = (W^{0.425} \times H^{0.725}) \times 0.007184$. Transmitral flow velocities were obtained from the apical 4-chamber view using pulsed Doppler with the 5 mm sampling volume placed just below the tips of the mitral leaflets. Peak flow velocity during the early diastolic filling phase (E wave) and during the atrial contraction (A wave) as well as the deceleration time (DT) and the isovolumetric relaxation time (IVRT) i.e. the time between aortic valve closure and mitral valve opening were measured. The right ventricular (RV) diameter was assessed at end-diastole from the apical 4-chamber view at basal level of the RV. All measurements were performed on a minimum of 3 cardiac cycles and mean values were recorded.

Spectral tissue Doppler

Spectral tissue Doppler (TD) velocities were obtained by placing a 5 mm sampling volume at the basal segment of the septal and lateral LV wall and at the basal lateral RV wall. Care was taken in order to keep the sample volume located in the ventricular myocardium throughout the heart cycle and the angle of incidence as parallel as possible to the longitudinal axis of myocardial motion. The manufacturers' default settings were kept unaltered (0 dB transmit gain and 3 dB receive gain). Accordingly, peak systolic (S'_{LV} and S'_{RV}) velocities as well as peak diastolic velocities during early diastole (E'_{LV} and E'_{RV}) and atrial contraction (A'_{LV} and A'_{RV}) were acquired and the mean values from the septal and lateral wall were obtained and analyzed.

Moreover, measurements of myocardial isovolumic relaxation time (IVRT′), isovolumetric contraction time (IVCT′) and ejection time (ET′) were obtained from the RV lateral basal wall and the myocardial performance index (MPI) was calculated according to the equation: $[(IVRT' + IVCT')/ET']$.

Myocardial deformation analysis

Myocardial deformation analysis was performed offline using the 2D strain software provided in the EchoPac software. The cardiac cycle providing the best visual assessment of the endocardial borders was selected and all the measurements performed by single operator. The endocardial border was outlined manually and adjusted to match the actual borders of the myocardium and the regions of interest were optimized so that their thickness represented the corresponding thickness of the LV segments. Using the 2D strain analysis application provided by the EchoPac, the LV was automatically subdivided in 18 segments and 2D longitudinal strain was analyzed for the LV from the 4-, 2- and 3-chamber views. Subsequently the global longitudinal 2D strain was obtained by averaging the segmental strains. Peak systolic longitudinal strain for LV and RV was calculated at the aortic valve closure. According to the recommendations the 2D images were recorded in order to provide a frame rate between 70-80 frames per second. RV 2D strain was measured by tracing the RV lateral wall. 2D strain was measured on images obtained at baseline and 30 minutes after the termination of the exercise test.

LV Elastance and Arterial Elastance measurements

Using echocardiography and Doppler derived flow variables, effective arterial elastance (E_a) and LV end-systolic elastance (E_{es}) were calculated at baseline and 30 min following maximal exercise. E_a constitutes a "lumped index" of LV afterload in the time-domain and is calculated as $E_a = LVESP/SV$ where LV end-systolic pressure (LVESP) was estimated as $LVESP = 0.9 \times SBP$ [16]. Arterial stiffness was defined as the reciprocal of compliance and assumed to be linearly related to pressure [17] and calculated as Stiffness = (SBP-DBP)/SV. Based on a two-element Windkessel model of the circulation with negligible central venous pressure, total peripheral resistance (TPR) was calculated as TPR = [DBP + (SBP-DBP)/3]/CO. [18] The relative importance of the components of E_a was studied after adjusting TPR for heart rate (HR) by dividing by the cardiac period (T).

E_{es} is defined as the slope of the line connecting the ESPVR of a run of heart beats recorded during a load intervention. Given its relative load-insensitivity, E_{es} is considered as the reference standard for measurements of LV contractility. E_{es} was estimated using the single-beat approach developed by Chen and co-workers [19]. Importantly, this method does not assume that the volume axis intercept of ESPVR is the origin of the diagram (0;0) but that the line can be extrapolated to intersect the volume axis at the point ($V_{0;0}$) [19].

Briefly, E_{es} was calculated as $E_{es(sb)} = [DBP - (E_{Nd(est)} \times LVESP)]/[SV \times E_{Nd(est)}]$ where $E_{Nd(est)}$ represents group-averaged normalized E_{es} values obtained as a function of EF and the ratio between SBP and DBP as described by the equation:

$$E_{Nd(est)} = 0.0275–0.165 \times EF + 0.3656 \times (DPB/SBP) + 0.515 \times E_{Nd(avg)}.$$

In this equation, $E_{Nd(avg)}$ is given by a seven-term polynomial function:

$$E_{Nd(avg)} = \sum_{i=0} a_i \times t_{Nd}^i$$

where summation is performed for i = 0 to 7, using values for a_i of [0.35695; -7.2266; 74.249; -307.39; 684.54; -856.92; 571.95; -159.1] respectively. The value of t_{Nd} was determined by the ratio of the pre-ejection period (R-wave to flow-onset) to the total systolic period (R-wave to end-flow), with the time at onset and termination of flow defined noninvasively from the pulsed Doppler waveform in LVOT.

Statistical analysis

All data are presented as mean ± SD and as a ratio for categorical data. Student's *t*-test and independent *t*-test were used when suitable for comparison of paired and unpaired data respectively. Normality was analyzed using Kolmogorov-Smirnov test. The Mann-Whitney rank sum test was employed for comparison of continues variables with skewed distribution. Spearman's rho and Pearson's correlation coefficient r was used as appropriate to examine the degree of correlation among variables.

Multiple regression analysis was performed for testing possible independent predictors of VO_2max. The statistical significance was set at a two tailed probability level of $p < 0.05$. All analyses were performed with SPSS for Windows, release 18.0 (SPSS Inc. Chicago, III).

Results

Baseline demographic, metabolic and cardiopulmonary characteristics

Demographic characteristics of the study population are provided in Table 1. As shown the participants of the two sexes were of similar age and body mass index (BMI). Not surprisingly, hemoglobin and creatinine levels were higher in males as was the SBP at rest when compared to the female participants ($p < 0.05$). However, NT pro-BNP and troponine levels did not differ significant between the subjects of the two sexes. Female subjects exhibited a lower SBP (119 ± 11 mmHg; mean ± SD) compared to male participants (130 ± 13 mmHg, $p < 0.05$), whereas DBP did not differ between sexes (Table 1).

Cardiopulmonary and metabolic responses to exercise

Maximum SBP during exercise was lower in female (171 ± 20 mmHg) than in male subjects (185 ± 17 mmHg, $p < 0.05$), whereas maximum HR was similar (females: 191 ± 9 bpm vs. males: 194 ± 7 bpm). CI at maximum exercise was lower in females (7.0 ± 1.0 $L/min/m_2$) than in males (8.3 ± 1.4 $L/min/m^2$, $p < 0.05$).

Table 1 Patient characteristics of the study population

Patient characteristics			
Parameters	**Male *(27)***	**Female *(24)***	**p-value**
Age (yrs)	17.0 ± 1.3	16.5 ± 1.8	ns
Height (cm)	179 ± 6	168 ± 5	<0.001
Weight (Kg)	69.7 ± 9.1	61.3 ± 9.2	0.002
BMI (kg/m^2)	21.7 ± 2.7	21.6 ± 2.8	ns
Training per week (hours)	8.8 ± 1.3	7.4 ± 1.6	0.002
SBP (mmHg)	130 ± 15	119 ± 7	0.03
DBP (mmHg)	70 ± 8	71 ± 9	ns
Creatinine (μmol/L)	78 ± 9	65 ± 10	<0.001
Hemoglobin (g/L)	147 ± 8	132 ± 6	<0.001
VO2max (mL/min/Kg)	49 ± 5	39 ± 5	<0.001
LV mass$_{index}$ (g/m^2)	88 ± 15	85 ± 18	ns

BMI denotes body mass index; SBP, systolic blood pressure; DBP, diastolic blood pressure; VO2max; maximal oxygen uptake during peak cardiopulmonary testing normalized to total body mass; LVmass$_{index}$, left ventricular mass normaliserad to body surface area.

RQ at maximum exercise was similar (females: 1.04 ± 0.06 vs. males: 1.05 ± 0.05, p > 0.05). VO_2max normalized to total body mass was lower in females (39.1 ± 5.1 mL/min/kg; 51.2 ± 6.8 mL/min/kg) compared to males (48.7 ± 5.5 mL/min/kg; p < 0.05).

Echocardiographic findings at baseline

None of the participants showed any evidence of structural or functional heart abnormality. Baseline echocardiographic characteristics are presented in Table 2. Despite larger EDVi and SVi (p < 0.05) in male participants, no differences were observed when comparing the LVEF. The RV end-diastolic diameter did not differ significantly between the participants of the two sexes when indexed to BSA ($p > 0.05$). TVI and 2D strain measurements recorded at baseline are presented in Table 2. As expected both male and female participants demonstrated excellent longitudinal LV and RV function as reflected by the high longitudinal myocardial velocities with similar values between the subjects of the two sexes ($p > 0.05$). The transmitral Doppler flow velocities and the DT were similar between the participants of the two sexes as were the MPI of the RV ($p > 0.05$).

On the other hand, LV longitudinal myocardial 2D strain and RV 2D strain was higher in females (LV global 2D strain: males: -20 ± 1%; females: -21 ± 2%; RV 2D strain: males: -29 ± 4% vs. females: -32 ± 5%, p < 0.05 in both cases).

Echocardiographic alterations in response to exercise

2D measurements obtained 30 minutes after the maximal cardiopulmonary test are shown in Table 2. Significant reductions in LVEDV and LVESV were observed in both sexes as compared to the baseline measurements.

Despite a significantly higher HR as compared to baseline, E'_{LV} was decreased following examination both at the septal and lateral wall ($p < 0.05$). Furthermore, male and female participants showed a reduction in global LV longitudinal 2D strain following exercise ($p < 0.05$). Early transmitral inflow velocities (E) were significantly lower compared to baseline measurements in both males and females. Similar to the observations for the LV, significant reduction in E'_{RV} and 2D strain$_{RV}$ were observed after the exercise in both sexes with higher values obtained in female participants as compared to males ($p < 0.05$). Furthermore, subjects of both sexes revealed a significant increase of the RV MPI $_{index}$ as a result of longer isovolumic myocardial phases and a shorter ejection period.

Measurements of LV and Arterial Elastance at baseline and in response to exercise

At baseline, LV systolic performance as evaluated by single beat E_{es} measurements demonstrated similar values in male and female participants (p > 0.005) with similar arterial load as estimated by E_a.

At peak exercise, CI was higher in male participants (8.3 ± 1.4 vs. 7.0 ± 1.0 L/min/m^2, p < 0001) and taking into account that maximal HR did not differ between sexes (194 ± 7 vs. 191 ± 9 bpm, p > 0.05), the sole factor responsible for this difference was a higher SVi in males compared to females (43 ± 7 vs. 37 ± 6 mL/m^2, p < 0001).

E_ai increased significantly compared to baseline values with participants of the two sexes displaying similar values (male: 4.0 ± 0.7; females 4.3 ± 0.8 mmHg/mL, p > 0.05) despite significantly higher systolic BP in males (males: 185 ± 17 mmHg; females 171 ± 20 mmHg, p < 0.001).

Following exercise, no significant differences in E_{es}, E_ai or E_a/E_{es} ratio were observed as compared to baseline values with higher E_{es} levels in female participants (p < 0.05, Table 2, Figures 1 and 2).

In order to investigate whether baseline LV and arterial elastance measurements correlated with baseline levels of NT-proBNP and troponine or changes in these measurements, regression analysis was performed failing to demonstrate a significant relation between the measurements.

Correlation analysis revealed that for the entire group, VO_2max normalized to the total body mass was significantly associated with resting EDVi (r = 0.3, p = 0.036) and inversely related with E_ai (r = -0.36, p = 0.01), but not with E_{es} (p > 0.05) or E_a/E_{es} ratio. However, when these correlations were tested for each sex separately the results differed. Specifically, in boys there was a strong inverse correlation between E_ai and VO_2max (r = -0.76, p < 0.001) (Figure 3). In the regression analysis performed including E_{es}, E_ai, E_a/E_{es} and EDVi, E_ai was identified as the only predictor of VO_2max standing for 55.5% of the variability in VO_2max. The regression equation

Table 2 Echocardiographic and hemodynamic measurements evaluated before and following exercise in female and male floor-ball players

Parameters	Pre-exercise		Post-exercise	
	Male *(n)*	Female *(n)*	Male *(n)*	Female *(n)*
HR (bmp)	71 ± 12† (27)	77 ± 10† (24)	78 ± 11 (27)	84 ± 11 (24)
Systolic BP (mmHg)	130 ± 15*† (27)	119 ± 7† (24)	122 ± 9* (27)	114 ± 7 (24)
Diastolic BP (mmHg)	70 ± 8† (27)	71 ± 9† (24)	68 ± 10 (27)	68 ± 7 (24)
LVEDD (mm)	51 ± 4*† (27)	48 ± 3† (24)	49 ± 2*(27)	46 ± 3 (24)
LVESD (mm)	34 ± 3† (27)	34 ± 4 (24)	33 ± 2 (27)	33 ± 3 (24)
LVEDV (mL)	121 ± 17*† (27)	92 ± 19† (24)	110 ± 18* (27)	86 ± 18 (24)
LVEDVi(mL/m^2)	65 ± 7*† (27)	54 ± 9† (24)	59 ± 8* (27)	50 ± 8 (24)
LVESV (mL)	49 ± 8† (27)	37 ± 9† (24)	48 ± 10 (27)	36 ± 11 (24)
SV (mL)	74 ± 11*† (27)	58 ± 9† (23)	64 ± 10* (27)	53 ± 9 (23)
SVi (mL/m^2)	40 ± 5*† (27)	34 ± 5† (23)	34 ± 5* (27)	31 ± 4 (23)
EF (%)	59 ± 4† (27)	60 ± 5† (24)	56 ± 5** (27)	60 ± 6 (24)
LA area (cm^2)	18 ± 3*† (27)	16 ± 3 (24)	17 ± 4 (27)	15 ± 3 (24)
2D Strain $_{LV}$	20 ± 1.5**† (27)	21.5 ± 2.4† (24)	17.9 ± 1.5* (27)	20.2 ± 2.7 (24)
S'_{LV} (cm/s)	9.0 ± 1.0 (25)	8.5 ± 1.1 (23)	8.7 ± 1.3 (25)	8.4 ± 1.1 (23)
E'_{LV} (cm/s)	15.2 ± 2.2† (25)	14.7 ± 2.6† (23)	13.9 ± 2.3 (25)	13.6 ± 2.9 (23)
A'_{LV} (cm/s)	6.9 ± 1.6 (25)	6.1 ± 1.4 (23)	6.3 ± 1.5 (25)	6.4 ± 1.7 (23)
IVRT' (ms)	62 ± 13 (26)	62 ± 13 (23)	61 ± 15 (26)	66 ± 14 (23)
E (m/s)	0.9 ± 0.2† (27)	1 ± 0.2† (24)	0.8 ± 0.1 (27)	0.9 ± 0.2 (24)
A (m/s)	0.4 ± 0.1 (27)	0.5 ± 0.1 (24)	0.5 ± +0.8 (27)	0.5 ± 0.1 (24)
DT (ms)	220 ± 52† (27)	203 ± 43† (24)	193 ± 51 (27)	188 ± 42 (24)
E_{es} (mmHg/mL)	2.9 ± 0.5 (27)	3.1 ± 0.6 (20)	2.7 ± 0.6* (27)	3.5 ± 1 (19)
E_a (mmHg/mL)	1.61 ± 0.23*† (27)	1.86 ± 0.31 (19)	1.74 ± 0.28 (27)	1.98 ± 0.39 (18)
E_ai (mmHg/mL/m^2)	3.0 ± 0.5*† (27)	3.1 ± 0.4 (19)	3.3 ± 0.7 (27)	3.3 ± 0.5 (18)
E_a/E_{es}	0.59 ± 0.1 (27)	0.63 ± 0.12 (18)	0.7 ± 0.33 (27)	0.59 ± 0.16 (18)
Stiffness (mmHg/mL)	0.82 ± 0.17 (27)	0.82 ± 0.25 (19)	0.86 ± 0.21 (27)	0.88 ± 0.2 (18)
TPR/T (mmHg/mL)	1.07 ± 0.21 (27)	1.21 ± 0.30 (19)	1.06 ± 0.17 (27)	1.16 ± 0.32 (18)
PCWP (mmHg)	9.4 ± 1.7** (26)	10.3 ± 1.7 (23)	9.2 ± 1.9** (27)	10.1 ± 1.6 (24)
RVEDD $_{basal}$ (mm)	37 ± 4** (27)	34 ± 4 (24)	37 ± 5* (27)	33 ± 3 (24)
RA area (cm^2)	15 ± 3**† (27)	13 ± 2† (24)	14 ± 3** (27)	12 ± 2 (24)
2D Strain $_{RV}$	29.6 ± 4.7† (27)	32.1 ± 4.5† (23)	27.9 ± 4.1 (27)	29.8 ± 3.2 (23)
S'_{RV} (cm/s)	14.4 ± 2.2 (27)	14.5 ± 2.0† (22)	14.4 ± 2.0 (27)	13.5 ± 1.7 (22)
E'_{RV} (cm/s)	17.3 ± 2.0† (27)	17.7 ± 3.3† (22)	15.4 ± 2.9 (27)	16.0 ± 4.0 (22)
A'_{RV} (cm/s)	10.1 ± 2.9 (26)	10.5 ± 2.8 (22)	9.5 ± 2.5 (26)	10.3 ± 3.4 (22)
MPI_{RV}	0.4 ± 0.2† (27)	0.4 ± 0.1† (24)	0.5 ± 0.1 (27)	0.5 ± 0.2 (24)

Values are expressed as mean ± SD. HR denotes heart rate; BP, blood pressure; LVEDD, left ventricular (LV) end-diastolic diameter; LVESD, LV end-systolic diameter; LVEDV; LV end-diastolic volume; LVEDVi, LVEDV indexed to body surface area; LVESV, LV end-systolic volume; SV, stroke volume; SVi, stroke volume indexed to body surface area; EF, ejection fraction; LA, left atrium; 2D $strain_{LV}$, 2-dimensional global LV strain; S'_{LV} E'_{LV} A'_{LV}, mean value of peak systolic, early and lateral diastolic longitudinal myocardial velocity respectively in basal LV septal and lateral wall; E, peak early transmitral flow velocity, A; peak transmitral flow velocity due to atrial contraction; DT; deceleration time; E_{es}; end-systolic LV elastance; E_a, arterial elastance; E_ai; arterial elastance normalized to body surface area; TPR/T, ratio between the total peripheral vascular resistance and the heart rate; PCWP, pulmonary capillary wedge pressure; RVEDD, right ventricular (RV) end-diastolic diameter at basal region of the RV; 2D $strain_{RV}$, 2-Dimensional strain at the lateral RV wall; RA, right atrium; S'_{RV}, E'_{RV} and A'_{RV}, mean value of peak systolic, early and lateral diastolic longitudinal myocardial velocity respectively in lateral RV wall; MPI_{RV}, RV myocardial performance index; *Denotes statistical significance of $p < 0.01$ between the sexes; **Denotes statistical significance of $p < 0.05$ between the sexes; †Denotes statistical significance of $p < 0.05$ between baseline and post exercise for the same sex.

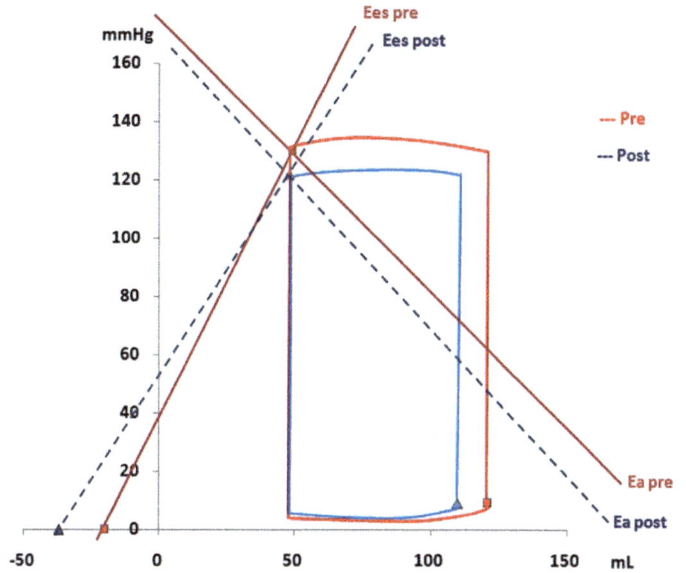

Figure 1 The pressure-volume relationship in male floor-ball players at baseline and following maximal cardiopulmonary testing. The slope of left ventricular (LV) end-systolic pressure and volume (ESPVR) relationship illustrates the LV contractility and was measured using single-beat LV elastance (E_{es}). The arterial elastance (E_a) was measured as the ratio between the LV end-systolic pressure and the stroke volume (SV). The figure illustrates the alterations in E_{es} and E_a prior (solid lines) and following the exercise (dashed lines).

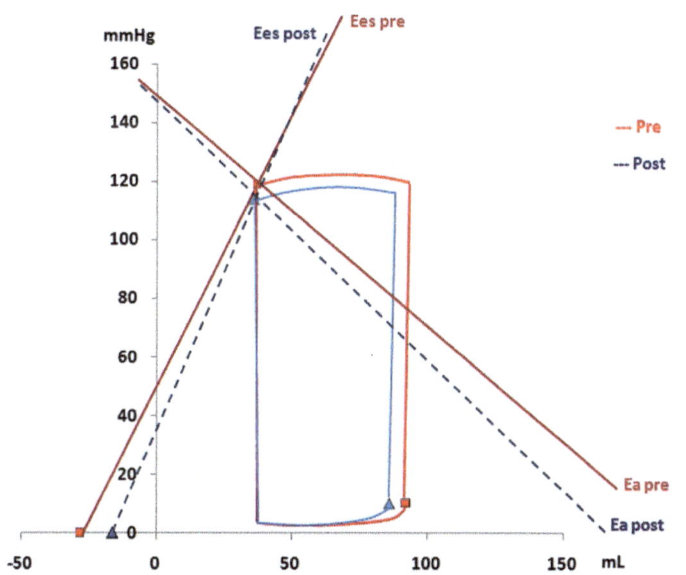

Figure 2 The pressure-volume relationship in female floor-ball players at baseline and following maximal cardiopulmonary testing. The slope of left ventricular (LV) end-systolic pressure and volume (ESPVR) relationship illustrates the LV contractility and was measured using single-beat LV elastance (E_{es}). The arterial elastance (E_a) was measured as the ratio between the LV end-systolic pressure and the stroke volume (SV). The figure illustrates the alterations in E_{es} and E_a prior (solid lines) and following the exercise (dashed lines).

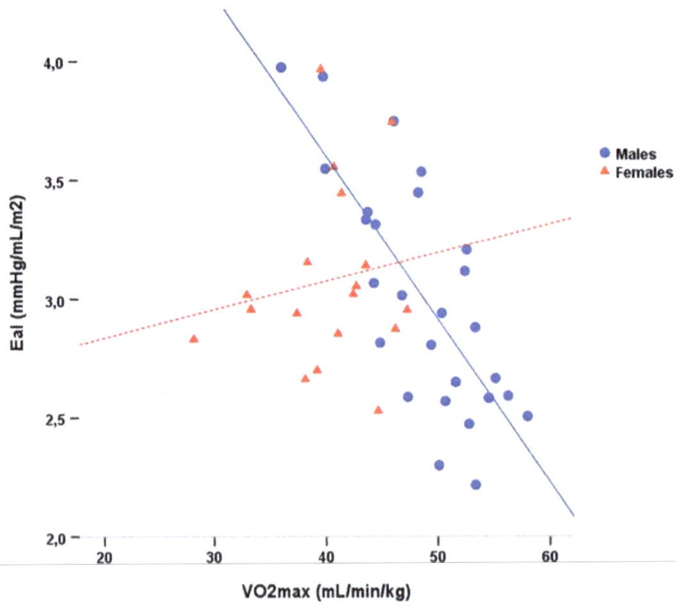

Figure 3 The relationship between the baseline arterial elastance normalized to body surface area (E_ai) and the maximal aerobic capacity as measured by VO2max normalized to the total body mass. As illustrated there was a strong inverse correlation between the E_ai and VO2max in male but not in female adolescents.

wasVO_2max = 73.7-8.34 × E_ai, with an overall model fit of r = 0.76, F (1, 25) = 33, p < 0.001. When the analysis was limited only to participants reaching RQ ≥ 1.05 at peak exercise the correlation pattern became even stronger with the E_ai in males being the only independent predictor standing for 65% of the explained variability in VO_2max. The regression equation in that case was VO_2max = 78.9-10.2 × E_ai, with an overall model fit of r = 0.83, F (1, 13) = 27, p < 0.001. On the other hand, in females VO_2max was not related with any of the tested variables (p > 0.05), (Figure 3).

Diastolic LV function and myocardial stiffness in response to exercise

Pulmonary capillary wedge pressure (PCWP) as estimated by the previously proposed equation [20] did not significantly change following the bout of maximal exercise testing in either sex. Similarly as shown in Figure 4, no changes in the slope of LVEDV to PCWP ratio were observed after exercise indicating unaltered LV end-diastolic stiffness.

Discussion

In this investigation we show that despite a significant reduction in longitudinal ventricular function, myocardial contractility remains essentially unaltered following a bout of maximal exercise testing in adolescent floorball players of both sexes. Furthermore, we demonstrate that the arterial load and the end-diastolic LV dimension at rest act as the only independent predictors of aerobic capacity in male but not in female participants.

The cardiopulmonary and metabolic responses to a maximal exercise testing have been well studied in adults and differences between sexes in this setting have been previously described [21]. Recently, we reported the results regarding the aerobic cardiopulmonary responses between males and females in the present cohort. Briefly, male and female adolescent participants exhibited comparable increases in HR and similar metabolic adaptation as pH, HCO3 -, lactate levels and the respiratory ratio (RQ) [22]. Additionally in terms of VO_2max, we showed that although females and males differ significantly when comparing values of VO_2max indexed to total body mass no differences were observed when VO_2max was normalized to estimated leg muscle mass [22].

Ventricular systolic performance in response to exercise

The issue of cardiac function in response to exercise has been previously investigated and there is growing body of evidence indicating that prolonged exercise may yield reduction in LV longitudinal performance [23-25]. Conversely, the effects of short bout of rigorous exercise on myocardial function are less clear [26]. In our cohort both the early diastolic velocities (E'_{LV}) and the longitudinal 2D strain declined following exercise which, taking into account that these two measurements constitute

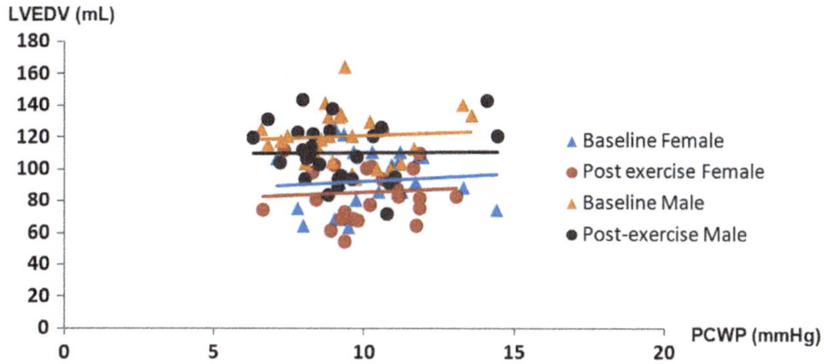

Figure 4 The end-diastolic pressure volume relationship (EDPVR) in male and female participants before and after maximal cardiopulmonary testing. The end-diastolic left ventricular (LV) pressure (LVEDP) was considered to equal the pulmonary wedge pressure and was estimated non-invasively by a previously described equation. LV end-diastolic stiffness illustrated by the EDPVR slope (solid lines) was similar for both sexes at baseline and was essentially unaltered following exercise.

sensitive markers of the LV function, implies attenuated LV performance at recovery following exercise [27,28]. However, when LV function was further evaluated using the end-systolic pressure-volume relationship (ESPVR), a method robust to load changes, LV contractility as estimated by E_{es} remained essentially unaltered in participants of both sexes following exercise. Whereas E'_{LV} as well as 2D strain have been proposed as being relatively load independent [29,30], later reports have demonstrated the influence of load alterations on these measurements [31,32]. In this context, the current findings suggest that the reductions in longitudinal LV strain and E'_{LV} may not explicitly represent reduction of the inherent myocardial contractility but might rather reflect exercise-induced changes in hemodynamic loading. Scott and associates in their study on triathletes demonstrated significant gender differences following prolonged strenuous exercise, with male participants exhibiting attenuated chronotropic and inotropic response to β-adrenergic stimulation [7]. The authors suggested that this might be partly the result of increased sympathetic response in males during exercise and a subsequent desensitization of cardiac β-receptors [7]. This gender-based disparity in β-receptor responsiveness has been observed in studies employing prolonged exercise [7,33]. Although the effect of short-duration maximal exercise on adrenergic cardiac receptors has not been yet investigated, possible similar influence could partly explain our findings as we demonstrate significantly higher E_{es} values in females compared to males post-exercise.

Similar to previous studies, we show a significant reduction of LVEDV in participants of both sexes after maximal exercise testing [34,35] whereas E/E'_{LV}, a well established surrogate of LA pressures, was essentially unaltered. These observations together with a significant reduction in E'_{LV}, a marker of early LV myocardial relaxation, advocate for a decrease in LV filling without a concomitant decrease in preload as expressed by LA pressures. Previous studies have suggested that the attenuation in LV filling following exercise could be the result of changes in myocardial relaxation and reduced suction effect during early diastole [36]. However, in our study, the lack of significant changes in myocardial relaxation as measured by IVRT′ does not support the notion of intrinsic exercise-induced alterations in early myocardial diastolic performance. On the other hand, there is growing evidence showing that RV function influences the LV mechanics and LV filling [36]. Employing TVI and 2D strain, it has been previously shown that following prolonged exercise, the longitudinal RV function is reduced [2]. Conversely, Poh and colleagues reported that strenuous exercise of short duration, resulted in augmented E'_{RV} as compared to baseline [26]. Opposed to this later study our findings show that both the RV strain and the early myocardial velocity of the RV free wall declined significantly following exercise, a discrepancy that might be the result of differences in study protocol. Indeed, in the present study the examination was performed 30 minutes after maximal cardiopulmonary testing and consequently the HR was similar to baseline whereas in the study of Poh et al. HR was significantly higher following exercise which has been shown to yield higher E'_{LV} [37]. Furthermore, the essentially unaltered RV dimensions together with a concomitant reduction in RV performance as measured by RV strain and E'_{RV}, suggests that the reduced LV filling might be the result of a reduction in the RV stroke volume rather than the consequence of a mere decrease in LV preload. In addition, as the two ventricles share a common septal wall, alterations in the RV function might influence LV diastolic function, impairing thus LV filling [36].

Aerobic capacity and hemodynamics

In line with previous reports, we demonstrate that male participants as compared to girls exhibited higher CI and aerobic capacity as measured by VO_2max adjusted to total body mass. The differences in aerobic response between the two sexes are discussed in detail in our previous report [22]. It have shown that the response of arterial load may vary during exercise, showing increase, decline or even remaining unaltered at peak exercise. In our study, only four participants (three females) demonstrated E_a reduction (1-10% decrease from baseline values) while the rest showed significant E_a increment (median increase 30%, range 3 to 131%). In a recent investigation on healthy adults no significant influence of age and sex on ΔE_ai was found [38]. In line with this observation, we show that male and female participants behave in a similar pattern regarding E_ai changes at peak exercise. In our cohort, ΔE_ai was inversely related with baseline E_ai and this relationship was very similar in the two sexes (ΔE_ai vs. E_ai rest; females: $r = -0.5$, $p = 0.003$, males $r = -0.51$, $r = 0.008$) which is in accordance with previous observations in healthy adults [38]. This implies that a more compliant arterial system at rest may shift to lesser degrees of compliance during exercise. Unfortunately the design of this study does not allow us to provide an answer to possible mechanisms that may contribute to this phenomenon.

There is increasing recognition on the importance of the arterio-ventricular interaction and the arterial load on the cardiac performance. Fahs et al. have recently described that the coupling ratio of arterial to ventricular elastance (E_a/E_{es}) is inversely related to the aerobic capacity as described by VO_2max [39] in female but not in male young endurance athletes. Based on this observation, we investigated whether baseline hemodynamic and echocardiographic variables could act as predictors of the aerobic capacity. In a model that included E_a, E_{es}, E_a/E_{es} as well as EDVi, we found that in the whole study group, E_ai at baseline significantly correlated with aerobic capacity and acted as the single independent predictor of VO_2max (beta = -0.41, model fit = 0.41, $p < 0.005$). However, it appears that sex influences this relationship as E_ai was a strong and the only predictor of the aerobic capacity in male participants (beta = -0.76, model fit = 0.76, $p < 0.001$) but lacked any significant correlation with VO_2max in females. When the analysis was limited to participants that exhibited RQ ≥1.05 at peak effort the correlation between E_ai and VO_2max became even stronger in males. Additionally, in male participants the degree of correlation between E_ai and VO_2max persisted even when VO_2max was adjusted for muscle leg mass, fat-free mass and trunk muscle mass ($r = -0.7$; $r = -0.74$, $r = 0.74$, $p < 0.001$ respectively) while no correlation was observed in females. Fahs and coauthors showed a weak inverse asssociation between E_a and VO_2max in their whole study cohort, but when sexes where separately examined no significant relationship was found between these parameters [39]. Similar to our findings, E_{es} failed to demonstrate significant association with aerobic capacity in that study [39]. The physiologic explanation for this discrepancy between sexes is unclear as the main determinants of E_ai i.e. the arterial stiffness, the TPR and the HR were similar in males and females prior and following exercise. Possible differential responses of the arterial system during exercise cannot be ruled out, as the design of the current study does not allow further interrogation regarding this issue. Previous investigations have indicated that in women there is mainly a parasympathetic regulation of the cardiovascular system at rest whereas in males the sympathetic activity is dominating both at rest [40] and during exercise [41], a disparity that may stand for the currently demonstrated discrepancy between sexes regarding the association of E_a and VO_2max in our study. A possible conditioning of the cardiovascular system during exercise might also contribute to the disparate relationship between E_ai and VO_2max in the two sexes as the frequency of training between sexes was significantly different with boys reporting more hours of training (9 ± 1 h/week) compared to females (7 ± 2 h/week).

Limitations

The present study was performed in adolescent floor ball athletes with an average of roughly 7 hours of physical exercise per week implying that the current results do not pertain to elite athletes. Additionally, although the participants of the two genders were matched according to age, we did not interrogate sexual maturation indices in our cohort which might constitute a confounder in the present study. A considerable part of study results were obtained using Doppler based methods. This implies that the results are subjected to possible suboptimal insonation angle. However, the impact of this possible influence is not considered to be significant as care was taken for the angle of incidence not to exceed 20 degrees. Measurements of cardiac output using inert gas are influenced in the presence of significant pulmonary or intracardiac shunting. The TTE examination did not reveal any signs of atrial or ventricular septal defect. However, we did not perform contrast echocardiography prior or during the exercise and thus the possibility of pulmonary shunting cannot be excluded and thus possible influence on the results of our study especially for cardiac output measurements during exercise cannot be fully excluded. Furthermore measurements of LV elastance were performed using the single-beat approach rather than conductance catheters which is considered the reference standard in this setting. However, the single beat method has been well validated against conductance catheters and provides reproducible results [19].

Conclusion

In conclusion, we demonstrate that LV myocardial responses to maximal cycle exercise did not differ between the female and male participants. Furthermore, we conclude that exercise induced reduction in ventricular function assessed by quantitative and Doppler measurements although comparable in both sexes may not indicate a decrease in intrinsic myocardial contractility. Additionally we show that arterial load at rest is a strong predictor of aerobic capacity in male but not female adolescent floorball players. Further studies are needed to investigate the differential effect of arterial load between the two sexes on maximal aerobic performance.

Competing interests

The authors declare that they have no competing interests.

Authors' contributions

ÅF has made substantial contribution for the data acquisition (information and subject recruitment, supervised and recorded data during exercise stress testing and blood sampling) and for the conception and design of the study. Has also been involved in the drafting of the manuscript as well as given final approval of the final version of the manuscript. CDS has made substantial contribution for data analysis (echocardiographic data analysis off-line) and interpretation (statistics); conception and design of the study. Has also been involved in the drafting and critical revision of the manuscript as well as given final approval of the final version of the manuscript. MÅ has made substantial contribution for the data acquisition (information and subject recruitment, supervised and recorded data during exercise stress testing and blood sampling) and for the conception and design of the study. Has also been involved in the drafting of the manuscript as well as given final approval of the final version of the manuscript. AS has made substantial contribution for data interpretation the conception and study design. Has also been involved in the drafting and critical revision of the manuscript as well as given final approval of the final version of the manuscript. LL has made substantial contribution for data interpretation; conception and design of the study. Has also been involved in the drafting and critical revision of the manuscript as well as given final approval of the final version of the manuscript. MS has made substantial contribution for the data acquisition and for the conception and design of the study. Has also been involved in the drafting of the manuscript as well as given final approval of the final version of the manuscript. AG has made substantial contribution for data acquisition (information and subject recruitment, supervised and recorded data during exercise stress testing and blood sampling, Innocor examination), analysis and interpretation; conception and design of the study. Has also been involved in the drafting and critical revision of the manuscript as well as given final approval of the final version of the manuscript. AM has made substantial contribution for data acquisition (echocardiographic examination and off-line analysis and interpretation (statistical analysis); conception and design of the study. Has also been involved in the drafting and critical revision of the manuscript as well as given final approval of the final version of the manuscript. All authors read and approved the final manuscript.

Authors' information

Åsa Fomin and Cristina DaSilva were equal first author contributors. Aristomenis Manouras and Anders Gabrielsen were equal senior author contributors.

Acknowledgements

This study was supported by the Swedish Heart-Lung foundation. We thank Eva Wallgren, Department of Cardiology, Karolinska Institutet for important technical and analytical support.

Author details

[1]Department of Medicine, Unit of Cardiology, Karolinska University Hospital, Stockholm, Sweden. [2]Department of Cardiology, Karolinska University Hospital, Stockholm, Sweden. [3]School of Technology and Health, Royal Institute of Technology, Stockholm, Sweden. [4]Department of Clinical Physiology and Cardiology, Karolinska University Hospital Huddinge, SE-141 86 Stockholm, Sweden.

References

1. Sarna S, Sahi T, Koskenvuo M, Kaprio J: **Increased life expectancy of world class male athletes.** *Med Sci Sports Exerc* 1993, **25**(2):237–244.
2. Neilan TG, Januzzi JL, Lee-Lewandrowski E, Ton-Nu TT, Yoerger DM, Jassal DS, Lewandrowski KB, Siegel AJ, Marshall JE, Douglas PS, Lawlor D, Picard MH, Wood MJ: **Myocardial injury and ventricular dysfunction related to training levels among nonelite participants in the Boston marathon.** *Circulation* 2006, **114**(22):2325–2333.
3. Sharma S, Zaidi A: **Exercise-induced arrhythmogenic right ventricular cardiomyopathy: fact or fallacy?** *Eur Heart J* 2012, **33**(8):938–940.
4. Douglas PS, O'Toole ML, Hiller WD, Hackney K, Reichek N: **Cardiac fatigue after prolonged exercise.** *Circulation* 1987, **76**(6):1206–1213.
5. Neilan TG, Ton-Nu TT, Jassal DS, Popovic ZB, Douglas PS, Halpern EF, Marshall JE, Thomas JD, Picard MH, Yoerger DM, Wood MJ: **Myocardial adaptation to short-term high-intensity exercise in highly trained athletes.** *J Am Soc Echocardiogr* 2006, **19**(10):1280–1285.
6. Hart E, Shave R, Middleton N, George K, Whyte G, Oxborough D: **Effect of preload augmentation on pulsed wave and tissue Doppler echocardiographic indices of diastolic function after a marathon.** *J Am Soc Echocardiogr* 2007, **20**(12):1393–1399.
7. Scott JM, Esch BT, Haykowsky MJ, Isserow S, Koehle MS, Hughes BG, Zbogar D, Bredin SS, McKenzie DC, Warburton DE: **Sex differences in left ventricular function and beta-receptor responsiveness following prolonged strenuous exercise.** *J Appl Physiol (1985)* 2007, **102**(2):681–687.
8. McManus AM, Armstrong N: **Physiology of elite young female athletes.** *Med Sport Sci* 2011, **56**:23–46.
9. Stamatakis E, Chaudhury M: **Temporal trends in adults' sports participation patterns in England between 1997 and 2006: the Health Survey for England.** *Br J Sports Med* 2008, **42**(11):901–908.
10. Carter JB, Banister EW, Blaber AP: **The effect of age and gender on heart rate variability after endurance training.** *Med Sci Sports Exerc* 2003, **35**(8):1333–1340.
11. Mitchell JH, Haskell W, Snell P, Van Camp SP: **Task Force 8: classification of sports.** *J Am Coll Cardiol* 2005, **45**(8):1364–1367.
12. Gabrielsen A, Videbaek R, Schou M, Damgaard M, Kastrup J, Norsk P: **Non-invasive measurement of cardiac output in heart failure patients using a new foreign gas rebreathing technique.** *Clin Sci (Lond)* 2002, **102**(2):247–252.
13. Damgaard M, Norsk P: **Effects of ventilation on cardiac output determined by inert gas rebreathing.** *Clin Physiol Funct Imaging* 2005, **25**(3):142–147.
14. Evangelista A, Flachskampf F, Lancellotti P, Badano L, Aguilar R, Monaghan M, Zamorano J, Nihoyannopoulos P: **European Association of Echocardiography recommendations for standardization of performance, digital storage and reporting of echocardiographic studies.** *Eur J Echocardiogr* 2008, **9**(4):438–448.
15. Lang RM, Bierig M, Devereux RB, Flachskampf FA, Foster E, Pellikka PA, Picard MH, Roman MJ, Seward J, Shanewise J, Solomon S, Spencer KT, St John Sutton M, Stewart W, American Society of Echocardiography's Nomenclature and Standards Committee; Task Force on Chamber Quantification; American College of Cardiology Echocardiography Committee; American Heart Association; European Association of Echocardiography, European Society of Cardiology: **Recommendations for chamber quantification.** *Eur J Echocardiogr* 2006, **7**(2):79–108.
16. Kelly RP, Ting CT, Yang TM, Liu CP, Maughan WL, Chang MS, Kass DA: **Effective arterial elastance as index of arterial vascular load in humans.** *Circulation* 1992, **86**(2):513–521.
17. Chemla D, Hebert JL, Coirault C, Zamani K, Suard I, Colin P, Lecarpentier Y: **Total arterial compliance estimated by stroke volume-to-aortic pulse pressure ratio in humans.** *Am J Physiol* 1998, **274**(2 Pt 2):H500–H505.
18. Chemla D, Antony I, Lecarpentier Y, Nitenberg A: **Contribution of systemic vascular resistance and total arterial compliance to effective arterial elastance in humans.** *Am J Physiol Heart Circ Physiol* 2003, **285**(2):H614–H620.

19. Chen CH, Fetics B, Nevo E, Rochitte CE, Chiou KR, Ding PA, Kawaguchi M, Kass DA: **Noninvasive single-beat determination of left ventricular end-systolic elastance in humans.** *J Am Coll Cardiol* 2001, **38**(7):2028–2034.
20. Nagueh SF, Middleton KJ, Kopelen HA, Zoghbi WA, Quinones MA: **Doppler tissue imaging: a noninvasive technique for evaluation of left ventricular relaxation and estimation of filling pressures.** *J Am Coll Cardiol* 1997, **30**(6):1527–1533.
21. Astrand PO: **Quantification of exercise capability and evaluation of physical capacity in man.** *Prog Cardiovasc Dis* 1976, **19**(1):51–67.
22. Fomin A, Ahlstrand M, Schill HG, Lund LH, Stahlberg M, Manouras A, Gabrielsen A: **Sex differences in response to maximal exercise stress test in trained adolescents.** *BMC Pediatr* 2012, **12**:127.
23. Neilan TG, Yoerger DM, Douglas PS, Marshall JE, Halpern EF, Lawlor D, Picard MH, Wood MJ: **Persistent and reversible cardiac dysfunction among amateur marathon runners.** *Eur Heart J* 2006, **27**(9):1079–1084.
24. Banks L, Sasson Z, Busato M, Goodman JM: **Impaired left and right ventricular function following prolonged exercise in young athletes: influence of exercise intensity and responses to dobutamine stress.** *J Appl Physiol* 2010, **108**(1):112–119.
25. George K, Oxborough D, Forster J, Whyte G, Shave R, Dawson E, Stephenson C, Dugdill L, Edwards B, Gaze D: **Mitral annular myocardial velocity assessment of segmental left ventricular diastolic function after prolonged exercise in humans.** *J Physiol* 2005, **569**(Pt 1):305–313.
26. Poh KK, Ton-Nu TT, Neilan TG, Tournoux FB, Picard MH, Wood MJ: **Myocardial adaptation and efficiency in response to intensive physical training in elite speedskaters.** *Int J Cardiol* 2008, **126**(3):346–351.
27. Gulati VK, Katz WE, Follansbee WP, Gorcsan J 3rd: **Mitral annular descent velocity by tissue Doppler echocardiography as an index of global left ventricular function.** *Am J Cardiol* 1996, **77**(11):979–984.
28. Oki T, Tabata T, Yamada H, Wakatsuki T, Mishiro Y, Abe M, Onose Y, Iuchi A, Ito S: **Left ventricular diastolic properties of hypertensive patients measured by pulsed tissue Doppler imaging.** *J Am Soc Echocardiogr* 1998, **11**(12):1106–1112.
29. Nagueh SF, Sun H, Kopelen HA, Middleton KJ, Khoury DS: **Hemodynamic determinants of the mitral annulus diastolic velocities by tissue Doppler.** *J Am Coll Cardiol* 2001, **37**(1):278–285.
30. Andersen NH, Terkelsen CJ, Sloth E, Poulsen SH: **Influence of preload alterations on parameters of systolic left ventricular long-axis function: a Doppler tissue study.** *J Am Soc Echocardiogr* 2004, **17**(9):941–947.
31. Opdahl A, Remme EW, Helle-Valle T, Lyseggen E, Vartdal T, Pettersen E, Edvardsen T, Smiseth OA: **Determinants of left ventricular early-diastolic lengthening velocity: independent contributions from left ventricular relaxation, restoring forces, and lengthening load.** *Circulation* 2009, **119**(19):2578–2586.
32. Burns AT, La Gerche A, D'Hooge J, MacIsaac AI, Prior DL: **Left ventricular strain and strain rate: characterization of the effect of load in human subjects.** *Eur J Echocardiogr* 2010, **11**(3):283–289.
33. Hart E, Dawson E, Rasmussen P, George K, Secher NH, Whyte G, Shave R: **Beta-adrenergic receptor desensitization in man: insight into post-exercise attenuation of cardiac function.** *J Physiol* 2006, **577**(Pt 2):717–725.
34. Seals DR, Rogers MA, Hagberg JM, Yamamoto C, Cryer PE, Ehsani AA: **Left ventricular dysfunction after prolonged strenuous exercise in healthy subjects.** *Am J Cardiol* 1988, **61**(11):875–879.
35. Whyte GP, George K, Sharma S, Lumley S, Gates P, Prasad K, McKenna WJ: **Cardiac fatigue following prolonged endurance exercise of differing distances.** *Med Sci Sports Exerc* 2000, **32**(6):1067–1072.
36. Esch BT, Scott JM, Haykowsky MJ, McKenzie DC, Warburton DE: **Diastolic ventricular interactions in endurance-trained athletes during orthostatic stress.** *Am J Physiol Heart Circ Physiol* 2007, **293**(1):H409–H415.
37. Peverill RE, Gelman JS, Mottram PM, Moir S, Jankelowitz C, Bain JL, Donelan L: **Factors associated with mitral annular systolic and diastolic velocities in healthy adults.** *J Am Soc Echocardiogr* 2004, **17**(11):1146–1154.
38. Chantler PD, Melenovsky V, Schulman SP, Gerstenblith G, Becker LC, Ferrucci L, Fleg JL, Lakatta EG, Najjar SS: **Use of the Frank-Starling mechanism during exercise is linked to exercise-induced changes in arterial load.** *Am J Physiol Heart Circ Physiol* 2012, **302**(1):H349–H358.
39. Fahs CA, Rossow LM, Yan H, Ranadive SM, Agiovlasitis S, Wilund KR, Baynard T, Fernhall B: **Resting and post exercise arterial-ventricular coupling in endurance-trained men and women.** *J Hum Hypertens* 2013, **27**(9):552–556.
40. Evans JM, Ziegler MG, Patwardhan AR, Ott JB, Kim CS, Leonelli FM, Knapp CF: **Gender differences in autonomic cardiovascular regulation: spectral, hormonal, and hemodynamic indexes.** *J Appl Physiol (1985)* 2001, **91**(6):2611–2618.
41. Ettinger SM, Silber DH, Collins BG, Gray KS, Sutliff G, Whisler SK, McClain JM, Smith MB, Yang QX, Sinoway LI: **Influences of gender on sympathetic nerve responses to static exercise.** *J Appl Physiol (1985)* 1996, **80**(1):245–251.

7

Effects of a home-exercise therapy programme on cervical and lumbar range of motion among nurses with neck and lower back pain: a quasi-experimental study

Tiina Freimann[1,2*], Eda Merisalu[3] and Mati Pääsuke[4]

Abstract

Background: Cervical and lumbar range of motion limitations are usually associated with musculoskeletal pain in the neck and lower back, and are a major health problem among nurses. Physical exercise has been evaluated as an effective intervention method for improving cervical and lumbar range of motion, and for preventing and reducing musculoskeletal pain. The purpose of this study was to investigate the effects of a home-exercise therapy programme on cervical and lumbar range of motion among intensive care unit nurses who had experienced mild to moderate musculoskeletal pain in the neck and or lower back during the previous six months.

Methods: A quasi-experimental study was conducted among intensive care unit nurses at Tartu University Hospital (Estonia) between May and July 2011. Thirteen nurses who had suffered musculoskeletal pain episodes in the neck and or lower back during the previous six months underwent an 8-week home-exercise therapy programme. Eleven nurses without musculoskeletal pain formed a control group.
Questions from the Nordic Musculoskeletal Questionnaire and the 11-point Visual Analogue Scale were used to select potential participants for the experimental group via an assessment of the prevalence and intensity of musculoskeletal pain. Cervical range of motion and lumbar range of motion in flexion, extension, lateral flexion and (cervical range of motion only) rotation were measured with a digital goniometer. A paired *t*-test was used to compare the measured parameters before and after the home-exercise therapy programme. A Student's *t*-test was used to analyse any differences between the experimental and control groups.

Results: After the home-exercise therapy, there was a significant increase ($p < 0.05$) in cervical range of motion in flexion, extension, lateral flexion and rotation, and in lumbar range of motion in lateral flexion. Cervical range of motion in flexion was significantly higher ($p < 0.01$) in the experimental group compared to the control group after therapy.

Conclusions: Our results suggest an 8-week intensive home-exercise therapy programme may improve cervical and lumbar range of motion among intensive care nurses. Further studies are needed to develop this simple but effective home-exercise therapy programme to help motivate nurses to perform such exercises regularly.

Trial registration: Current Controlled Trials ISRCTN19278735. Registered 27 November 2015.

Keywords: Cervical range of motion, Lumbar range of motion, Musculoskeletal pain, Exercise therapy

* Correspondence: tiina.freimann@kliinikum.ee
[1]Tartu University Hospital, Puusepa 8, Tartu 51014, Estonia
[2]Department of Public Health, Medical Faculty, University of Tartu, Ravila 14a, Tartu 50411, Estonia
Full list of author information is available at the end of the article

Background

Cervical range of motion (CROM) and lumbar range of motion (LROM) limitations are usually associated with musculoskeletal pain (MSP) in the neck and lower back, and is a major health problem among intensive care unit (ICU) nurses [1, 2]. Earlier studies have indicated a high frequency of neck and lower back pain among Estonian nurses [3], necessitating a search for appropriate intervention methods to improve CROM and LROM in order to prevent and reduce neck and lower back pain among nurses.

Physical exercise has been evaluated as an effective intervention method for improving CROM and LROM [4], and for reducing MSP in the neck and lower back [5, 6]. Many authors have emphasized that such programmes should be conducted with sufficient frequency, intensity and duration, plus appropriate ergonomic counselling and supervision [7, 8]. Ergonomic interventions without physical exercise may be ineffective in preventing or reducing MSP [9, 10], possibly because of insufficient or inconsistent implementation of ergonomic practices [11]. Some studies have supported physical activity programmes in the workplace as being more effective intervention methods compared to home-exercise programmes [6]. However, Jakobsen and et al. [12] found the effects of physical exercise on musculoskeletal pain did not depend on whether exercises were conducted at the workplace or during leisure time at home. Moreover, Kuukkanen et al. [13] found that supervised home exercises led to reduced lower back pain and these positive effects persisted for more than five years after the exercise programme was compleated. Some studies have found positive results of physical exercise when the training period lasted longer than 10 weeks [8].

The literature review by Dawson et al. [14] provides conflicting evidence regarding the efficacy of physical exercise to prevent lower back pain among nurses. At present there is no simple and cost-effective physical exercise programme for improving cervical and lumbar ROM, and reducing neck and lower back pain, among nurses.

The aim of our study was to investigate the effects of an 8-week home-exercise therapy programme that included ergonomic counselling and supervision, on CROM and LROM among ICU nurses who had suffered episodes of mild to moderate MSP in the neck and or lower back during the previous six months. We hypothesized that our specially designed home-exercise therapy programme could improve cervical and lumbar range of motion to reduce neck and lower back pain among ICU nurses.

Methods

Subjects and settings

This case control series study was conducted among ICU nurses ($n = 96$) at Tartu University Hospital (Estonia) between May and July 2011. Twenty-two female intensive care nurses from three different ICUs fulfilled the eligibility criteria for the experimental group, and thirteen completed the 8-week home-exercise therapy programme. The other nine participants gave up due to health reasons, a change of residence or a lack of time. Eleven nurses fulfilled the eligibility criteria for the control group and registered to participate in the study. A participant flowchart is provided in Fig. 1. The study was approved by the Research Ethics Committee of the University of Tartu (protocol number 202 T-19) and conducted in accordance with the Helsinki Declaration. All subjects were informed about the purpose and content of the study and provided written consent.

Inclusion criteria for the experimental group were: having worked full time for at least a year in the ICU; being under 40 years of age; having a body mass index <32; having experienced mild to moderate pain in the cervical and or lumbar regions during the previous six months. Inclusion criteria for the control group were:

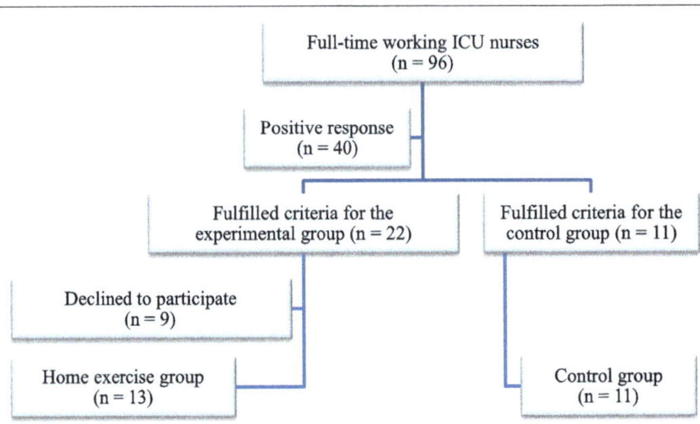

Fig. 1 Participant flowchart

being under 40 years of age; having a body mass index <32; experiencing no MSP during the previous six months. Exclusion criteria for both groups were acute orthopaedic and or neurological diseases and pregnancy.

The exercise therapy programme

The home-exercise therapy programme was chosen for the experimental group because of its simplicity and low cost compared with workplace exercise programmes [15]. It was important that the participants would be able to perform the exercises by themselves, i.e. without continuous supervision by a physiotherapist. Based on previous studies [4, 16, 17], effective stretching and strengthening exercises for the cervical and lumbar region were included in the exercise therapy programme (Fig. 2).

The experimental group underwent 8-weeks of exercise therapy, with the frequency and intensity of the exercises increasing every two weeks. The training load progressively increased according to the principle of the gradual rising of loads [18]. The participants were asked to perform exercises as one to three sets of 8–10 repetitions. Exercises 4a, 4b and 12 (both feet) were performed with 2–3 repetitions per set. The goal for subjects was to perform exercises once a day, six days a week, for 8 weeks. Each session lasted from 20 min in the first two weeks to 60 min in the last two weeks. The control group were asked to continue their normal life.

Before the start of the home-exercise programme, the experimental group underwent training with the guidance of a physiotherapist regarding the specific ergonomic considerations and correct techniques for performing the exercises at home. Ergonomic guidance was also given for correct working postures and patient handling tasks. The experimental group received written materials that included photographs depicting the correct techniques of the exercise therapy. After four weeks the experimental group met with a programme supervisor (physiotherapist), who examined their technique and resolved any problems related to the programme.

Data collection

A questionnaire was prepared for the selection of potential participants, which included questions from the Nordic Musculoskeletal Questionnaire (NMQ) [19] and the 11-point Visual Analogue Scale (VAS) [20]. The prevalence and intensity of MSP lasting for longer than a day in the neck and or lower back during the previous six

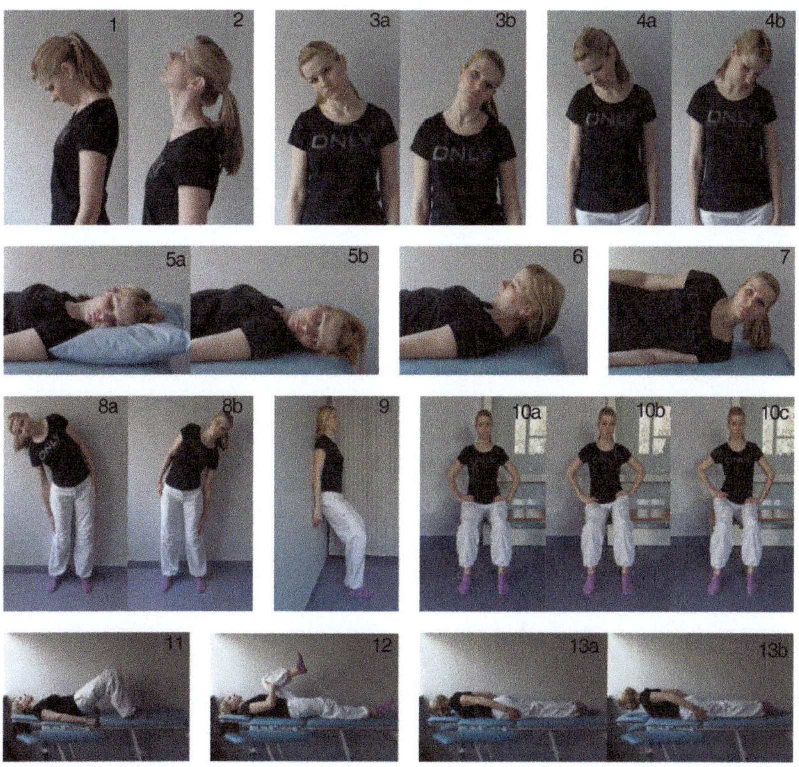

Fig. 2 Examples of the stretching and strengthening exercises used in the home-exercise therapy programme. * The subject of this figure gave consent for these photos to be reproduced here

months was assessed [20]. Mild to moderate MSP constituted the inclusion criteria for the experimental group. Throughout the programme the experimental group completed a training diary, which contained a detailed description of time spent on each session, the exercises conducted and a description of any other aerobic training not included in the study programme. The control group continued their normal life and did not keep an exercise diary.

Measurements

CROM in flexion, extension, lateral flexion and rotation, and LROM in flexion, extension and lateral flexion, were measured using a digital goniometer (AcumarTM Digital Inclinometer, Version 5.0), which is an objective and reliable method [21–23] recommended by international clinical guidelines [24, 25]. All CROM and LROM measurements in the experimental group were taken before and after the 8-week exercise therapy programme; measurements for the control group were taken at the same time as the second measurements for the experimental group. All the measurements were made by the same physical therapist and researcher to achieve a high reliability of measurements [22]. The best of three performances was used for each flexion, extension and rotation measurement.

Statistical analysis

Statistical analyses were carried out using the Statistical Package for the Social Sciences (SPSS) Version 18.0. First, descriptive statistics were used to analyse the data. The means and standard deviations of each measurement per group were calculated. A paired *t*-test was used to compare CROM and LROM before and after the home-exercise therapy programme; a Student's *t*-test was used to examine any differences between the experimental and control groups. The significance level for all tests was set at $p < 0.05$.

Results

The age ranges of the experimental and control groups were 23–37 ($n = 13$) and 22–39 ($n = 11$) years old respectively. Both groups were homogeneous ($p > 0.05$) for the anthropometric variables measured (Table 1).

Eight of the nurses in the experimental group had experienced both neck and lower back pain, two of them only neck pain and three only lower back pain. The mean pain intensity score (using the 11-point VAS) over the six months was 4.1 (SD 2.5). According to their training diaries, the experimental group conducted home-exercise therapy on average five times per week over the 8-week period, with the duration of exercising ranging from 20 min per session in the first two weeks to 60 min per session in the last two weeks.

Table 1 Comparison of age and anthropometric parameters in the experimental and control groups

Features	Experimental group ($n = 13$)		Control group ($n = 11$)		
	Mean	SD	Mean	SD	p
Age (yrs)	29.2	5.1	31.1	5.1	0.414
Height (cm)	165.6	4.8	167.5	3.6	0.191
Weight (kg)	66.5	2.4	67.8	3.0	0.885
BMI (kg/m^2)	24.2	0.9	24.2	1.1	0.977

Table 2 presents the means and standard deviations for CROM and LROM for each group, *p*-values for the comparison of variables before and after the exercise therapy program and differences between the experimental and control groups. Statistically significant differences were found in the experimental group's CROM values before and after therapy. There was a significant increase in cervical flexion (26 %; 14.7°; $p = 0.000$), extension (18 %; 10.7°; $p = 0.002$), right lateral flexion (15 %; 6.0°; $p = 0.002$), left lateral flexion (14 %; 5.9°; $p = 0.012$), right rotation (10 %; 8.5°; $p = 0.002$) and left rotation (9 %; 7.4°; $p = 0.010$). After therapy CROM in flexion was significantly higher in the experimental group compared to the control group (11 %; 6,5°; $p = 0.004$). Significant increases in lumbar right lateral flexion (20 %; 5.5°; $p = 0.003$) and left lateral flexion (17 %; 5.1°; $p = 0.009$) after therapy were also found.

Discussion

This study evaluated the effects of an 8-week home-exercise therapy programme on CROM and LROM among ICU nurses. We found a significant increase in cervical flexion, extension, lateral flexion and rotation, and in lumbar lateral flexion, after therapy. The largest increase in range of motion was found for cervical flexion; after 8-weeks, this value approached the age-specific normal CROM value of 58–60° [26]. Our study results showed the exercise therapy programme had a greater effect on CROM compared to LROM. Therefore, the types of exercises needed to achieve better results in both CROM and LROM within a single therapy programme should be explored further. Our study results are difficult to compare with previous findings due to differences in study designs, exercise therapy programmes and outcome measurements. Only in some previous studies are CROM and or LROM compared before and after an exercise therapy programme. Tseng et al. [27] examined the effects of range-of-motion exercise on the upper and lower extremities and found positive effects in enhancing physical and psychological functions of older people after a stroke. More evidence is available concerning the positive effects of regular exercise on musculoskeletal symptoms [28–30]. Alexandre et al. [29] suggested that regular exercise can reduce

Table 2 Cervical and lumbar range of motion values in the experimental and control groups and *p*-values for the comparison of differences within and between groups

	Experimental group			Control group		
	Mean[a] (SD)	Mean[b] (SD)	p	Mean (SD)	p[c]	p[d]
Cervical ROM						
Flexion	42.3 (8.1)	57.0 (7.0)	0.000	50.5 (7.6)	0.109	0.004
Extension	49.5 (10.7)	60.2 (9.2)	0.002	58.4 (13.5)	0.080	0.704
Lateral flexion (right)	34.8 (4.5)	40.8 (5.5)	0.002	37.6 (6.2)	0.133	0.203
Lateral flexion (left)	35.5 (6.6)	41.4 (7.8)	0.012	39.9 (7.1)	0.107	0.634
Rotation (right)	75.7 (8.7)	84.2 (6.4)	0.002	83.2 7.3)	0.323	0.731
Rotation (left)	78.4 (8.8)	85.8 (7.6)	0.010	84.8 (6.1)	0.354	0.766
Lumbar ROM						
Flexion	62.2 (9.8)	61.2 (7.2)	0.698	60,0 (7.9)	0.275	0.691
Extension	22.4 (7.9)	23.6 (5.9)	0.528	28.2 (7.6)	0.090	0.113
Lateral flexion (right)	21.9 (4.7)	27.4 (2.2)	0.003	27.2 (7.4)	0.045	0.925
Lateral flexion (left)	24.5 (6.0)	29.6 (3.6)	0.009	27.6 (5.4)	0.142	0.272

[a]experimental subjects before therapy; [b]experimental subjects after therapy; [c]experimental subjects before therapy compared to controls; [d]experimental subjects after therapy compared to controls
$p < 0.05$ constituted significant differences within and between groups

musculoskeletal symptoms in nursing personnel. However, Dehlin et al. [31] found no effect of eight weeks of physical exercise on lower back pain. The negative results in their study could be explained by the low frequency of physical exercises, because in the study exercise was performed only twice a week and may thereby have been insufficient to decrease MSP. Cleland et al. [32] found that thoracic spine manipulation together with cervical range of motion exercise was more beneficial for patients with neck pain than exercise only. Since neck and lower back pain are often associated with CROM and LROM limitations, the results of previous studies allowed us to make assumptions about how physical exercise led to CROM and LROM improvements. After the exercise therapy programme in our study, six participants were completely pain-free; and on mean pain intensity in the neck and lower back of the other seven participants was significantly lower than before (0.7 (SD 0.7).

Our method of investigation had the advantage of using well-known instruments for collecting MSP self-evaluations (NMQ and VAS); however Numerical Pain Rating Scale (NPRS) have been found to be more clinimetrically reliable than VAS [33, 34]. We also used an objective and reliable method for collecting CROM and LROM measurements (AcumarTM Digital Inclinometer, Version 5.0) [21–23]. Additionally, as all CROM and LROM measurements were made by the same physical therapist, a high reliability of measurements can be assumed [22].

The main limitations of this study were related to the number of subjects and quasi-experimental design of the study. Due to the small population of volunteer ICU nurses, it was difficult to find a sufficient sample size of subjects with suitable characteristics for randomization. In general, the major problem with quasi-experimental designs is that the experimental and control group might not be similar in terms of the demographic parameters selected for intervention and comparison. This lack of recruitment numbers required the control group to be from an asymptomatic population. However, the experimental and control group in our study were homogeneous for age, height, weight and BMI (Table 1). Our study was limited to investigating the effects of a home-exercise therapy programme on CROM and LROM. Other intervention strategies (e.g. participatory ergonomics) that could increase the effectiveness of any programme should also be taken into consideration [35]. As the aetiology of cervical and lumbar disorders is multifactorial, a combination of intervention programmes for intensive care nurses should be studied in the future [36]. However, as the cost-effectiveness of any intervention method is an important consideration, it would be ideal to find effective and low-cost interventions [15].

According to the training diaries nine of the experimental subjects participated in other aerobic training, such as cycling, running, walking, swimming, rollerblading and rowing, on average two times a week. Aerobic training outside of the exercise therapy programme was negatively associated with total CROM. This association might show possible over-training and or physical overload in the cervical spine, which may have influenced the effectiveness of the programme. In the future, randomized controlled trials are recommended to investigate the effects of exercise therapy programmes on CROM and LROM with and without other types of aerobic training. Consideration of the duration of the exercise program, initiating at 20 min and increasing to 60 min, may also need to be considered in terms of participant demand.

Our study results confirm that home-exercise programmes are useful for improving cervical and lumbar range of motion. To achieve better results in mobility of lumbar flexion and extension parameters, specific exercises individually adapted for each person need to be implemented in further studies. Although Alexandre et al. [29] suggest that a standard programme of exercises conducted twice a week with an ergonomic approach could reduce musculoskeletal symptoms in nursing personnel, an individual approach could be more effective. Jakobsen et al. [12] found that performing physical exercise at the workplace together with colleagues may be more motivating for some employees.

Conclusions

The present study indicated that CROM increased in all studied directions and that LROM increased in lateral flexion after the completion of an 8-week home-exercise therapy programme designed for intensive care nurses with MSP. We conclude that the used home-exercise therapy programme seemed to be effective for improving CROM and to a lesser extent LROM. Further studies are needed to develop this simple but effective home-exercise therapy programme to help motivate nurses to perform such exercises regularly. This study may contribute to the knowledge base within this area, however further research is required in larger samples, possibly with a symptomatic control group and more clinically rigorous outcome measures.

Abbreviations

CROM: Cervical range of motion; LROM: Lumbar range of motion; MSP: Musculoskeletal pain; ICU: Intensive care unit; NMQ: Nordic Musculoskeletal Questionnaire; VAS: Visual Analogue Scale.

Competing interests

The authors declare that they had no competing interests.

Authors' contributions

TF devised the study, performed the statistical analysis and drafted the manuscript. MP designed the study, coordinated the data collection and helped to draft the manuscript. EM was involved in writing the manuscript. All authors read and approved the final manuscript.

Acknowledgements

This research received no specific grant from any funding agency in the public, commercial or not-for-profit sectors. Tiina Freimann's studies were supported by the European Social Fund's Doctoral Studies and Internationalisation Programme DoRa, administered by the Archimedes Foundation. We would like to thank Kaari Annama for collecting the data and Inge Ringmets for consultation on the statistical analysis.

Author details

[1]Tartu University Hospital, Puusepa 8, Tartu 51014, Estonia. [2]Department of Public Health, Medical Faculty, University of Tartu, Ravila 14a, Tartu 50411, Estonia. [3]Institute of Technology, Estonian University of Life Sciences, Kreuzwaldi 56, Tartu 51014, Estonia. [4]Institute of Exercise Biology and Physiotherapy, University of Tartu, Ravila 14a, Tartu 50411, Estonia.

References

1. Bos E, Krol B, Star L, Groothoff J. Risk factors and musculoskeletal complaints in non-specialized nurses, IC nurses, operation room nurses, and X-ray technologists. Int Arch Occup Environ Health. 2007;80:198–206.
2. June KJ, Cho SH. Lumbar pain and work-related factors among nurses in intensive care units. J Clin Nurs. 2010;20:479–87.
3. Freimann T, Coggon D, Merisalu E, Animägi L, Pääsuke M. Risk factors for musculoskeletal pain amongst nurses in Estonia: cross-sectional study. BMC Musculoskelet disord. 2013;14:334.
4. Häkkinen A, Kautiainen H, Hannonen P, Ylinen J. Strength training and stretching versus stretching only in the treatment of patients with chronic NP: a randomised one-year follow-up study. Clin Rehabil. 2008;22:592–600.
5. Linton SJ, van Tulder MW. Preventive interventions for back and neck pain problems: what is the evidence? Spine. 2001;26:778–87.
6. Proper KI, Koning M, van der Beek AJ, Hildebrandt VH, Bosscher RJ, van Mechelen W. The effectiveness of worksite physical activity programs on physical activity, physical fitness, and health. Clin J Sport Med. 2003;13:106–17.
7. Henchoz Y, So AKL. Exercise and nonspecific low back pain: a literature review. Joint Bone Spine. 2008;75:533–9.
8. Coury HJCG, Moreira RFC, Dias NB. Evaluation of the effectiveness of workplace exercise in controlling cervical, shoulder and lumbar pain: a systematic review. Bras J Physioter. 2009;13:461–79.
9. Hartvigsen J, Lauritzen S, Lings S, Lauritzen T. Intensive education combined with low tech ergonomic intervention does not prevent low back pain in nurses. Br Med J. 2005;62:13–7.
10. Driessen MT, Proper KI, van Tulder MW, Anema JR, Bongers PM, van der Beek AJ. The effectiveness of physical and organisational ergonomic interventions on low back pain and neck pain: a systematic review. Occup Environ Med. 2010;67:277–85.
11. Driessen MT, Proper KI, Anema JR, Bongers PM, van der Beek AJ. Process evaluation of a participatory ergonomics programme to prevent low back pain and neck pain among workers. Implement Sci. 2010;5:65.
12. Jakobsen MD, Sundstrup E, Brandt M, Kristensen AZ, Jay K, Stelter R, et al. Effect of workplace- versus home-based physical exercise on pain in healthcare workers: study protocol for a single blinded cluster randomized controlled trial. BMC Musculoskelet Disord. 2014;15:119.
13. Kuukkanen T, Mälkia E, Kautiainen H, Pohjolainen T. Effectiveness of a home exercise programme in low back pain: a randomized five-year follow-up study. Physiother Res Int. 2007;12:213–24.
14. Dawson AP, McLennan SN, Schiller SD, Jull GA, Hodges PW, Stewart S. Experimentals to prevent back pain and back injury in nurses: a systematic review. Occup Environ Med. 2007;64:642–50.
15. Palmer KT, Harris EC, Linaker C, Barker M, Lawrence W, Cooper C, et al. Effectiveness of community- and workplace-based experimental to manage musculoskeletal-related sickness absence and job loss: a systematic review. Rheumatology. 2012;51:230–42.
16. Hayden JA, van Tulder MW, Tomlinson G. Systematic review: strategies for using exercise therapy to improve outcomes in chronic low back pain. Ann Intern Med. 2005;142:776–85.
17. Page P. Current concepts in muscle stretching for exercise and rehabilitation. Int J Sports Phys Ther. 2012;7:109–19.
18. Kraemer WJ, Adams K, Cafarelli E, Dudley GA, Dooly C, Feigenbaum MS, et al. American College of Sports Medicine Position Stand: Progression Models in Resistance Training for Healthy Adults. Med Sci Sports Exerc. 2002;34:364–80.
19. Kuorinka I, Jonsson B, Kilbom A, Vinterberg H, Biering-Sorensen F, Andersson G, et al. Standardised Nordic questionnaire for the analysis of musculoskeletal symptoms. Appl Ergon. 1987;18:233–7.
20. Scott J, Huskisson EC. Vertical or horizontal visual analogue scales. Ann Rheum Dis. 1979;38:560.
21. Fitzgerald GK, Wynveen KJ, Rheault W, Rothschild B. Objective assessment with establishment of normal values for lumbar spinal range of motion. Phys Ther. 1983;63:1776–81.

22. Youdas JW, Carey JR, Garrett TR. Reliability of measurements of cervical spine range of motion – comparison of three methods. Phys Ther. 1991;71:98–104.
23. Saur PMM, Ensink FBM, Frese K, Seeger D, Hildebrandt J. Lumbar range of motion: reliability and validity of the inclinometer technique in the clinical measurement of trunk flexibility. Spine. 1996;21:1331–8.
24. Childs J, Cleland J, Elliott J, Teyhen DS, Wainner RS, Whitman JM, et al. NP: clinical practice guidelines linked to the international classification of functioning, disability, and health from the Orthopaedic Section of the American Physical Therapy Association. J Orthop Sports Phys Ther. 2008;38:A1–34.
25. Delitto A, George SZ, Van Dillen L, Whitman JM, Sowa G, Shekelle P, et al. LBP Clinical Practice Guidelines Linked to the International Classification of Functioning, Disability, and Health from the Orthopaedic Section of the American Physical Therapy Association. J Orthop Sports Phys Ther. 2012;42:A1–57.
26. Swinkels RAHM, Swinkels-Meewisse IEJCM. Normal values for cervical range of motion. Spine. 2014;5:362–7.
27. Tseng CN, Chen CCH, WU SC, Lin LC. Effects of range-of-motion exercise programme. J Adv Nurs. 2006;57:181–91.
28. Skargren E, Oberg B. Effects of an exercise program on musculoskeletal symptoms and physical capacity among nursing staff. Scand J Med Sci Sports. 1996;6:122–30.
29. Alexandre NMC, de Moraes MAA, Correa Filho HR, Jorge SA. Evaluation of a program to reduce back pain in nursing personnel. Rev Saude Publica. 2001;35:356–61.
30. Yuan SC, Chou MC, Hwu LJ, Chang YO, Hsu WH, Kuo HW. An intervention program to promote health-related physical fitness in nurses. J Clin Nurs. 2008;18:1404–11.
31. Dehlin O, Berg S, Andersson GB, Grimby G. Effect of physical training and ergonomic counselling on the psychological perception of work and on the subjective assessment of low-back insufficiency. Scand J Rehabil Med. 1981;3:1–9.
32. Cleland JA, Mintken PE, Carpenter K, Fritz JM, Glynn P, Whitman J, et al. Examination of a clinical prediction rule to identify patients with neck pain likely to benefit from thoracic spine thrust manipulation and a general cervical range of motion exercise: multi-center randomized clinical trial. Phys Ther. 2010;90:1239–50.
33. Hjermstad MJ, Fayers PM, Haugen DF, Caraceni A, Hanks GW, et al. Studies comparing Numerical Rating Scales, Verbal Rating Scales, and Visual Analogue Scales for assessment of pain intensity in adults: a systematic literature review. J Pain Symptom Manage. 2011;41:1073–93.
34. Jensen RE, Rothrock NE, DeWitt EM, Spiegel B, Tucker CA, et al. The role of technical advances in the adoption and integration of patient-reported outcomes in clinical care. Med Care. 2015;53:153–9.
35. Hignett S. Intervention strategies to reduce musculoskeletal injuries associated with handling patients: a systematic review. Occup Environ Med. 2003;60:e6 (http://www.occenvmed.com/cgi/content/full/60/9/e6).
36. Horneij E, Hemborg B, Jensen I et al. No significant differences between intervention programmes on neck, shoulder and low back pain: a prospective randomized study among home-care personnel. J Rehabil Med. 2001;33:170–6.

8

Ice swimming – 'Ice Mile' and '1 km Ice event'

Beat Knechtle[1,2*], Thomas Rosemann[2] and Christoph A. Rüst[2]

Abstract

Background: Ice swimming for 1 mile and 1 km is a new discipline in open-water swimming since 2009. This study examined female and male performances in swimming 1 mile ('Ice Mile') and 1 km ('1 km Ice event') in water of 5 °C or colder between 2009 and 2015 with the hypothesis that women would be faster than men.

Methods: Between 2009 and 2015, 113 men and 38 women completed one 'Ice Mile' and 26 men and 13 completed one '1 km Ice event' in water colder than +5 °C following the rules of International Ice Swimming Association (IISA). Differences in performance between women and men were determined. Sex difference (%) was calculated using the equation ([time for women] – [time for men]/[time for men] × 100). For 'Ice Mile', a mixed-effects regression model with interaction analyses was used to investigate the influence of sex and environmental conditions on swimming speed. The association between water temperature and swimming speed was assessed using Pearson correlation analyses.

Results: For 'Ice Mile' and '1 km Ice event', the best men were faster than the best women. In 'Ice Mile', calendar year, number of attempts, water temperature and wind chill showed no association with swimming speed for both women and men. For both women and men, water temperature was not correlated to swimming speed in both 'Ice Mile' and '1 km Ice event'.

Conclusions: In water colder than 5 °C, men were faster than women in 'Ice Mile' and '1 km Ice event'. Water temperature showed no correlation to swimming speed.

Background

Official open-water ultra-distance swimming races at the world class level have been held since 2000 [1–3] apart from the 'English Channel Swim' which has been held as a solo swim since 1875 [4].

Sex differences are lower in swimming compared to running [5]. In elite pool swimmers competing in breaststroke, backstroke, medley and freestyle up to 1500 m, women reduced the gap to men with increasing race distance [6–10]. In long-distance open-water swimming from 5 to 25 km, women reduced the gap to men in 10 km, but not in 25 km [3]. In longer distances, however, women were able to reduce the sex difference in races such as 'La Traversée Internationale du Lac St-Jean' held in Canada between 1955 and 2012 [11] and 'Maratona del Golfo Capri-Napoli' held in Italy from 1954 to 2013 [12].

In open-water swimming, women are also able to beat men [13, 14]. Two recent studies investigating female and male open-water swimmers described for the first time that women were able to swim faster than men [13, 14]. In the 46-km 'Manhattan Island Marathon Swim' held in water temperatures below +20 °C, the best women were ~13 % faster than the best men [13]. It was argued that the low water temperature and the higher body fat in women were the most likely reasons that women were able to beat men [13]. Similarly to the 'Manhattan Island Marathon Swim', the fastest women crossed the 'Catalina Channel' faster than the fastest men [14].

Women might outperform men in open-water swimming due to greater proportions of body fat – *e.g.,* better buoyancy or insulation. Female swimmers have more adipose tissue than male swimmers [15] and the distance between the centre of buoyancy and the centre of mass is larger for men compared to women [15]. Both the centre of buoyancy and mass are more caudal in women compared to men [15]. Higher body fat (*i.e.,* thicker skinfold thicknesses and more subcutaneous fat) helps to endurance longer in cold water [16–18]. It has been shown in several instances that subjects with higher body fat were able to stay longer in cold water [16–18]. The longer swimming times of subjects with higher body

* Correspondence: beat.knechtle@hispeed.ch
[1]Gesundheitszentrum St. Gallen, Vadianstrasse 26 9001, St. Gallen, Switzerland
[2]Institute of Primary Care, University of Zurich, Zurich, Switzerland

fat were attributed largely to their greater buoyancy enabling them to keep their heads above water during the early hyperventilation [19].

Ice swimming is a new discipline within open-water swimming. In ice swimming, Lynne Cox [20] and Lewis Pugh [21] are the two pioneers with the first and most outstanding achievements. Lynne Cox swam in 1975 the 16-km Cook Strait in New Zealand at 10 °C, in 1987 the Bering Strait from the island of Little Diomede (Alaska) to Big Diomede (former Soviet Union) in 2:05 h:min at 6–7 °C and in 2002 in Antarctica from the ship 'Orlova' to Neko Harbor 1.96 km in 25:00 min:sec [20]. Lewis Pugh swam in 2007 across the Geographic North Pole for 1 km at −1.7 °C in 18:50 min:sec, and in 2010 1 km in 2 °C for 22:51 h:min across Lake Pumori, a glacial lake on Mount Everest at 5'300 m above sea level [21].

Based upon these achievements of Lynne Cox [20] and Lewis Pugh [21], Ram Barkai from South Africa founded in 2009 the 'International Ice Swimming Association' (IISA) [22]. The IISA introduced the 'Ice Mile' as its ultimate achievement of swimming in ice cold water. An 'Ice Mile' is defined as swimming 1 mile (1.609 km) in water of +5 °C or colder [22]. The swimmer must complete the mile unassisted using only a pair of swimming goggles, a swimming cap and a standard swimming suit [22]. The IISA has defined how an ice swimmer can complete an official 'Ice Mile' [23]. Following the IISA, the swim distance must be at least 1 one mile or 1609.3 m [23]. The swim must be in water of a temperature of 5 °C or lower and measured as follows [23]: The water temperature must be measured for at least 10 min between 127 and 508 mm below the water surface, the water temperature must be established by using the average reading obtained from three digital thermometer readings with a temperature accuracy of ±1 °C. The thermometers must be water submerged thermometers and no laser or infra-red thermometers are allowed. The official water temperature must be measured no more than 30 min before the start of the swim. The swim must be followed by independent observers [23]. In 2014, IISA introduced the '1 km Ice event' covering 1 km in addition to the 'Ice Mile'. The event allows for swimmers to compete in icy waters of +5 °C or less under IISA rules for 1000 m. Swimming times in 'Ice Mile' and '1 km Ice event' are recorded since 2009 and 2014, respectively [22].

Little is known about swimming performance in ice cold water; one study regarding performance of two men [16] and no published data regarding performance of women exists. The present study investigated the performances for female and male swimmers in 'Ice Mile' and '1 km Ice event' since 2009. The first man completing an official 'Ice Mile' was Ram Barkai on January 31, 2009, in Lake Zurich, Switzerland, in 43:00 h:min. The first woman achieved an 'Ice Mile' on July 23, 2011, in Fraserburg, South Africa in 26:45 h:min. Although the swim time for the women was faster than the time for the man, Ram Barkai was swimming 2.2 km, longer than the official distance of an 'Ice Mile'. Based upon the fact that Lynne Cox was the first person to swim in icy water [20] before the first man [21] and the recent findings that women were able to beat men in open-water swimming in low water temperatures (<20 °C) [13, 14], we hypothesized that women would be faster than men in both 'Ice Mile' and '1 km Ice event'. We also considered repeated finishes in our analysis since it was hypothesized that extensive previous experience was important for successful ice swimming [16, 17].

Methods

Ethics

All procedures used in the study were approved by the Institutional Review Board of Kanton St. Gallen, Switzerland with a waiver of the requirement for informed consent of the participants given the fact that the study involved the analysis of publicly available data.

Data sampling and data analysis

The data set for this study was obtained from the website of the 'International Ice Swimming Association' (IISA) [22]. The last access to the database was March 29, 2015. On the IISA website, the results of successful swims are presented with date, name of the athletes, sex, water temperature, and wind chill. Performance time was extracted from the database. Since some 'Ice Miles' were longer than one mile, we converted all performance times in 'Ice Mile' and '1 km Ice event' to swimming speed in km/h.

Statistical analysis

Each set of data was tested for normal distribution (D'Agostino and Pearson omnibus normality test) and for homogeneity of variances (Levene's test) before statistical analyses. Sex difference in percent (%) was calculated using the equation ([swim time for women] – [swim time for men]/[swim time for men] × 100). To find differences between two groups, a Student's t-test was used in case of normal distributed data (with Welch's correction in case of unequal variances) and a Mann–Whitney test was used in case of not normal distributed data. A mixed-effects regression model with swimmer as random variable to consider swimmers who completed several events was used to analyse changes in swimming speed across years. We included sex, experience (*i.e.*, number of previous successful swims), water temperature, wind chill and calendar year as fixed variables. We also considered interaction effects between sex, experience, water temperature and wind chill. The final model was selected by means of Akaike information Criterion (AIC). A potential correlation between water temperature and swimming speed was tested using Pearson correlation coefficients. Statistical analyses were performed using IBM SPSS Statistics (Version 22, IBM SPSS, Chicago, IL, USA) and GraphPad Prism (Version 6.01, GraphPad Software, La Jolla, CA, USA). Significance was accepted at $p < 0.05$ (two-sided for *t*-tests). Data are given as mean ± standard deviation (SD).

Results

'Ice Mile'

From 2009 to 2015, data from 169 swimmers (123 men and 46 women) were available. Men were faster than women for the three fastest, the ten fastest and when all women and men were compared (Table 1). Water temperature in 'Ice Mile' was +3.76 ± 1.39 °C, varying from −1.0 to +5.0 °C. Water temperature and swimming speed showed no correlation for men ($r^2 = 0.0037$, $p = 0.520$, Fig. 1) and women ($r^2 = 0.0288$, $p = 0.307$, Fig. 2). Calendar year, number of attempts, water temperature and wind chill were not associated with swimming speed for women and men (Table 2). Swimming speed showed no changes across calendar years for men ($r^2 = 0.19$, $p = 0.329$) and women ($r^2 = 0.70$, $p = 0.077$). The sex difference in swimming speed between the annual fastest women and men remained unchanged ($r^2 = 0.12$, $p = 0.576$) between 2011 and 2015 where men were 0.37 ± 0.09 km/h (17.9 ± 5.3 %) faster than women (Fig. 3).

'1 km Ice event'

Data from 78 swimmers (53 men and 25 women) were available. All data were from winter 2015; therefore, no analyses for trends across calendar years were possible. Men were faster than women for the three and the ten fastest (Table 1). Water temperature in '1 km Ice event' was +3.79 ± 0.84 °C, varying from +3.1 °C to +4.8 °C. Water temperature and swimming speed were not associated in men ($r^2 = 0.094$, $p = 0.306$, Fig. 4) and women ($r^2 = 0.023$, $p = 0.452$, Fig. 5).

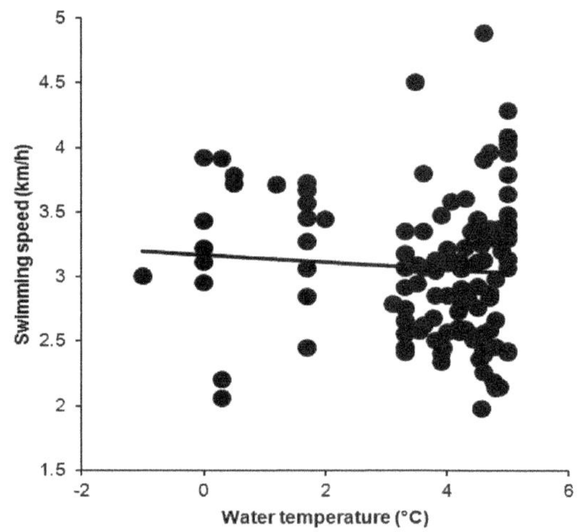

Fig. 1 Correlation between water temperature and swimming speed for men in 'Ice Mile'

Sex difference

We compared the sex difference between 'Ice Mile' and '1 km Ice event' for the fastest swimmers. For the three fastest in 'Ice Mile' and '1 km Ice event', the sex differences were 16.1 ± 2.3 % and 10.3 ± 0.8 %, respectively. The difference of 5.8 ± 1.6 % between the two events was statistically significant ($p = 0.024$). For the ten fastest in 'Ice Mile' and '1 km Ice event', the sex differences were 16.9 ± 4.0 % and 21.1 ± 8.3 %, respectively. The sex difference of 4.2 ± 7.1 % for the ten fastest in '1 km Ice event' and 'Ice Mile' was not statistically significantly different ($p > 0.05$).

Discussion

This study investigated the performance and the sex difference in performance for women and men completing an official 'Ice Mile' and '1 km Ice event' with the hypothesis that women would be faster than men in 'Ice Mile' and '1 km Ice event'. The main findings were, (*i*), the fastest men were faster than the fastest women in

Table 1 The fastest women and men with sex difference for 'Ice Mile' and '1 km Ice event'

'Ice Mile'					
Women (km/h)		Men (km/h)	Difference (km/h)	Difference (%)	Significance
Three fastest	3.92 ± 0.21	4.56 ± .030	0.63 ± 0.11	16.1 ± 2.3	$p = 0.010$
Ten fastest	3.56 ± 0.31	4.16 ± 0.31	0.59 ± 0.12	16.9 ± 4.0	$p < 0.0001$
All	2.82 ± 0.53	3.06 ± 0.54	0.24 ± 0.01	8.5 ± 1.8	$p < 0.0001$
'1 km Ice event'					
Three fastest	4.02 ± 0.13	4.44 ± 0.15	0.41 ± 0.50	10.3 ± 0.8	$p = 0.0024$
Ten fastest	3.53 ± 0.36	4.25 ± 1.55	0.71 ± 0.22	21.1 ± 8.3	$p < 0.0001$
All	2.92 ± 0.58	3.39 ± 0.57	0.47 ± 0.01	13.8 ± 1.7	$p < 0.0001$

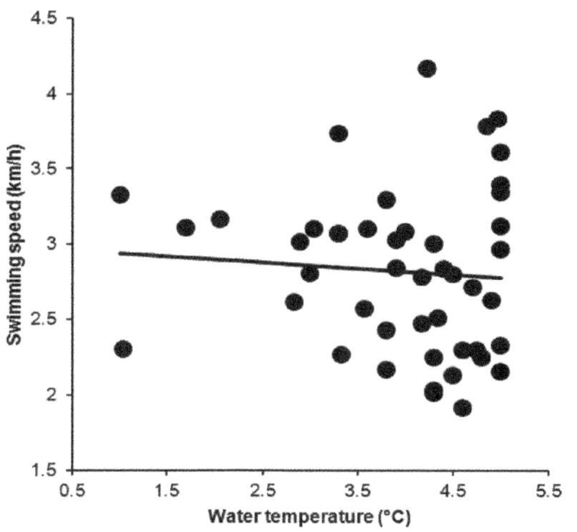

Fig. 2 Correlation between water temperature and swimming speed for women in 'Ice Mile'

'Ice Mile' and '1 km Ice event', (*ii*), the sex difference remained unchanged across calendar years in 'Ice Mile' and, (*iii*), no correlation existed between water temperature and swimming speed for women and men in 'Ice Mile' and '1 km Ice event'.

The fastest men were faster than the fastest women

A first important finding was that women were not faster than men as hypothesized. Based upon previous findings where women were faster than men in the 'Manhattan Island Marathon Swim' [13] and the 'Catalina Channel Swim' [14] where athletes competed at water temperatures < 20 °C we hypothesized that women would be faster than men in swimming in ice cold water. However, the fastest men were faster than the fastest women in both 'Ice Mile' and '1 km Ice event'. We based our assumption that women would be faster than men in ice swimming on previous reports that female open-water ultra-distance swimmers have more body fat than male swimmers [24]. A study investigating body composition in open-water swimmers in the 26.4-km 'Marathon Swim' in Lake Zurich, Switzerland, showed that men (18.8 ± 4.5 % body fat) had ~12 % less percent body fat than women (30.7 ± 3.7 % body fat) [24].

Most probably, percent body fat is not the most important predictor for a fast swim time in open-water swimming. In female and male open-water ultra-endurance swimmers in the 26.4-km 'Marathon Swim' in Lake Zurich, Switzerland, a potential association between anthropometric characteristics and race time was investigated [25]. For men, body height, Body Mass Index (BMI), length of arm, and swimming speed during training were related to race time after bivariate analysis. For women, swimming speed during training was associated with race time. In the multivariate analysis, BMI and swimming speed during training were related to race time for men [25]. Body fat percentage was not predictive for women and men in open-water distance swimming at moderate water temperatures (>20 °C) [25] and also in ice swimming.

Another potential explanation could be differences in body core temperature between women and men during open-water distance swimming [26]. In a 10-km open-water swimming competition held at a water temperature of ~21 °C, the drop in body core temperature was more pronounced in women (4.2 ± 0.7 °C) than in men (2.7 ± 0.8 °C) [26]. In men, race time was inversely related to pre-competition body temperature [26]. Differences in body composition between women and men might be of

Table 2 Coefficients and standard errors (SE) from a multivariable regression model. Interactions between variables are also presented

Parameter	Estimate	SE	df	*t*	*p*-value
Constant term	30.61	22.39	141.26	1.36	0.17
Female	0.23	0.17	129.30	1.29	0.19
Calendar year	−0.01	0.01	141.25	−1.32	0.18
Number of attempts	0.007	0.01	82.60	0.62	0.53
Water temperature	−0.005	0.01	59.42	−0.48	0.63
Wind chill	0.002	0.002	82.47	0.86	0.38
Female × Number of attempts	−0.12	0.09	61.70	−1.31	0.19
Female × Water temperature	−0.04	0.03	148.47	−1.40	0.16
Female × Wind chill	−0.03	0.03	143.75	−1.07	0.28
Water temperature × × Wind chill	0.0003	0.001	75.83	0.31	0.75
Female × Water temperature × Wind chill	0.006	0.008	149.11	0.80	0.42
Female × Number of attempts × Water temperature × Wind chill	0.002	0.002	55.64	0.95	0.34
Female × Number of attempts × Water temperature × Wind chill	$-8.5 \times E^{-5}$	0.0005	37.5	−0.16	0.87

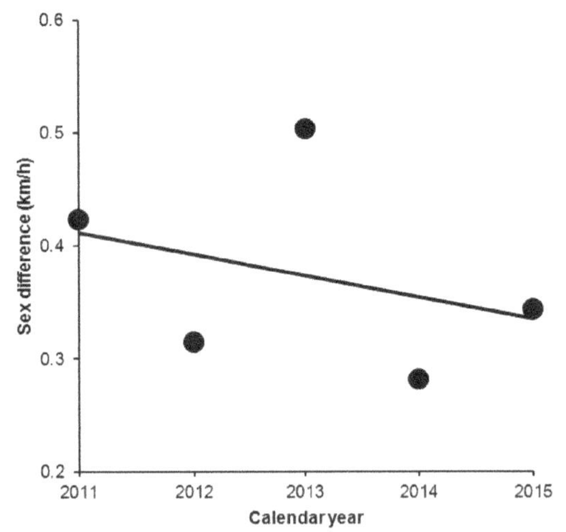

Fig. 3 Sex difference between the annual fastest women and men in 'Ice Mile' between 2011 and 2015

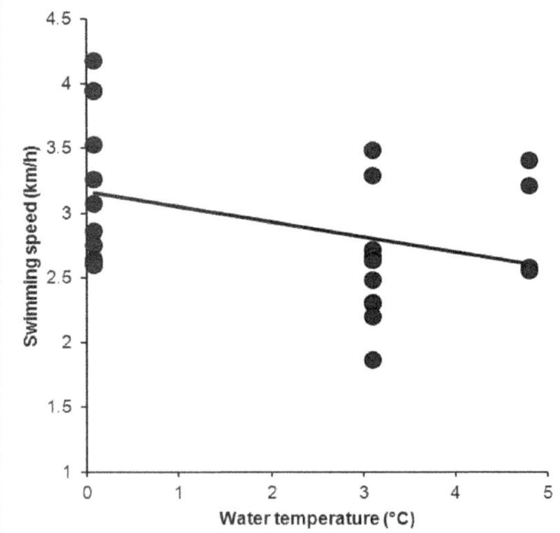

Fig. 5 Correlation between water temperature and swimming speed for women in '1 km Ice event'

importance [18, 27]. In a 19.2-km open water swimming race, longer race duration was associated with an increased risk of hypothermia, and higher BMI was associated with a decreased risk of hypothermia [27]. In swimmers competing in water temperature below 11 °C, athletes with lower body fat finished their swims after less time in the water than those with thicker skinfold thickness. The rectal temperatures were, however, not significantly lower [18]. In the present study investigating women and men swimming 1 mile and 1 km in water below 5 °C, the duration of the swims was rather short

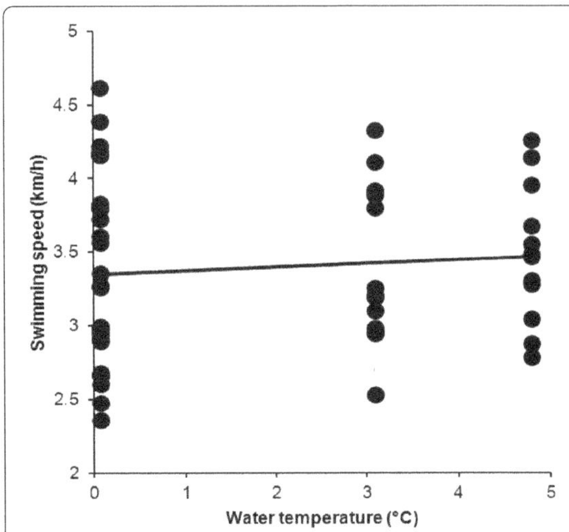

Fig. 4 Correlation between water temperature and swimming speed for men in '1 km Ice event'

and body core temperature might not have dropped seriously.

Sex difference in performance

The first woman completed in 2011 an official 'Ice Mile'. Between 2011 and 2015, the sex difference in the annual fastest women and men in 'Ice Mile' remained unchanged at ~18 %. For the three and the ten fastest in 'Ice Mile', the sex difference was ~16–17 %. For '1 km Ice event', however, the sex differences for the three and ten fastest were ~10 % and ~21 %, respectively.

The sex difference in swimming speed has been investigated in several studies for pool [5, 28–31] and open-water [1, 11–13, 32–34] swimmers. In master pool swimmers aged from 35 to 70 years, the percent sex difference in freestyle swimming from 50 m to 1500 m became progressively smaller with increasing distance from 50 m (19 ± 1 %) to 1500 m (11 ± 1 %) [5]. When swimming performances in different disciplines and strokes were investigated, men were generally ~8.9 % faster than women [31]. Although two very recent studies showed that women were able to beat men in open-water swimming [13, 14], men were generally faster than women in pool [6, 29] and open-water [1, 11, 12, 33, 34] swimming. However, in some studies, women were able to achieve similar performances to men in open-water swimming [28, 32].

The sex differences in these ice swimmers were higher compared to sex differences reported for pool [6, 29] and open-water [1, 3] swimmers competing at moderate water temperatures (~20 °C). For pool swimmers competing at world-class level (*i.e.,* finalists in Olympic Games and World Championships) in different strokes and distances up to 1500 m, the sex difference was at ~9–10 % [6]. For freestyle swimming from 50 m to 1500 m, the sex difference was unchanged at ~9 % [29]. In elite 10-km open-water swimmers competing at world-class level, the sex difference was at ~7 % [1]. In the annual fastest swimmers competing in FINA World Cup races from 2000 to 2012 in 5 km, 10 km and 25 km, the sex differences in swimming speed remained at ~7 %, ~6 % and ~9 %, respectively [3]. The sex difference for the three fastest ice swimmers (~10 %) was comparable to the findings for freestyle pool swimmers up to 1,500 m [29], but increased to ~21 % for the ten fastest ever. Differences in body composition [24] and body core temperature [26] between women and men might explain these differences.

Between 2011 and 2015, the annual fastest men were ~18 % faster than the annual fastest women. Women reduced the gap to men in open-water ultra-distance swimming in the last years [11, 12]. The short period of five calendar years was the most likely reason for the unchanged sex difference. Other studies investigated time periods of decades where women considerably reduced the gap to men [11, 12, 34].

For these short distances of 1 mile and 1 km, men might profit from their higher skeletal muscle mass to swim faster than women. In the 26.4-km 'Marathon Swim' in Lake Zurich, Switzerland, men (42.0 ± 3.2 kg) had 12.6 kg more skeletal muscle mass than women (29.4 ± 2.9 kg) [24]. Another potential explanation could be the different numbers of women and men. The number of men competing in these events was considerably higher compared to the number of women. The ratio was 2.67 in 'Ice Mile' (123 men and 46 women) and 2.12 in '1 km Ice event' (53 men and 25 women). Therefore, it is equally possible that this large difference may explain some of the observed high sex differences. However, we compared the sex difference between 'Ice Mile' and '1 km Ice event' for the three and ten fastest swimmers. If/when this sport becomes more popular and more elite athletes start competing (especially women), the sex gap is likely to reduce. This is most likely the best explanation for sex differences. Future studies might then compare all women to all men to find the true sex difference without selection to the fastest swimmers. Indeed, the sex difference decreased in 'Ice Mile' from 16.9 % to 8.5 % when the ten fastest and all swimmers were considered, and from 21.1 % to 13.8 % in '1 km Ice event' in the ten fastest and all swimmers (Table 1).

No correlation between water temperature and swimming speed

A second important finding was that no correlation existed between water temperatures and swimming speed. Most probably the small range between nearly 0 and +5 °C gave no room for changes in swimming speed. Tipton et al. [35] investigated ten volunteers during three self-paced breaststroke swims in a variable-speed swimming flume at +25 °C, +18 °C, and +10 °C for a maximum of 90 min. Apart from oxygen consumption, rectal temperature, also swimming speed and angle, and stroke rate and length were measured. Swimming efficiency and length of stroke decreased more and rate of stroke and swim angle increased more in water of 10 °C than in warmer water.

Limitations and implications for future research

A limitation of this study is the short time frame of 5 years and the low number of female swimmers. We assume that the sex difference will be lower with a higher number of successful women. Future studies should measure body fat in both women and men and body core temperature during the swims.

Conclusion

In ice swimming in water colder than +5 °C, men were faster than women in 1 mile ('Ice Mile') and 1 km ('1 km Ice event'). Between 2011 and 2015, the sex difference remained unchanged in 'Ice Mile' at ~18 %. In 'Ice Mile', calendar year, number of attempts, water temperature and wind chill showed no relation with swimming speed for women and men. For 'Ice Mile' and '1 km Ice event', swimming speed showed no correlation to water temperature for women and men.

Competing interests

The authors declare that they have no competing interests.

Authors' contributions

BK collected all data and drafted the manuscript. CR performed the statistical analyses and helped in drafting the manuscript. TR revised the manuscript critically for important intellectual content. All authors read and approved the final manuscript.

References

1. Vogt P, Rüst CA, Rosemann T, Lepers R, Knechtle B. Analysis of 10 km swimming performance of elite male and female open-water swimmers. Springerplus. 2013;2:603.
2. Zingg MA, Rüst CA, Rosemann T, Lepers R, Knechtle B. Analysis of swimming performance in FINA World Cup long-distance open water races. Extrem Physiol Med. 2014;3:2.
3. Zingg MA, Rüst CA, Rosemann T, Lepers R, Knechtle B. Analysis of sex differences in open-water ultra-distance swimming performances in the FINA World Cup races in 5 km, 10 km and 25 km from 2000 to 2012. BMC Sports Sci Med Rehabil. 2014;6:7.
4. Knechtle B, Rosemann T, Rüst CA. Participation and performance trends by nationality in the 'English Channel Swim' from 1875 to 2013. BMC Sports Sci Med Rehabil. 2014;6:34.
5. Senefeld J, Joyner MJ, Stevens A, Hunter SK. Sex differences in elite swimming with advanced age are less than marathon running. Scand J Med Sci Sports. 2015. doi:10.1111/sms.12412 [Epub ahead of print].
6. Wild S, Rüst CA, Rosemann T, Knechtle B. Changes in sex difference in swimming speed in finalists at FINA World Championships and the Olympic Games from 1992 to 2013. BMC Sports Sci Med Rehabil. 2014;6:25.

7. Wolfrum M, Rüst CA, Rosemann T, Lepers R, Knechtle B. Changes in breaststroke swimming performances in national and international athletes competing between 1994 and 2011 -a comparison with freestyle swimming performances. BMC Sports Sci Med Rehabil. 2014;6:18.
8. Wolfrum M, Knechtle B, Rüst CA, Rosemann T, Lepers R. Sex-related differences and age of peak performance in breaststroke versus freestyle swimming. BMC Sports Sci Med Rehabil. 2013;5:29.
9. Wolfrum M, Rüst CA, Rosemann T, Lepers R, Knechtle B. The effect of course length on individual medley swimming performance in national and international athletes. J Hum Kinet. 2014;42:187–200.
10. Wolfrum M, Knechtle B, Rüst CA, Rosemann T, Lepers R. The effects of course length on freestyle swimming speed in elite female and male swimmers - a comparison of swimmers at national and international level. Springerplus. 2013;2:643.
11. Rüst CA, Knechtle B, Rosemann T, Lepers R. Women reduced the sex difference in open-water ultra-distance swimming - La Traversée Internationale du Lac St-Jean, 1955–2012. Appl Physiol Nutr Metab. 2014;39:270–3.
12. Rüst CA, Lepers R, Rosemann T, Knechtle B. Will women soon outperform men in open-water ultra-distance swimming in the 'Maratona del Golfo Capri-Napoli'? Springerplus. 2014;3:86.
13. Knechtle B, Rosemann T, Lepers R, Rüst CA. Women outperform men in ultradistance swimming: the Manhattan Island Marathon Swim from 1983 to 2013. Int J Sports Physiol Perform. 1983;2014(9):913–24.
14. Knechtle B, Rosemann T, Rüst CA. Women cross the 'Catalina Channel' faster than men. SpringerPlus. 2015;4:332.
15. McLean SP, Hinrichs RN. Sex differences in the centre of buoyancy location of competitive swimmers. J Sports Sci. 1998;16:373–83.
16. Knechtle B, Christinger N, Kohler G, Knechtle P, Rosemann T. Swimming in ice cold water. Ir J Med Sci. 2009;178:507–11.
17. Rüst CA, Knechtle B, Rosemann T. Changes in body core and body surface temperatures during prolonged swimming in water of 10 °C - a case report. Extrem Physiol Med. 2012;1:8.
18. Keatinge WR, Khartchenko M, Lando N, Lioutov V. Hypothermia during sports swimming in water below 11 degrees C. Br J Sports Med. 2001;35:352–3.
19. Keatinge WR, Prys-Roberts C, Cooper KE, Honour AJ, Haight J. Sudden failure of swimming in cold water. Br Med J. 1969;1(5642):480–3.
20. Website of Lynne Cox, www.lynnecox.org, last accessed August 1, 2015
21. Website of Lewis Pugh, http://lewispugh.com, last accessed August 1, 2015
22. Website of 'International Ice Swimming Association' (IISA), www.internationaliceswimming.com, last accessed August 1, 2015
23. Website with rules of IISA, www.internationaliceswimming.com/wp-content/uploads/2014/09/IISA-Rules-Swim-Rules.pdf, last accessed August 1, 2015
24. Weitkunat T, Knechtle B, Knechtle P, Rüst CA, Rosemann T. Body composition and hydration status changes in male and female open-water swimmers during an ultra-endurance event. J Sports Sci. 2012;30:1003–13.
25. Knechtle B, Baumann B, Knechtle P, Rosemann T. Speed during training and anthropometric measures in relation to race performance by male and female open-water ultra-endurance swimmers. Percept Mot Skills. 2010;111:463–74.
26. Castro RR, Mendes FS, Nobrega AC. Risk of hypothermia in a new Olympic event: the 10-km marathon swim. Clinics (Sao Paulo). 2009;64:351–6.
27. Brannigan D, Rogers IR, Jacobs I, Montgomery A, Williams A, Khangure N. Hypothermia is a significant medical risk of mass participation long-distance open water swimming. Wilderness Environ Med. 2009;20:14–8.
28. Eichenberger E, Knechtle B, Rüst CA, Knechtle P, Lepers R, Rosemann T. No gender difference in peak performance in ultra-endurance swimming performance - analysis of the 'Zurich 12-h Swim' from 1996 to 2010. Chin J Physiol. 1996;2012(55):346–51.
29. Rüst CA, Rosemann T, Knechtle B. Sex difference in age and performance in elite Swiss freestyle swimmers competing from 50 m to 1,500 m. Springerplus. 2014;3:228.
30. Tanaka H, Seals DR. Age and gender interactions in physiological functional capacity: insight from swimming performance. J Appl Physiol (1985). 1997;82:846–51.
31. Thibault V, Guillaume M, Berthelot G, Helou NE, Schaal K, Quinquis L, et al. Women and men in sport performance: the gender gap has not evolved since 1983. J Sports Sci Med. 2010;9:214–23.
32. Eichenberger E, Knechtle B, Knechtle P, Rüst CA, Rosemann T, Lepers R. Best performances by men and women open-water swimmers during the 'English Channel Swim' from 1900 to 2010. J Sports Sci. 2012;30:1295–301.
33. Eichenberger E, Knechtle B, Knechtle P, Rüst CA, Rosemann T, Lepers R, et al. Sex difference in open-water ultra-swim performance in the longest freshwater lake swim in Europe. J Strength Cond Res. 2013;27:1362–9.
34. Fischer G, Knechtle B, Rüst CA, Rosemann T. Male swimmers cross the English Channel faster than female swimmers. Scand J Med Sci Sports. 2013;23:e48–55.
35. Tipton M, Eglin C, Gennser M, Golden F. Immersion deaths and deterioration in swimming performance in cold water. Lancet. 1999;354:626–9.

9

Effects of conditioning hops on drop jump and sprint performance: a randomized crossover pilot study in elite athletes

Jakob Kümmel[1*], Julian Bergmann[1], Olaf Prieske[2], Andreas Kramer[1], Urs Granacher[2] and Markus Gruber[1]

Abstract

Background: It has previously been shown that conditioning activities consisting of repetitive hops have the potential to induce better drop jump (DJ) performance in recreationally active individuals. In the present pilot study, we investigated whether repetitive conditioning hops can also increase reactive jump and sprint performance in sprint-trained elite athletes competing at an international level.

Methods: Jump and sprint performances of 5 athletes were randomly assessed under 2 conditions. The control condition (CON) comprised 8 DJs and 4 trials of 30-m sprints. The intervention condition (HOP) consisted of 10 maximal repetitive two-legged hops that were conducted 10 s prior to each single DJ and sprint trial. DJ performance was analyzed using a one-dimensional ground reaction force plate. Step length (SL), contact time (CT), and sprint time (ST) during the 30-m sprints were recorded using an opto-electronic measurement system.

Results: Following the conditioning activity, DJ height and external DJ peak power were both significantly increased by 11 % compared to the control condition. All other variables did not show any significant differences between HOP and CON.

Conclusions: In the present pilot study, we were able to demonstrate large improvements in DJ performance even in sprint-trained elite athletes following a conditioning activity consisting of maximal two-legged repetitive hops. This strengthens the hypothesis that plyometric conditioning exercises can induce performance enhancements in elite athletes that are even greater than those observed in recreationally active athletes.. In addition, it appears that the transfer of these effects to other stretch-shortening cycle activities is limited, as we did not observe any changes in sprint performance following the plyometric conditioning activity.

Keywords: Post-activation potentiation, Performance gains, Reactive movement, Plyometric exercise

Background

The muscle's capability of generating high forces is dependent on its contractile history and can be acutely enhanced following voluntary contractions at maximal or near-maximal intensities [1]. These short-term enhancements can be observed on a behavioral and mechanistic level. In fact, acute conditioning-induced performance enhancements were reported for jumping and sprinting activities [2]. Most frequently, heavy resistance exercise protocols (e.g., squats with high loads) or maximal voluntary isometric contractions of the lower limb muscles have been used as conditioning activities to elicit athletes' performance gains in jumping and sprinting tasks.

A few studies used plyometric exercise as a conditioning stimulus in order to increase countermovement jump (CMJ) [3–11], DJ [8, 12, 13], sprint [6, 11] and back squat performance [14]. It has been discussed that plyometrics have a high potential as a potentiating exercise to enhance athletes' sport-specific performance due to similarities in their technical structure (e.g. explosive force or power) with sport-specific skills [10]. Terzis and colleagues for example have shown that 5 consecutive DJs significantly improved immediate following squat

* Correspondence: jakob.kuemmel@uni-konstanz.de
[1]Sensorimotor Performance Lab, Department of Sport Science, University of Konstanz, 78476 Konstanz, Germany
Full list of author information is available at the end of the article

underhand front shot throwing distance by ~5 % [15], and 3 consecutive CMJs to elongate shot put distance by ~3 % [16]. Read and colleagues even found that CMJs increase subsequent golf club velocity of a golf swing [17]. In contrast, tuck jumps failed to improve the round kick force in karate athletes [10], and the 10 m and 20 m sprint performance of soccer players [6].

Those divergent findings related to the potentiating effect of plyometrics on subsequent performance enhancements have been attributed to the wide variety and diversity of methodological issues concerning the potentiating protocol, such as e.g. the level of activation during the conditioning [5], different resting periods [6, 18], and subsequent activities [9, 10]. These issues have a major effect on the concurrent incidence of potentiating mechanisms (e.g. activation of higher order motor units or enhanced contractile properties) and exhausting mechanisms (e.g. neuromuscular fatigue) on the subsequent performance [1].

Another point that has been discussed to affect the response to conditioning exercise is the training status and the strength level of the athletes [5]. There is evidence that human muscles with shorter twitch contraction times and a higher percentage of type II fibers exhibit a greater potentiating effect [19], proposing that strength and or power trained athletes whose muscles contain a greater type II muscle fiber cross sectional area benefit to a larger extent from the potentiating effect compared to their less active peers [2, 20]. A systematic review and meta-analysis on the potentiating effects on athletes' performances revealed beneficial effects up to 6 % [21]. However two recently published studies found evidence for augmented lower body performance up to 12 % in recreationally active men, by means of 10 maximal repetitive reactive jumps (2 leg hops) prior to a subsequent DJ [12, 13]. It is unresolved whether athletes that are highly trained in strength and power activities can also benefit from this type of conditioning exercise. Further, there is limited information available whether those performance gains can be transferred to other stretch-shortening cycle movements. Therefore, the aim of this pilot study was to investigate whether a conditioning activity consisting of 10 repetitive hops can increases jump and sprint performance in highly strength and sprint-trained athletes who compete on an international level.

Methods

A total number of 6 athletes participated in this study. However, one athlete could not participate in all measurements due to other reasons, thus he was treated as a drop out. Finally, 5 athletes completed the protocol of the present study (2 women and 3 men, means ± standard deviation (SD), age women: 23 ± 8 years, height women: 181 ± 3 cm, body mass women: 79 ± 8 kg; age men: 21 ± 2 years, height men 186 ± 14 cm, body mass men 99 ± 19 kg).

All participants were highly sprint-trained elite athletes competing on an international level. In addition, these athletes were well experienced in performing drop jumps since it was part of their daily training and testing routine. All of them gave their written informed consent to the experimental procedures. The study was conducted in accordance with the Declaration of Helsinki and approved by the local ethics committee of the University of Konstanz.

The athletes were tested on two separate days with at least one day of rest in between. DJ and sprint performance was assessed under two conditions in a random sequence on separate testing days, but always at the same time of day for each athlete to prevent any circadian effects. The PAP condition (HOP) afforded athletes to perform 10 repetitive reactive hops prior to each single DJ and each single 30 m sprint. The control condition (CON) included the same tests as in the PAP condition, however without any prior conditioning activity. The order of the sprint and DJ performance measurements was counterbalanced between all participants.

Prior to both experimental conditions (HOP, CON), the athletes performed a warm-up consisting of 25 heel rises, 45 s of submaximal repetitive two leg jumps (hops), and 15 squats as it was part of their general warm-up procedure prior to performance. Afterwards, they performed 3 DJs from a drop height of 46 cm to ensure consistent jumping technique in the subsequent tests. Participants had to jump barefoot, hands akimbo, and the heels did not touch the floor. In addition, they were instructed to conduct all hops and DJs with short ground contact times and maximal rebound jump height. Following this familiarization protocol, participants executed 8 DJs with a rest of 1 min between each DJ. During the HOP condition, the athletes executed 10 maximal hops 10 s prior to each jump (Bergmann interval) [12]. A break of 10 min was allowed between DJs and sprints. The 4 sprints were executed from an upright starting position on an indoor tartan track with the athletes wearing spiked shoes. Between each single sprint there was a resting period of 5 min. The athletes were asked to choose the sprint start on their own within the time frame of 10-20 s after the 10 hops were completed.

A force plate (Leonardo Mechanograph®, Novotec Medical, Pforzheim, Germany; sampling frequency 800 Hz) was used to record vertical ground reaction force and to quantify DJ performance. Contact times (CT_{DJ}), rebound flight times (FT), peak forces (F_{max}), and mechanical external concentric peak power relative to the individual athletes' body mass (P_{max}) were then calculated (Leonardo Mechanography Research Edition®

software, Novotec Medical, Pforzheim, Germany). The performance index (PI) was calculated by dividing FT by CT_{DJ}. Rebound jump height (JH) was determined by the following formula: $JH = {}^{1}/_{8} \cdot g \cdot FT^2$ (g = gravitational constant).

An opto-electronic measurement system (OptoJump next®, MicroGate®, Bolzano, Italy) was used to quantify sprint performance over a distance of 30 m (spatial resolution: 0.01 m; sampling frequency: 1000 Hz). This system recorded the split sprint time over distances of 10 m, 20 m, and 30 m (ST_{10}, ST_{20}, and ST_{30}). In addition, step length (SL) as well as contact times (CT_{Sprint}) were measured during the first 10 meters of the sprint trials.

The mean values of 8 DJs and 4 sprints from each condition were used to compare performance variables between HOP and CON. Due to the limited number of study participants, differences between CON and HOP regarding JH and sprint performance (ST_{10}, ST_{20}, ST_{30}, SL, and CT_{Sprint}) were analysed using the non-parametric Wilcoxon signed-rank test for paired samples.

Additionally, dependent t-tests for paired samples were calculated to reveal intra-individual differences in the 8 drop jumps between CON and HOP. To do so, JH, CT_{DJ}, P_{max}, F_{max}, and PI of the 8 jumps from both conditions were compared within each athlete. Group data are presented as mean values ± SD. Test-retest reliability was determined by means of a 2-way mixed model calculation for the intraclass correlation coefficient (ICC) on consistency [22] of each of the sprint and jump variables between the CON and HOP condition. Level of significance was set to $p < 0.05$.

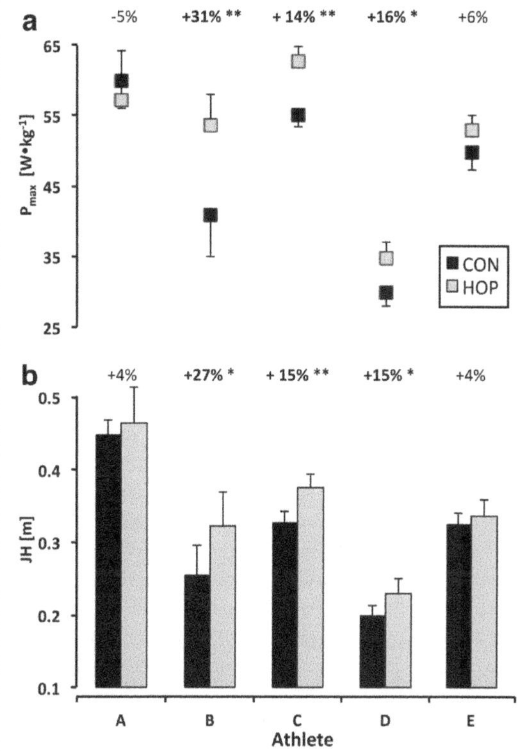

Fig. 1 The individual mean (±SD) P_{max} (**a**) and JH (**b**) of 8 DJs under the control (CON; black squares/bars) and PAP (HOP; gray squares/bars) condition. P_{max} revealed higher values in the same 3 athletes that exhibited higher rebound jump heights in the HOP condition. In athlete E, P_{max} curtly failed to reach the level of significance ($p = 0.05$). Percentage differences related to the control condition are depicted above the bars of each single athlete. Asterix indicating significant within-subject differences (* $p < 0.05$ and ** $p < 0.01$) between CON and HOP. Nota bene, JH increased in each single athlete after the conditioning stimulus, however it was significant only in 3 out of 5

Results

The Wilcoxon signed-rank test for paired samples revealed a significant increase in mean jump height (11 %; $p < 0.05$) in the HOP (0.35 m) compared to the CON (0.31 m) condition (ICC_{JH}: 0.98, $p < 0.01$). The mean JH over the 8 DJs increased for each single athlete in the HOP compared to the CON condition (see Fig. 1). However, when analyzing the JH of each athlete's jumps in the two conditions with dependent t-tests for paired samples, these differences were significant in 3 out of 5 athletes (B, C, D; ICC_{Pmax}: 0.93, $p < 0.05$). The same 3 athletes reached a significantly higher P_{max} during the 8 DJs in the HOP compared to the CON condition (see Fig. 1). One of the two remaining participants (E) showed a tendency for a higher P_{max} value in the HOP compared to the CON condition ($p = 0.051$). Of note, athlete A showed a lower P_{max} value in the HOP condition compared to CON. The same athlete exhibited a significant longer CT_{DJ} in the HOP condition (13 %, $p < 0.05$), whereas athlete B had a shorter CT_{DJ} (10 %, $p < 0.05$, see Table 1; ICC_{CT}: 0.88, $p < 0.05$). The PI increased individually between 6-24 % and this difference was significant for athletes B, C and D (ICC_{PI}: 0.89, $p < 0.05$). In contrast to P_{max}, no significant differences were found for F_{max} between the two experimental conditions in all analyzed participants (ICC_{Fmax}: 0.94; $p < 0.01$).

The mean values of ST_{10}, ST_{20}, and ST_{30} differed by less than 1 % (ICC_{ST10}: 0.97; ICC_{ST20}: 0.99; ICC_{ST30}: 0.99, $p < 0.01$) and no significant differences were found between the two experimental conditions (Table 2). Similarly, step lengths (ICC_{SL1}: 0.73, $p = 0.12$; ICC_{SL2}: 0.91, $p < 0.01$) as well as contact times (ICC_{CT1}: 0.93; ICC_{CT1}: 0.86, $p < 0.05$) showed no significant changes between the HOP and CON conditions.

Table 1 Individual mean values (±SD) of the parameters performance index (PI), contact time (CT_{DJ}), and peak forces (F_{max}) for 8 DJs under the CON and HOP condition

Athlete	PI		CT_{DJ} [s]		F_{max} [kN]	
	CON	PAP	CON	PAP	CON	PAP
A	3.1 ± 0.2	2.9 ± 0.4	0.194 ± 0.012	0.219 ± 0.022*	6.3 ± 0.6	6.9 ± 0.4
B	2.7 ± 0.3	3.4 ± 0.2**	0.169 ± 0.011	0.152 ± 0.013*	6.3 ± 0.4	6.3 ± 0.5
C	3.4 ± 0.1	3.7 ± 0.1**	0.150 ± 0.005	0.149 ± 0.007	6.5 ± 0.3	6.1 ± 0.4
D	2.1 ± 0.2	2.3 ± 0.1*	0.195 ± 0.014	0.186 ± 0.007	6.3 ± 0.3	6.0 ± 0.2
E	3.0 ± 0.1	3.2 ± 0.2	0.170 ± 0.008	0.164 ± 0.012	8.0 ± 0.3	8.0 ± 0.8
Mean (±SD)	2.9 ± 0.5	3.1 ± 0.5	0.176 ± 0.019	0.174 ± 0.029	6.7 ± 0.6	6.7 ± 0.6

An asterix indicates significant within-subject differences between the two experimental conditions (* $p < 0.05$ and ** $p < 0.01$). Group mean values (±SD) are presented in the bottom row

Discussion

In the present pilot study, we were able to demonstrate that 10 maximal repetitive hops can significantly increase performance in subsequent drop jumps in sprint-trained elite athletes competing on an international level. Thus, this study delivers further evidence for the high potential of plyometrics as a conditioning exercise to enhance lower limb performance, which is demonstrated by the significant increase in rebound jump height and peak power. However, the same conditioning activity failed to induce significant changes in 30-m sprint performance. More specifically, neither the 10 m and 20 m sprint time nor the kinematics of the first 10 m were affected by this type of conditioning activity. This result indicates a highly specific effect of the conditioning activity that fails to transfer into another complex sport specific task.

We used 10 maximal hops as conditioning with a rest of 10 s between pre-activation and performance assessment, as this protocol has been shown to induce remarkable performance increases in previous studies on recreational subjects [12, 13]. Reactive hops are characterized by high ground reaction forces, which have to be counteracted by the muscles of the lower limbs in a limited period of time in order to provide a basis for energy storage and recoil during the movement [23, 24]. These high forces were found to be sufficient to elucidate post-activation potentiation in the triceps surae muscle as well as increase DJ height [12]. This incorporates findings of previous studies that used conditioning exercise with a similar movement pattern and force characteristic to potentiate jump performances [4, 8]. Studies that used other types of plyometrics such as tuck jumps [5, 6, 10] or drop landings [25] either failed or reached only little potentiating effects on subsequent jump performance. Reasons for this are discussed to be the high load of the condition stimulus that masks the potentiating effect by concurrence of fatigue [5, 6], a failure in transferring the potentiating effect to higher power output [25], and a relatively low-force intensity being unable to induce a postactivation potentiation [6, 25]. We posit the latter point to be the major responsible reason for the equivocal findings of the abovementioned studies. The ground reaction forces that have been reported to appear during tuck jumps and depth jumps in athletes reach 3.6 times the athlete's body mass [26]. Against this, there are indications in the literature for hops to reach values about 5 times their body mass [27, 28] and the athletes of the present study even reached an average peak ground reaction force of 7.5 times their body mass. Hence the results of the present study underpin reactive jumps to be the favorable plyometric conditioning activity when

Table 2 Individual and group mean values (±SD) of the split sprint times over distances of 10 m, 20 m, and 30 m (ST_{10}, ST_{20}, and ST_{30}) of the 4 30-m-sprints under the CON and HOP conditions

Athlete	ST_{10} [s]		ST_{20} [s]		ST_{30} [s]	
	CON	PAP	CON	PAP	CON	PAP
A	1.60	1.60	2.73	2.74	3.79	3.83
B	1.63	1.63	2.80	2.82	3.92	3.95
C	1.70	1.72	2.95	2.97	4.14	4.20
D	1.88	1.83	3.19	3.12	4.44	4.35
E	1.76	1.81	3.11	3.15	4.36	4.42
Mean (±SD)	1.71 ± 0.10	1.72 ± 0.10	2.96 ± 0.20	2.96 ± 0.18	4.13 ± 0.26	4.15 ± 0.25

jump performance should be enhanced. This attempt of explanation for the divergent findings is further supported by the results of Masamoto et al. [14]. They have evidence for 2 DJs to increase the lower limb performance of a squat exercise after a rest of 30 s, whereas 3 tuck jumps had no impact on this exercise.

Contradicting this theory, Esformes at al. failed to show any potentiating effect of reactive jumps, including speed bounce and reactive hops, on subsequent CMJs [3]. A finding that was attributed to the low recruitment of muscle fibers during the conditioning activity. Besides the fact that the authors did not measure electromyographic activity during the conditioning exercise, this explanation deems to be insufficient since it is widely accepted that reactive movements have a high level of motor unit recruitment due to the pronounced contribution of the short-latency stretch-reflex component in the eccentric part of the movements [29–31]. We suppose that this is rather a matter of either less reactiveness in the execution of the vertical bounds or an exceeding resting period between the conditioning and performance assessment. Given that the muscles' potentiated twitch peak torque is highest immediately following the conditioning activity and disappears in the proximate 5 min [12, 19], it is expected that performance increases might as well be largest immediately after a conditioning activity. This has been confirmed by two recently published original works, which provide evidence for the largest performance gains to occur immediately after (i.e. 10 s and 1 min, respectively) maximal repetitive hops [13, 32]. However, Lesinski et al. reported in their meta-analysis that the highest athletic performance increases occur after a rest interval of 6 - 10 min when moderate to heavy resistive exercises has been applied as conditioning exercise [21]. Bringing both points together, this might indicate a different time course of the net effect between potentiation and fatigue for a conditioning stimulus delivered by means of heavy resistance exercises versus a plyometric conditioning activity such as repetitive reactive hops. An exceeding resting period could be another reason for the missing effect of reactive conditioning exercise on improved jump performances in the study of Esformes and colleagues [3].

In line with previous findings in recreationally active participants [12], we found a significant increase in DJ performance of 11 % after the conditioning hops compared to CON. Since we used a similar conditioning and rest protocol as Bergmann et al. [12], it appears possible to argue that well-trained strength and sprint athletes competing on an international level can benefit from this kind of conditioning activity to a similar extent as compared to recreationally active individuals at least with regards to reactive movements. Due to the low sample size, we also analyzed individual changes in DJ performance after conditioning hops compared to control. Three out of 5 athletes (2 men, 1 w) showed significant improvements in JH following the conditioning activity. Increases ranged between 15 % and 27 % (Fig. 1). The two remaining athletes showed small changes in jump height (both +4 %), failing the level of significance. From these individual results we deduce that some reactively trained athletes can benefit remarkably from this kind of conditioning activity. In a study of Weber and colleagues, varying responses to a certain type of conditioning were attributed to the inhomogeneity of the participants [33]. Even though the authors did not intend to investigate individual responses to this kind of conditioning, they found individual performance gains from roughly +15 % to 0 % and even negative values were observed in two athletes. From studies using electrically evoked muscle twitches, it is known that the muscle fiber type distribution is an important factor determining the potentiating responses [19, 34]. Power-trained athletes should have a higher twitch response potentiation compared to endurance-trained athletes [35], as sprint-trained athletes exhibit a greater proportion of type two fibers in their muscles [36]. Due to the fact that all participants in the present study had a very high performance level with regard to lower limb explosive strength, which is demonstrated by the short sprint times (Table 2) and the high P_{max} values (Fig. 1), differences in fiber type composition appear to be an insufficient explanation for the inter-subject variability of the potentiation response. Apart from physiological factors, the demands of the testing task might have been different for each athlete. The DJ height was set to 46 cm for all participants, since the individual optimal DJ height could not be estimated in a prior session due to athletes' time constraints. For the two athletes who had no significant improvements after conditioning, the drop height might have been higher than their individual optimal drop height [37, 38], thus reducing their mechanical power output [39] and possibly diminishing the potentiating effect [20].

Another interesting finding of this pilot study concerns changes in the biomechanical variables of the DJ movement. While for the conditioned DJs the JH, P_{max} and PI increased, whereby F_{max} remained unchanged. This is in accordance with findings from French et al., who observed that these changes were not associated with significant changes in ground contact time [40]. Hence, increased JH following the conditioning activity seems to be the result of an elevated force-time curve. Further analyses of the individual DJ performance revealed a significant increase of P_{max} in 3 athletes who had an augmented JH subsequent to the conditioning activity. Likewise, increases in external P_{max} have been reported by Chiu et al. in squat and CMJs following a conditioning activity of 5 squats at 90 % of the 1 repetition maximum [41]. An increased external concentric peak power is the result of a higher force during the concentric phase of the movement [42]. Since we were not able to detect any significant changes in F_{max} and CT, an elevated force level is a likely agent for the increased impulse during the concentric phase [40]. Even though some studies reported elevated F_{max} values in jumps following a conditioning activity [32, 40, 41], the present pilot study indicates that after hops, it is the overall shape of the ground reaction force rather than F_{max}, which potentiates the DJ performance.

Several mechanisms are discussed to be responsible for enhanced performance following a conditioning activity. Intrinsic properties, such as changes in the muscle architecture or a higher Ca^{2+} sensitivity of the muscle fibers as well as recruitment of higher order motor units might cause the increased jump performance subsequent to the conditioning hops [1]. However, there is evidence that changes in neuronal output following the conditioning hops are not a likely mechanism responsible for the performance enhancements in subsequent DJs [12]. Several authors have proposed that the viscoelastic properties of the muscle-tendon unit might change subsequent to heavy resistance exercises [20] or plyometric conditioning [32]. In turn, this may result in a change in leg stiffness, allowing a higher contribution of passive tension to the overall force production during the concentric part of a stretch shortening cycle movement. In fact, it is known that there is an optimal leg stiffness value to maximize the external concentric peak power output during a DJ [39]. Therefore, it is possible that the significantly higher P_{max} in the athletes with considerably increased JH was due to changes in leg stiffness that brought it closer to the individual optimum, thus allowing a higher force contribution from the stretch-shortening cycle to the concentric propulsion phase of the DJ [20].

In contrast to other studies that used conditioning activities to enhance sprint performance [21], we were not able to demonstrate a decrease in sprint time (i.e., improved performance) in the present pilot study by means of a plyometric conditioning. Two studies reported a shorter sprint time of up to 3 % when using heavy loaded squats (60 % to 90 % of 1-RM) combined with resting intervals of 4 to 5 min as a conditioning stimulus [18, 43]. To our knowledge, only one study was able to show that plyometric exercises used as a conditioning activity can increase athletes' sprint performance [44]. These authors used alternated-leg bounding either with or without an additional load (+10 % of the body mass). They reported up to 3 % shorter sprint times following weighted jumps compared to the control condition without prior conditioning activity, and smaller improvements with unloaded jumps. As the muscular load during alternate-leg bounds is higher compared to hops on two legs, it is possible that hops without additional load do not put sufficient load on the relevant muscles, which might be crucial for improved sprint performance. Nevertheless, the considerable performance gains in the DJs are in clear contrast to the lack of improvement in sprint performance. How can this high task specificity be explained? The results of training studies investigating the effects of different kinds of plyometrics on improvements in sprint performance suggest that plyometric training increases external leg power output during jumps, but has little or no effect on sprint performance [45]. This poor transfer was ascribed to contraction velocity specificity and differences in the movement between jumping and sprinting, requiring a different inter- and intramuscular coordination [45]. Therefore, a type of jump that is more similar to the movement during the acceleration phase of a sprint would probably yield better results when used as a conditioning activity. For example, CMJ height is related to the maximal sprint velocity [46, 47] and a good predictor of sprint performance, particularly over the first 30 m [48]. This may be due to the tendency that CMJs rely more on concentric muscle actions that generate energy, whereas reactive jumps with short ground contact times such as DJs and repetitive hops rely more on the stretch-shortening cycle and energy storage [49, 50]. Consequently, squat jumps and CMJs might be more suitable as performance-enhancing conditioning activities during the acceleration phase of a sprint than DJs or repetitive hops. And although the latter are closer to the movement in the constant speed phase of a sprint, they might not even be able to improve performance in this later phase, as the muscle activity in the preceding acceleration phase might interfere with any potential potentiating effects.

Conclusion

Findings from this pilot study imply that in sprint-trained elite athletes 10 maximal repetitive hops can substantially increase performance in subsequent DJs. Compared to previous studies, the DJ results of the present study highlight the potential of a plyometric conditioning exercise to increase lower limb strength and power output, which can even can be effective in sprint trained elite-athletes. Equivocal findings related to plyometrics might arise from varying loads that have to be counteracted by the muscles during the conditioning exercises.

This type of conditioning activity did not affect sprint performance. We presume that the hops did not provide a sufficient conditioning stimulus for the muscle groups that primarily determine sprint performance.

The performance gains of the present study were most likely associated with an improved concentric propulsion phase of the DJs, making the stiffness of the muscle-tendon complex one likely candidate for the observed jump performance enhancement. Therefore, reactive hops might be more suitable as a warm-up routine prior to competitions in disciplines whose performances are rather determined by the stretch-shortening cycle, e.g. jump disciplines.

Abbreviations

1-RM: one repetition maximum; CMJ: countermovement jump; CON: control condition; CT_{sprint} / CT_{DJ}: ground contact time during sprinting/of a drop jump; DJ: drop jump; F_{max}: peak ground reaction force in vertical direction; FT: rebound flight time; G: gravitational constant; HOP: hops conditions; ICC: intraclass correlation coefficient; JH: rebound jump height; P_{max}: external concentric peak power; PI: performance index; SD: standard deviation; SL: step length; ST_{10}/ ST_{20}/ ST_{30}: sprint time over a distance of 10 m, 20 m, 30 m.

Competing interests

The authors declare that they have no competing interests.

Authors' contributions

JK was involved in the data collection, data analysis and manuscript preparation. JB was responsible for the original study design and contributed to all parts of the work of this study. AK was responsible for the data analysis and interpretation of the drop jump data and he helped to draft the manuscript. OP was responsible for the data acquisition and data analysis of the sprint data. MG and UG were involved in the theoretical conceptualization and in the interpretation of the study data. All authors commented on the draft, read and approved the final manuscript.

Acknowledgements

This study was funded by a grant of the German Federal Institute of Sports Science (BISp) (IIA1-070802/13) based on a decision of the German Federal Parliament (Deutscher Bundestag). The BISp provided the funding for the present study but was not involved in the analysis, interpretation or the right to approve or disapprove publication of the research.

Author details

[1]Sensorimotor Performance Lab, Department of Sport Science, University of Konstanz, 78476 Konstanz, Germany. [2]Division of Training and Movement Sciences, Faculty of Human Sciences, University of Potsdam, 14469 Potsdam, Germany.

References

1. Tillin MNA, Bishop D. Factors modulating post-activation potentiation and its effect on performance of subsequent explosive activities. Sports Med. 2009;39(2):147–66.
2. Hodgson M, Docherty D, Robbins D. Post-activation potentiation. Sports Med. 2005;35(7):585–95.
3. Esformes JI, Cameron N, Bampouras TM. Postactivation potentiation following different modes of exercise. J Strength Cond Res. 2010;24(7):1911–6.
4. Chen Z-R, Wang Y-H, Peng H-T, Yu C-F, Wang M-H. The acute effect of drop jump protocols with different volumes and recovery time on countermovement jump performance. J Strength Cond Res. 2013;27(1):154–8.
5. Tsolakis C, Bogdanis GC, Nikolaou A, Zacharogiannis E. Influence of type of muscle contraction and gender on postactivation potentiation of upper and lower limb explosive performance in elite fencers. J Sports Sci Med. 2011;10(3):577.
6. Till KA, Cooke C. The effects of postactivation potentiation on sprint and jump performance of male academy soccer players. J Strength Cond Res. 2009;23(7):1960–7.
7. Donti O, Tsolakis C, Bogdanis GC. Effects of baseline levels of flexibility and vertical jump ability on performance following different volumes of static stretching and potentiating exercises in elite gymnasts. J Sports Sci Med. 2014;13(1):105.
8. De Villarreal ESS, González-Badillo JJ, Izquierdo M. Optimal warm-up stimuli of muscle activation to enhance short and long-term acute jumping performance. Eur J Appl Physiol. 2007;100(4):393–401.
9. Tsolakis C, Bogdanis GC. Acute effects of two different warm-up protocols on flexibility and lower limb explosive performance in male and female high level athletes. J Sports Sci Med. 2012;11(4):669.
10. Margaritopoulos S, Theodorou A, Methenitis S, Zaras N, Donti O, Tsolakis C. The effect of plyometric exercises on repeated strength and power performance in elite karate athletes. J Phys Educ Sport. 2015;15(2):310.
11. Dello IA, Padulo J, Eliakim A, Gottlieb R, Bareli R, Meckel Y. Post activation potentiation effects on vertical and horizontal explosive performances of young handball and basketball athletes. J Sports Med Phys Fitness. 2015; Sep 23 [Epub ahead of print].
12. Bergmann J, Kramer A, Gruber M. Repetitive hops induce postactivation potentiation in triceps surae as well as an increase in the jump height of subsequent maximal drop jumps. PLoS One. 2013;8(10):e77705.
13. Bergmann J, Kramer A, Gruber M. Reaktive hoppings als direkte vorbereitung auf maximale niedersprünge. Leistungssport. 2014;44(3):19–24.
14. Masamoto N, Larson R, Gates T, Faigenbaum A. Acute effects of plyometric exercise on maximum squat performance in male athletes. J Strength Cond Res. 2003;17(1):68–71.
15. Terzis G, Spengos K, Karampatsos G, Manta P, Georgiadis G. Acute effect of drop jumping on throwing performance. J Strength Cond Res. 2009;23(9): 2592–7.
16. Terzis G, Karampatsos G, Kyriazis T, Kavouras SA, Georgiadis G. Acute effects of countermovement jumping and sprinting on shot put performance. J Strength Cond Res. 2012;26(3):684–90.
17. Read PJ, Miller SC, Turner AN. The effects of postactivation potentiation on golf club head speed. J Strength Cond Res. 2013;27(6):1579–82.
18. McBride J, Nimphius S, Erickson T. The acute effects of heavy-load squats and loaded countermovement jumps on sprint performance. J Strength Cond Res. 2005;19(4):893–7.
19. Hamada T, Sale DG, MacDougall JD, Tarnopolsky MA. Postactivation potentiation, fiber type, and twitch contraction time in human knee extensor muscles. J Appl Physiol. 2000;88(6):2131–7.
20. Maloney SJ, Turner AN, Fletcher IM. Ballistic exercise as a pre-activation stimulus: a review of the literature and practical applications. Sports Med. 2014; 44(10):1347-59.
21. Lesinski M, Muehlbauer T, Büsch D, Granacher U. Akute Effekte der Postaktivierungspotenzierung auf Kraft-und Schnelligkeitsleistungen bei Sportlern. Sportverletz Sportschaden. 2013;27(03):147–55.
22. Shrout PE, Fleiss JL. Intraclass correlations: uses in assessing rater reliability. Psychol Bull. 1979;86(2):420.
23. Farley CT, Blickhan R, Saito J, Taylor CR. Hopping frequency in humans: a test of how springs set stride frequency in bouncing gaits. J Appl Physiol. 1991;71(6):2127–32.
24. Farley CT, Morgenroth DC. Leg stiffness primarily depends on ankle stiffness during human hopping. J Biomech. 1999;32(3):267–73.
25. Hilfiker R, Hübner K, Lorenz T, Marti B. Effects of drop jumps added to the warm-up of elite sport athletes with a high capacity for explosive force development. J Strength Cond Res. 2007;21(2):550–5.
26. Jensen RL, Ebben WP. Quantifying plyometric intensity via rate of force development, knee joint, and ground reaction forces. J Strength Cond Res. 2007;21(3):763–7.
27. Kramer A, Ritzmann R, Gollhofer A, Gehring D, Gruber M. A new sledge jump system that allows almost natural reactive jumps. J Biomech. 2010;43(14):2672–7.
28. Kramer A, Ritzmann R, Gruber M, Gollhofer A. Four weeks of training in a sledge jump system improved the jump pattern to almost natural reactive jumps. Eur J Appl Physiol. 2012;112(1):285–93.
29. Komi PV. Stretch-shortening cycle. In Komi P, editor. Strength Power Sport. Oxford: Balckwell Science; 2008. p.184-201.
30. Komi PV. Stretch-shortening cycle: a powerful model to study normal and fatigued muscle. J Biomech. 2000;33(10):1197–206.
31. Zuur AT, Lundbye-Jensen J, Leukel C, Taube W, Grey MJ, Gollhofer A, et al. Contribution of afferent feedback and descending drive to human hopping. J Physiol. 2010;588(5):799–807.

32. Tobin DP, Delahunt E. The acute effect of a plyometric stimulus on jump performance in professional rugby players. J Strength Cond Res. 2014;28(2):367–72.
33. Weber KR, Brown LE, Coburn JW, Zinder SM. Acute effects of heavy-load squats on consecutive squat jump performance. J Strength Cond Res. 2008;22(3):726–30.
34. Hamada T, Sale DG, MacDougall JD, Tarnopolsky MA. Interaction of fibre type, potentiation and fatigue in human knee extensor muscles. Acta Physiol Scand. 2003;178(2):165–73.
35. Pääsuke M, Saapar L, Ereline J, Gapeyeva H, Requena B, Ööpik V. Postactivation potentiation of knee extensor muscles in power-and endurance-trained, and untrained women. Eur J Appl Physiol. 2007;101(5):577–85.
36. Macdougall JD. Hypertrophy and hyperplasia. Strength and Power in Sport. London: Blackwell; 2008.
37. Walsh M, Arampatzis A, Schade F, Brüggemann G. The effect of drop jump starting height and contact time on power, work performed, and moment of force. J Strength Cond Res. 2004;18(3):561–6.
38. Bobbert, Huijing PA, van Ingen Schenau GJ. Drop jumping. II. The influence of dropping height on the biomechanics of drop jumping. Med Sci Sports Exerc. 1987;19(4):339-46.
39. Arampatzis A, Schade F, Walsh M, Brüggemann G-P. Influence of leg stiffness and its effect on myodynamic jumping performance. J Electromyogr Kinesiol. 2001;11(5):355–64.
40. French DN, Kraemer WJ, Cooke CB. Changes in dynamic exercise performance following a sequence of preconditioning isometric muscle actions. J Strength Cond Res. 2003;17(4):678–85.
41. Chiu LZF, Fry AC, Weiss LW, Schilling BK, Brown LE, Smith SL. Postactivation potentiation response in athletic and recreationally trained individuals. J Strength Cond Res. 2003;17(4):671–7.
42. Knudson DV. Correcting the use of the term "power" in the strength and conditioning literature. J Strength Cond Res. 2009;23(6):1902–8.
43. Rahimi R. The acute effects of heavy versus light-load squats on sprint performance. Facta Univ-Ser: Phys Educ Sport. 2007;5(2):163–9.
44. Turner AP, Bellhouse S, Kilduff LP, Russell M. Post-activation potentiation of sprint acceleration performance using plyometric exercise. J Strength Cond Res. 2014. doi:10.1519/JSC.0000000000000647.
45. Young WB. Transfer of strength and power training to sports performance. Int J Sports Physiol Perform. 2006;1(2):74.
46. Kale M, Asci A, Bayrak C, Acikada C. Relationships among jumping performances and sprint parameters during maximum speed phase in sprinters. J Strength Cond Res. 2009;23(8):2272–9. doi:10.1519/JSC.0b013e3181b3e182.
47. Smirniotou A, Katsikas C, Paradisis G, Argeitaki P, Zacharogiannis E, Tziortzis S. Strength-power parameters as predictors of sprinting performance. J Sports Med Phys Fitness. 2008;48(4):447–54.
48. Cronin JB, Hansen KT. Strength and power predictors of sports speed. J Strength Cond Res. 2005;19(2):349–57.
49. Bobbert, Mackay M, Schinkelshoek D, Huijing P, van Ingen Schenau G. Biomechanical analysis of drop and countermovement jumps. Eur J Appl Physiol Occup Physiol. 1986;54(6):566-73.
50. Fukashiro S, Komi PV, Järvinen M, Miyashita M. In vivo achilles tendon loading'during jumping in humans. Eur J Appl Physiol Occup Physiol. 1995;71(5):453–8.

10

The feasibility and effectiveness of high-intensity boxing training versus moderate-intensity brisk walking in adults with abdominal obesity

Birinder S Cheema[1,2*], Timothy B Davies[1], Matthew Stewart[1], Shona Papalia[1] and Evan Atlantis[3,4]

Abstract

Background: High-intensity interval training (HIIT) performed on exercise cycle or treadmill is considered safe and often more beneficial for fat loss and cardiometabolic health than moderate-intensity continuous training (MICT). The aim of this pilot study was to assess the feasibility and effectiveness of a 12-week boxing training (HIIT) intervention compared with an equivalent dose of brisk walking (MICT) in obese adults.

Methods: Men and women with abdominal obesity and body mass index >25 kg/m^2 were randomized to either a boxing group or a brisk walking (control) group for 12 weeks. Each group engaged in 4 training sessions per week, equated for total physical activity. Feasibility outcomes included recruitment rates, assessment of training intensities, adherence and adverse events. Effectiveness was assessed pre and post intervention via pertinent obesity-, cardiovascular-, and health-related quality of life (HRQoL) outcomes.

Results: Nineteen individuals expressed an interest and 63% (n = 12) consented. Recruitment was slower than anticipated (1.3 participants/week). The boxing group trained at a significantly higher intensity each week versus the brisk walking group ($p < 0.05$). Two participants in the boxing group experienced an adverse event; both continued to exercise with modifications to the exercise program. No other adverse events were noted. The boxing group attended more sessions (79% vs. 55%) and had a lower attrition rate (n = 0 vs. n = 2) than the walking group. Analysis of covariance revealed that the boxing group significantly improved body fat percentage ($p = 0.047$), systolic blood pressure ($p = 0.026$), augmentation index (AIx; $p < 0.001$), absolute VO_{2max} ($p = 0.015$), and Physical Functioning ($p = 0.042$) and Vitality ($p = 0.024$) domains of HRQoL over time. The walking group did not improve any clinical outcomes, and experienced a worsening of Vitality ($p = 0.043$).

Conclusions: Boxing training (HIIT) in adults with abdominal obesity is feasible and may elicit a better therapeutic effect on obesity, cardiovascular, and HRQoL outcomes than an equivalent dose of brisk walking (MICT). Robustly designed randomized controlled trials are required to confirm these findings and inform clinical guidelines and practice for obesity treatment.

Trial registration: Trial registration: ACTRN12615000007538

Keywords: High-intensity interval training, Exercise, Body composition, Weight loss, Fat loss, Exercise, Health, Quality of life

* Correspondence: B.Cheema@uws.edu.au
[1]School of Science and Health, University of Western Sydney, Locked Bag 1797, Penrith, 2751 Campbelltown, New South Wales, Australia
[2]The National Institute of Complementary Medicine, University of Western Sydney, Campbelltown, NSW 2650, Australia
Full list of author information is available at the end of the article

Background

Obesity is a major risk factor for many chronic non-communicable diseases, and the prevalence of this condition in the global population has doubled since 1980 [1]. Recent data suggest that approximately 36.9% of men and 29.8% of women worldwide are categorically obese [2]. The high and rising prevalence of obesity is associated with increased rates of cardiovascular diseases, cancers [3], type 2 diabetes and chronic kidney disease [1], placing tremendous strain on healthcare systems and national economies [4]. Individuals with obesity also suffer from low health-related quality of life (HRQoL) [5] and increased mortality [6] versus their healthy peers. Innovative and efficient strategies for treating excess body fat are still needed, and could result in significant health and economic benefits.

Current physical activity guidelines [7,8] recommend 150 to >250 minutes per week of moderate-intensity continuous training (MICT) such as brisk walking to target overweight/obesity and maintain an optimal body weight. These physical activity guidelines are similar to those recommended by the World Health Organization for general health [9]. However, randomized controlled trials (RCT) suggest that brisk walking interventions (≥12 weeks) elicit only a small beneficial effect on body weight and adiposity outcomes in overweight and obese adults [10-12]. Hence, this modality of exercise, despite being recommended [7,8], may not be particularly effective for inducing clinically meaningful reductions in body fat.

High-intensity interval training (HIIT) involves alternating brief (6 s-4 min) high intensity (≥75% VO_{2max}) and lower intensity workloads or rest throughout an exercise session. This shorter duration of exercise may be a more efficient alternative for eliciting fat loss than MICT. Studies in patients with cardiac and metabolic diseases [13-17] have consistently shown that HIIT (≥12 weeks) performed on a cycle or treadmill ergometer is safe, and can result in greater improvements of cardiorespiratory fitness (VO_{2max}), endothelial function (i.e. atherosclerosis), insulin signalling and left ventricular morphology and function versus MICT matched for training load or volume (frequency/duration). Studies have also shown that HIIT can significantly increase HRQoL [13,18]. There is preliminary evidence suggesting that HIIT can elicit significantly greater reductions of adiposity than MICT in overweight and obese cohorts [19-21]. However, this evidence is less consistent and indicates a need for further research.

Boxing training typically involves high intensity intervals of 2 to 3 minutes combined with shorter intervals of rest. Therefore, boxing training is recognized as a metabolically demanding mode of HIIT [22]. Despite its popularity in practice, no study to date has investigated the use of boxing training as a mode of HIIT for the management of obesity and related health outcomes. Therefore, the aim of this pilot study was to assess the feasibility and effectiveness of a 12-week boxing training (HIIT) intervention compared with an equivalent dose of brisk walking (MICT) in adults with abdominal obesity. Feasibility outcomes included recruitment rates, assessment of training intensities, adherence and adverse events, and effectiveness was assessed pre and post intervention *via* pertinent obesity, cardiovascular, and HRQoL outcomes.

Methods

Study design

A parallel group design that randomized participants to a boxing group or brisk walking (control) group was utilized. Outcome measures were assessed prior to and following a 12-week intervention period. Post intervention testing was completed >72 hr after the final exercise session. A blinded assessor with *International Society for the Advancement of Kinanthropometry* (*ISAK*) accreditation collected all anthropometric (obesity) data. Randomization assignments were computer-generated (www.randomization.com) and stratified by gender, by an investigator not involved in data collection; assignments were given to participants in sealed envelopes upon the completion of baseline testing. The University of Western Sydney Human Research Ethics Committee approved all procedures, and informed consent was received from all participants.

Participants

Participants were recruited over a nine-week period from June 3 to August 2, 2013 by means of flyer advertisements, university staff email lists and social media (Facebook). The aim was to recruit two participants per week, on average. *Eligibility criteria*: adult (>18 years); body mass index (BMI) >25 kg/m^2; abdominal obesity as a risk factor for cardiometabolic disease according to the International Diabetes Federation (i.e. waist circumference >94 cm in men and >80 cm in women) [23]; available to complete four exercise sessions per week; able to communicate in English; willingness and cognitive ability to provide written informed consent. *Exclusion criteria:* physically active (i.e. engaging in greater than 3 sessions of moderate-intensity exercise per week); current or history of ischaemic heart disease, cerebrovascular disease, type 2 diabetes mellitus, advanced metabolic disease (e.g. chronic kidney disease) or uncontrolled pulmonary disease.

Interventions

Boxing

Participants in the boxing group were prescribed four, 50-min sessions of supervised boxing training per week.

A boxing instructor assisted in designing the program. All sessions were fully supervised by qualified personnel. The interval-based exercises were preceded by a 5 min warm-up of continuous skipping at a self-selected intensity. Intervals were prescribed at 2:1 (i.e. 2 min of high-intensity activity followed by 1 min of rest (standing or pacing) between intervals and exercises). Three intervals of each of the following five exercises were performed for a total of 30 min of high-intensity effort: (1) heavy bag, (2) focus mitts, (3) circular body bag, (4) footwork drills, and (4) skipping. The total amount of physical activity (excluding warm up and rest periods) was computed as 30 min × 6 metabolic equivalents (MET) per minute = 180 MET min [24]. During the high-intensity bouts, participants were instructed to exercise at a rating of perceived exertion of 15-17/20 ("hard" to "very hard") with the goal of achieving >75% of age-predicted maximal heart rate (i.e. 220-age; HR_{max}).

Training intensity Heart rate was monitored using a Polar Heart Rate monitor (Polar® RS800sd Kempele, Finland) and was recorded at the completion of each high-intensity interval; these values were averaged across each week, and reported as percentage of age-predicted HR_{max}.

Walking

Participants in the walking group were prescribed four, 50-min sessions of brisk walking per week. These sessions were unsupervised and completed in any location convenient to the participant (e.g. within their own neighbourhood, etc.). Participants were instructed to begin each session with a 5-min gradual warm-up and walk as quickly as possible for the remainder of the session (45 min). The total amount of physical activity (excluding warm up) was computed as 45 min × 4 metabolic equivalents (MET) per minute = 180 MET-min [24].

Training intensity Participants were taught how to manually monitor their heart rate and record the measure pre-, mid- and post-exercise. These data were recorded in a training journal. The mid-exercise readings were averaged across each week, and reported as percentage of age-predicted HR_{max}.

Adherence and adverse events

Adherence was defined as the number of training sessions attempted divided by the number offered multiplied by 100%. Adverse events were documented by means of a structured, open-ended questions administered weekly, in person or *via* telephone or email.

Clinical outcome measures

Obesity outcomes

Waist circumference was measured in a horizontal plane, midway between the inferior margin of the ribs and the superior border of the iliac crest, according to standard protocol [25]. Height and weight were measured with calibrated scale (A&D Company Ltd., Japan) and stadiometer (Holtain Ltd., Crymych, UK), respectively, and BMI was computed from these measures [25]. Six skinfold sites (i.e. triceps, subscapular, supraspinale, abdominal, front thigh and medial calf) were recorded using Holtain callipers (Holtain Ltd., Crymych, UK) if the skinfold was ≤40 mm and Slim-guide callipers (Creative Health Products, Plymouth, USA) if the skinfold was >40 mm. Body fat percentage was computed from the six skinfold sites using validated equations [26].

Cardiovascular outcomes

Resting blood pressure (systolic/diastolic) and heart rate were assessed manually at the brachial and radial artery, respectively, with the participant in a seated position according to standard protocols [27]. Arterial stiffness was assessed using the SphygmoCor System (AtCor Medical Pty, Sydney, Australia). This system derives the central aortic pressure waveform noninvasively from the pulse pressure recorded at a peripheral site. Participants were seated for a 10-min period, then radial pulse pressure waveform recording were obtained using a hand-held, high fidelity tonometer (Millar Instruments, Houston, Texas). The aortic pressure waveforms are comprised of a forward wave caused by left ventricular contraction and a reflected wave due to backflow arising from regions of increased impedance in the peripheral vessels. The resultant of these two pressures is known as the augmentation index (AIx) which was recorded. The SphygmoCor algorithm normalises AIx to a heart rate of 75 beats per minute. This method is highly reproducible [28] and has been used extensively to evaluate arterial stiffness in healthy [29,30] and chronically diseased cohorts [31]. Population norms for AIx range from −23.27% to 63.07% in adults (aged 18–86 years) with larger values indicating greater arterial stiffness [32].

Cardiorespiratory fitness (VO_{2max}) was assessed *via* indirect calorimetry (Jaeger Metabolic Gas Analysers, Viasys Healthcare, Germany) using a standard ramp protocol on a laboratory treadmill (LE 200 CE, Viasys Health Care, USA). O_2 and CO_2 sensors were calibrated prior to each test using high-grade calibration gas with certified gas concentrations (O_2 = 16%, CO_2 = 5%, N_2 = balance). The protocol began at a pre-determined, comfortable walking speed for 3 minutes; the grade was increased by 2% each minute thereafter until volitional fatigue.

HRQoL outcomes

The *Medical Outcomes Trust Short Form-36 Health Survey (Version 1.0)* (SF-36) [33] was used to evaluate Physical Functioning, General Health and Vitality domains of HRQoL. Higher scores, ranging from 0–100, denote higher HRQoL.

Statistical analyses

Analyses were performed using the Statistical Package for the Social Sciences (IBM©, SPSS Version 19.0). All data were inspected visually and statistically for normality (skewness and kurtosis between −1 and +1). Analyses were completed according to intention-to-treat strategy, using the last-observation-carry-forward imputation method for any missing data. Within group changes over time were evaluated by paired t-tests. Group x time effects were determined by analysis of covariance (ANCOVA) of the post-treatment score controlling for the baseline score and potential confounding variables identified by comparing groups at baseline. Cohen's *d* effect sizes were calculated to explore the effectiveness of the intervention and provide data to inform sample size calculations in future studies. Effect sizes were interpreted according to the conventions of small (0.20), moderate (0.50), or large (0.80). A p value of <0.05 was considered indicative of statistical significance.

Results

Recruitment and flow of participants

Nineteen individuals (n = 19) expressed an interest in the study and five individuals were deemed ineligible due to a medical condition, or not meeting the waist circumference or physical activity criteria (Figure 1). Fourteen individuals were deemed eligible, however two elected not to participate due to inconvenience. Twelve individuals provided written informed consent, completed baseline testing and were randomized into the boxing training (n = 6) or walking (n = 6) groups. Recruitment rate was slower than expected (12 participants/9 weeks of recruitment = 1.3 participants recruited per week). Two female participants in the walking group withdrew: one due to a pre-existing knee injury requiring surgery (week 2) and one for personal reasons (week 5).

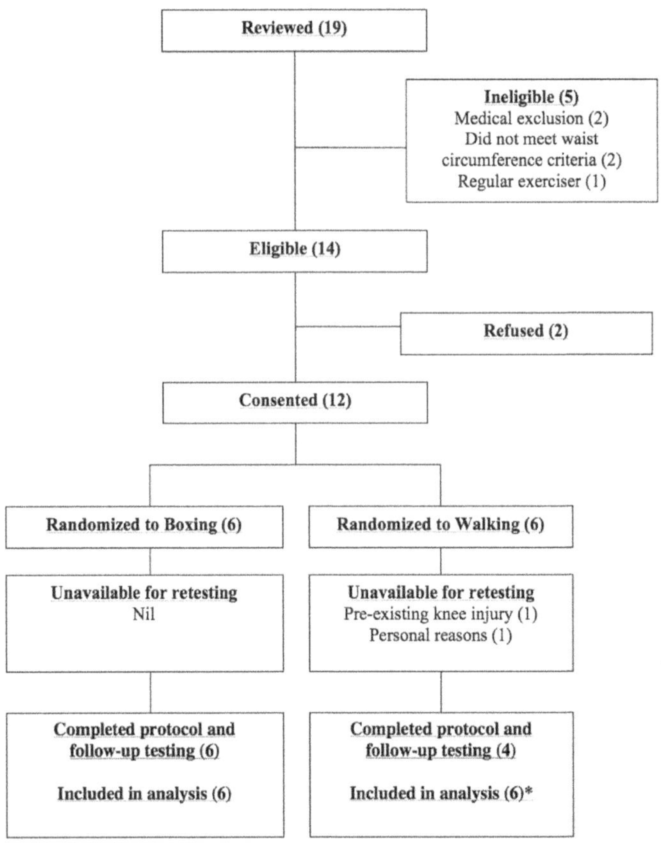

Figure 1 Flow of participants through the trial. *Baseline data carried forward for 2 participants lost to follow-up.

Baseline data were carried forward for both participants for analyses (intention-to-treat).

Baseline characteristics

No statistically significant differences were noted between groups at baseline (Table 1). However, due to clinically important differences in age and waist circumference, these variables were included as covariates in all ANCOVA models. The cohort ranged in age from 19 to 72 years, BMI ranged from 26.4 to 40.3 kg/m^2 and all participants fulfilled the criterion for abdominal obesity [23]. Common comorbidities included hypertension (n = 3) and asthma (n = 2).

Training intensity

Mean training heart rate during the 12-week intervention period ranged from 86-89% and 64-77% of age-predicted HR_{max} in the boxing and walking groups, respectively (Figure 2). The boxing group trained at a significantly higher intensity versus the walking group in each week ($p < 0.05$).

Adherence and adverse events

Adherence to training was 79 ± 15% and 55 ± 43% in the boxing and walking groups, respectively, inclusive of the two participants in the walking group who withdrew (Figure 1). Excluding these participants, attendance in the walking group was 82 ± 12%. The difference in attendance between groups was not significant inclusive- (p = 0.24) or exclusive (p = 0.75) of the two participants who dropped out. Five participants in the boxing group and 3 participants in walking group attended more than 70% of their prescribed exercise sessions.

A female participant in the boxing group experienced tennis elbow in week 1 that may have been due to the intervention. She remained in the study by substituting kicking and elbow striking in place of punching. A male participant in the boxing group experienced a strain of the gastrocnemius muscle in week 8, which may have been induced by skipping. The participant substituted rowing for skipping while his calf muscle recovered. Neither participant missed a training session due to their injury. No additional adverse events were noted.

Table 1 Baseline characteristics of the total cohort and groups

Characteristic	Total cohort (n = 12)	Boxing (n = 6)	Walking (n = 6)
Age (y)	39 (17)	43 (19)	36 (15)
Women:Men	7:5	3:3	4:2
Body weight (kg)	90.7 (16.3)	95.7 (21.0)	85.6 (9.1)
Height (cm)	169.6 (8.2)	172.3 (7.7)	166.8 (8.4)
BMI (kg/m^2)	31.4 (4.4)	32.0 (5.9)	30.8 (2.6)
Waist circumference (cm)	104.7 (14.4)	111.0 (18.0)	98.4 (6.2)
Body fat percentage (%)	35.4 (11.3)	33.5 (10.1)	37.3 (13.1)

Data continuous variables reported as mean (standard deviations).

Outcomes

Obesity outcomes

Within and between group analyses are presented in Table 2. The boxing group reduced body fat percentage over time with a small to medium effect that reached statistical significance (Cohen's $d = 0.41$; p = 0.047). Waist circumference, body mass and BMI was also reduced in the boxing group with small to medium effect (Cohen's $d = 0.29$-0.48); however, these effects did not achieve statistical significance. The walking group reduced body fat percentage over time with a small effect (Cohen's $d = 0.21$; p = 0.17) with no other effects noted. No group x time interaction effects were noted for waist circumference, body mass, BMI, or body fat percentage.

Cardiovascular outcomes

The boxing group reduced resting systolic- and diastolic blood pressure, heart rate, augmentation index, and pulse pressure over time with a medium to large effect (Cohen's $d = 0.69$-1.50); reductions in AIx ($p < 0.001$) and systolic blood pressure (p = 0.026) reached statistical significance. By contrast, the walking group unexpectedly increased pulse pressure, AIx, and systolic blood pressure over time with a small to large effect (Cohen's $d = 0.33$-0.93) though none of these changes reached statistical significance (Table 2). Small to medium group x time interaction effects indicating positive adaptation in the boxing group versus the walking group were noted for AIx (Cohen's $d = 0.41$; p = 0.064) and resting systolic- (Cohen's $d = 0.33$; p = 0.10) and diastolic blood pressure (Cohen's $d = 0.26$; p = 0.16).

The boxing group improved relative- (Cohen's $d = 1.28$; p = 0.06) and absolute VO_{2max} (Cohen's $d = 0.41$; p = 0.015) over time with a large and medium effect, respectively. The effect for absolute VO_{2max} was statistically significant. The control group did not improve these measures over time. No group x time interaction effects were noted for VO_{2max} measures.

HRQoL outcomes

The boxing group improved Physical Functioning (Cohen's $d = 0.98$; p = 0.042), General Health (Cohen's $d = 1.45$; p = 0.07) and Vitality (Cohen's $d = 0.74$; p = 0.024) domains of HRQoL over time with large effects. The effects for Physical Functioning and Vitality were significant. By contrast, the walking group significantly reduced Vitality over time with a moderate effect (Cohen's $d = 0.30$; p = 0.043) and did not experience a change in the other two domains. Small to moderate group x time interaction effects favouring the boxing group were noted each of these HRQoL

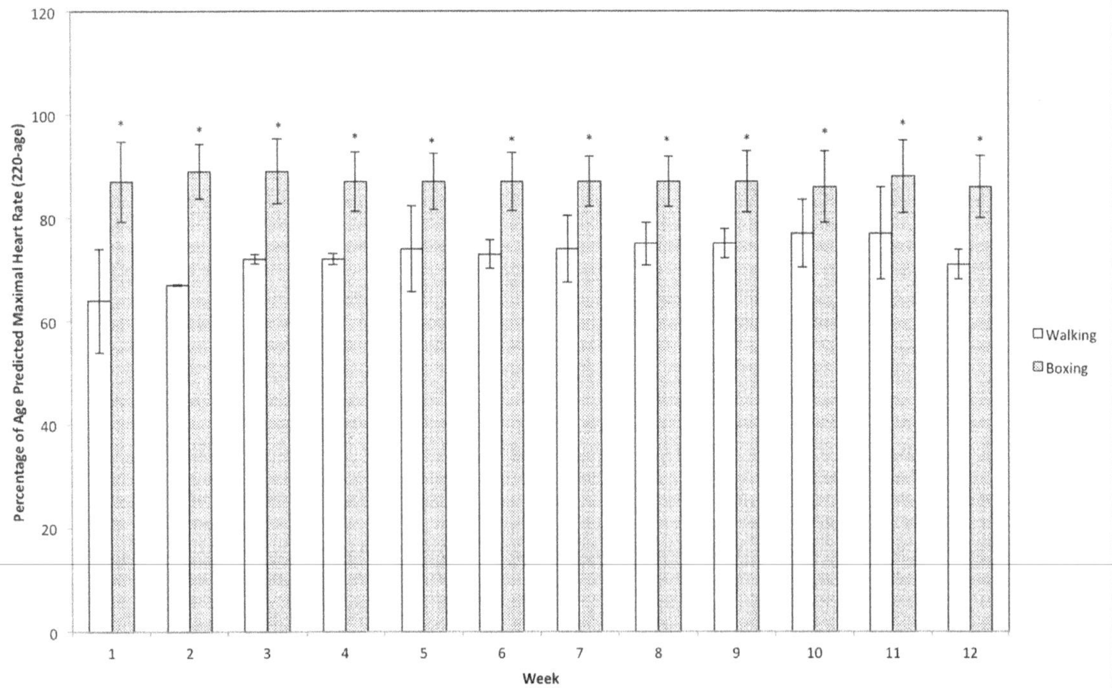

Figure 2 Mean training heart rate in the boxing and walking groups. *Significant difference versus the walking group.

domains (Cohen's d = 0.22-0.54) with the effect for Vitality reaching statistical significance (p = 0.02).

Sensitivity and post hoc analyses

Group x time sensitivity analyses were performed without imputation of missing data from the two participants in the walking group who withdrew and did not undergo final assessment. The outcomes of these analyses did not differ with primary analyses except that AIx was significantly improved in the boxing group versus the walking group over time (Cohen's d = 0.58; p = 0.046).

To determine the effect of higher adherence on treatment effects, group x time *post hoc* analyses were performed using data from participants who completed >70% of the boxing (n = 5) or walking (n = 3) intervention. The outcomes of these analyses did not differ with the primary analyses.

Discussion

This is the first pilot study to assess the feasibility and effectiveness of a 12-week boxing training (HIIT) intervention compared with an equivalent dose of brisk walking (MICT) in 12 obese adults. Our recruitment rate was slower than anticipated. There is some evidence to suggest that boxing might be perceived as a high-risk activity [34], and methods to facilitate recruitment and retention, perhaps involving appropriate survey instruments [35] should be considered in the development of future trials. No serious adverse events were noted and the boxing group attended more exercise sessions and had a lower attrition rate than the walking group, suggesting that this form of HIIT may be feasible to administer in this cohort. Limitations of this pilot study included the small sample size (n = 12), lack of a non-exercising control group, the lack of direct supervision of the walking group, and the lack of monitoring of dietary and physical activity changes, which are key confounding variables. These limitations must be considered in the development of future RCT.

Obesity outcomes

The boxing group significantly reduced body fat percentage (−13.2%; p = 0.047) and experienced a small-to-moderate (non-significant) reduction of waist circumference (−5.3%) body mass (−4.1%) and BMI (−4.0%) over time. Collectively, these adaptations indicate reduced body adiposity, which is associated with a reduced risk of chronic diseases (i.e. insulin resistance, type 2 diabetes, cancers, and cardiovascular diseases) and associated mortality [36-38]. It is difficult to quantify the clinical significance of these changes given our small sample size and pooling of data for men and women. Stevens et al. [39] suggest that ≥5% weight loss is clinically meaningful. The boxing group approached this level of change (−4.1%) while no change was noted in the walking group (−0.3%). A longer training

Table 2 Summary of within and between group changes on clinical outcomes

Outcome measures	Boxing (n = 6)					Walking (n = 6)					*P* (between groups)	*Effect size* (between groups)
	Week 0	Week 16	%Change	*P*	Effect size (within group)	Week 0	Week 16	%Change	*P*	Effect size (within group)		
Obesity outcomes:												
Waist circumference (cm)	111.1 (18.0)	104.4 (12.2)	−5.3 (7.7)	0.19	0.48	98.4 (6.2)	97.8 (6.7)	−0.6 (2.7)	0.61	0.10	0.86	0.004
Body mass (kg)	95.7 (21.0)	90.8 (15.1)	−4.1 (7.0)	0.23	0.29	85.6 (9.1)	85.4 (9.4)	−0.3 (1.2)	0.63	0.02	0.93	0.001
BMI (kg/m^2)	32.0 (5.9)	30.5 (4.0)	−4.0 (7.3)	0.25	0.33	30.8 (2.6)	30.7 (3.0)	−0.3 (1.8)	0.78	0.03	1	0
Body fat percentage (%)	33.5 (10.1)	29.5 (11.1)	−13.2 (10.6)	0.047	0.41	37.3 (13.1)	35.0 (11.3)	−5.4 (7.5)	0.17	0.21	0.95	0.004
Cardiovascular outcomes:												
Resting HR (beats/min)	66 (4)	62 (6)	−6 (8)	0.10	0.86	75 (12)	74 (11)	−1 (4)	0.43	0.09	0.34	0.13
Resting SBP (mmHg)	137 (12)	123 (8)	−10 (7)	0.026	1.50	127 (4)	129 (8)	+2 (5)	0.45	0.34	0.10	0.33
Resting DBP (mmHg)	89 (8)	82 (9)	−8 (8)	0.074	0.90	89 (7)	89 (5)	0 (7)	1	0	0.16	0.26
Augmentation Index (%)	17.0 (15.4)	7.2 (15.7)	−126.7 (128.4)	<0.001	0.69	12.0 (18.5)	16.8 (12.6)	+41.4 (95.2)	0.41	0.33	0.064	0.41
Pulse Pressure (mmHg)	47 (9)	41 (5)	−10 (23)	0.28	0.90	38 (3)	41 (4)	+9 (14.0)	0.22	0.93	0.36	0.12
VO_2max (ml/kg min)	27.9 (2.4)	32.5 (5.0)	+16.9 (18.6)	0.06	1.28	29.0 (6.4)	28.8 (8.0)	−1.1 (16.3)	0.93	0.03	0.34	0.13
VO_2max (L/min)	2.691 (0.688)	2.970 (0.802)	+10.2 (6.7)	0.015	0.41	2.490 (0.691)	2.454 (0.761)	−1.6 (16.5)	0.78	0.05	0.22	0.21
HRQoL outcomes:												
Physical Functioning	92.5 (6.1)	96.7 (2.6)	+4.7 (4.4)	0.042	0.98	91.7 (11.7)	90.8 (8.0)	−0.12 (9.3)	0.81	0.10	0.11	0.32
General Health	53.3 (8.8)	65.0 (8.9)	+25.2 (32.1)	0.07	1.45	65.8 (20.1)	62.5 (25.1)	−7.3 (16.8)	0.44	0.15	0.21	0.22
Vitality	50.0 (28.5)	66.3 (191)	+54.8 (49.9)	0.024	0.74	68.8 (32.6)	59.7 (33.8)	−19.1 (28.3)	0.043	0.30	0.02	0.54

Data expressed as mean (standard deviation). *Abbreviations*: *BMI* body mass index, *HR* heart rate, *SBP* systolic blood pressure, VO_{2peak} peak oxygen consumption. Effect size = Cohen's *d*.

duration (>12 weeks) or more frequent training (>4 sessions/wk) may have induced more favourable adaptation of obesity outcomes.

Studies in overweight and obese participants have consistently shown that HIIT performed on treadmill or cycle ergometer (12–26 weeks) can reduce BMI, waist circumference, body weight and body fat percentage versus a no-exercise control [17]. However, the effect of HIIT versus MICT on adiposity outcomes remains equivocal with many studies demonstrating an equivalent effect [17,40] and other studies showing a superior [19,20] or inferior effect [41] of HIIT. These inconsistent data may be due to the heterogeneity of HIIT interventions (e.g. intervals have ranged from 6 s to 4 min [21]), cohorts (e.g. age, level of obesity), and methods use to equate the HIIT and MICT prescriptions across studies. Further research is therefore warranted [21]. No significant group x time interaction effects were noted for obesity outcomes in the present study. However, within group changes suggest a need for a well-powered study of boxing training (HIIT) versus brisk walking (MICT) to explore these comparisons further. Such studies should also investigate the effect of various prescriptions (dosages) of HIIT on these outcomes. Based on the percentage change score data for abdominal obesity (waist circumference) in the boxing group (−5.3 ± 7.7%) and walking group (−0.6 ± 2.7%), we estimate that approximately 50 participants (25 per group) would provide 80% power to detect a statistically significant difference between groups on this outcome measure.

Cardiovascular outcomes

The boxing group significantly reduced resting systolic blood pressure (−10%; $p = 0.026$) and AIx (−126.7%; $p < 0.001$) and increased absolute VO_{2max} (+10.2%; $p = 0.015$) while experiencing large effects (Cohen's d >0.86) and trends toward reduced resting heart rate (−6%; $p = 0.10$) and diastolic blood pressure (−8%; $p = 0.074$) and relative VO_{2max} (+16.9%; $p = 0.06$). No adaptations were noted in the walking group, and trends toward group x time interaction were noted for AIx ($p = 0.064$), and resting systolic- ($p = 0.10$) and diastolic blood pressure ($p = 0.16$).

Our findings suggest that the boxing intervention induced favourable adaptations of the central and peripheral cardiovascular system. HIIT has consistently been shown to increase VO_{2max} more than MICT in healthy adults [42], and those with cardiometabolic diseases [14,17,43]. Increased VO_2max and reduced resting heart rate can likely be attributed to a training-induced increase in stroke volume [44], which can be influenced by factors such as the reversal of left ventricular remodelling and increased ejection fraction (*via* increased end-diastolic volume and reduced end-systolic volume) [14]. Further, the improvement of systolic- and diastolic blood pressure and AIx in the boxing group indicates a reduction in total peripheral resistance (i.e. reversal of atherosclerosis) which is likely accompanied by improved endothelial function [45]. The underlying mechanism for these adaptations is the vascular shear stress induced by higher intensity exercise [46]. Numerous studies have shown that central and peripheral adaptations to exercise in sedentary and chronically diseased cohorts are superior with HIIT (on cycle or treadmill) as compared to MICT [13,16,18]. The changes experienced by the boxing group in the present study may be clinically significant, and therefore require further investigation.

HRQoL outcomes

The boxing group increased Vitality (+54.8%; $p = 0.024$), Physical Functioning (+4.7%; $p = 0.042$) and General Health (+25.2; $p = 0.07$) domains of HRQoL with a large effect (Cohen's $d = 0.74\text{-}1.45$) over time. By contrast, the walking group experienced a significant reduction in Vitality (−19.1%; $p = 0.043$) and experienced no change in the other two domains. A significant group x time effect favouring the boxing group was noted for Vitality ($p = 0.02$). Few studies have investigated the effect of HIIT on HRQoL. Significant improvements in SF-36 Physical Functioning and General Health domains of HRQoL have been noted in a previous study prescribing 12 weeks of HIIT performed on a treadmill in 88 men and women with essential hypertension [18]. Further, a study by Wisloff et al. [13], showed a statistically significant increase in the global domain of HRQoL in heart failure patients prescribed 12 weeks of HIIT versus MICT performed on treadmill. Our findings suggest that boxing training is effective for increasing several domains of HRQoL. There is a need to further explore the potential physiological mechanisms that contribute to the improvement of HRQoL and related psychological outcomes (e.g. emotion, motivation, life satisfaction, etc.) in response to HIIT in individuals who are sedentary and obese. Further, studies have shown that low HRQoL is associated with obesogenic dietary behaviours and work-productivity losses [47]; therefore, HIIT may be able to positively adapt these outcomes as well. Accordingly, robust RCT are required to further investigate the effects of boxing training on HRQoL and the clinical significance of these data.

Conclusion

Boxing training (HIIT) in adults with abdominal obesity is feasible and may elicit a better therapeutic effect on obesity, cardiovascular- and HRQoL outcomes than an equivalent dose of brisk walking (MICT). Robustly designed randomized controlled trials are required to confirm these findings and inform clinical guidelines and practice for obesity treatment.

Competing interests

The authors declare that they have no competing interests.

Authors' contributions

BSC conceived and designed the study, led the statistical analyses, and drafted the manuscript. TBD was involved in the acquisition of data, delivery of interventions, and drafting the manuscript. MS provided consultation regarding the design of the boxing intervention. SP was involved in the acquisition of data and drafting the manuscript. EA provided consultation regarding study methodology and was involved in drafting the manuscript. All authors have read and approved the final manuscript.

Acknowledgements

This research was supported by honours project research funding provided by the University of Western Sydney. We sincerely thank Sean Raftry and Catherine Phillips for organizing equipment and providing technical support for this study.

Author details

[1]School of Science and Health, University of Western Sydney, Locked Bag 1797, Penrith, 2751 Campbelltown, New South Wales, Australia. [2]The National Institute of Complementary Medicine, University of Western Sydney, Campbelltown, NSW 2650, Australia. [3]School of Nursing and Midwifery, University of Western Sydney, Campbelltown, New South Wales, Australia. [4]School of Medicine, University of Adelaide, Adelaide, South Australia, Australia.

References

1. World Health Organization. Global status report on noncommunicable diseases 2010. Geneva: World Health Organization; 2011.
2. Ng M, Fleming T, Robinson M, Thomson B, Graetz N, Margono C, et al. Global, regional, and national prevalence of overweight and obesity in children and adults during 1980-2013: a systematic analysis for the Global Burden of Disease Study 2013. Lancet. 2014;384(9945):766–81.
3. Bhaskaran K, Douglas I, Forbes H, Santos-Silva I, Leon DA, Smeeth L. Body-mass index and risk of 22 specific cancers: a population-based cohort study of 5.24 million UK adults. Lancet. 2014;384(9945):755–65.
4. Bloom DE, Cafiero ET, Jane-Llopis E, Abrahams-Gessel S, Bloom LR, Fathima S, et al. The Global Economic Burden of Noncommunicable Diseases. In: Geneva: World Economic Forum; 2011.
5. Jia H, Lubetkin EI. The impact of obesity on health-related quality-of-life in the general adult US population. J Public Health (Oxford, England). 2005;27(2):156–64.
6. Flegal KM, Kit BK, Orpana H, Graubard BI. Association of all-cause mortality with overweight and obesity using standard body mass index categories: a systematic review and meta-analysis. JAMA. 2013;309(1):71–82.
7. Donnelly J, Blair S, Jakicic J, Manore M, Rankin J, Smith B. American College of Sports Medicine Position Stand. Appropriate physical activity intervention strategies for weight loss and prevention of weight regain for adults. Med Sci Sports Exerc. 2009;41(2):459.
8. Haskell W, Lee I, Pate R, Powell K, Blair S, Franklin B, et al. Physical activity and public health: updated recommendations for adults from the American College of Sports Medicine and the American Heart Association. Circulation. 2007;116:1081–93.
9. World Health Organization. Global recommendations on physical activity for health. Geneva: World Health Organization; 2010.
10. Richardson CR, Newton TL, Abraham JJ, Sen A, Jimbo M, Swartz AM. A meta-analysis of pedometer-based walking interventions and weight loss. Annals Family Med. 2008;6(1):69–77.
11. Murphy MH, Nevill AM, Murtagh EM, Holder RL. The effect of walking on fitness, fatness and resting blood pressure: a meta-analysis of randomised, controlled trials. Prev Med. 2007;44(5):377–85.
12. Thorogood A, Mottillo S, Shimony A, Filion KB, Joseph L, Genest J, et al. Isolated aerobic exercise and weight loss: a systematic review and meta-analysis of randomized controlled trials. Am J Med. 2011;124(8):747–55.
13. Wisloff U, Stoylen A, Loennechen JP, Bruvold M, Rognmo O, Haram PM, et al. Superior cardiovascular effect of aerobic interval training versus moderate continuous training in heart failure patients a randomized study. Circulation. 2007;115(24):3086–94.
14. Cornish AK, Broadbent S, Cheema BS. Interval training for patients with coronary artery disease: a systematic review. Eur J Appl Physiol. 2011;111(4):579–89.
15. Rognmo O, Hetland E, Helgerud J, Hoff J, Slordahl SA. High intensity aerobic interval exercise is superior to moderate intensity exercise for increasing aerobic capacity in patients with coronary artery disease. Eur J Cardiovasc Prev Rehabil. 2004;11(3):216–22.
16. Tjønna AE, Lee SJ, Rognmo Ø, Stølen TO, Bye A, Haram PM, et al. Aerobic interval training versus continuous moderate exercise as a treatment for the metabolic syndrome: a pilot study. Circulation. 2008;118(4):346–54.
17. Kessler HS, Sisson SB, Short KR. The potential for high-intensity interval training to reduce cardiometabolic disease risk. Sports Med. 2012;42(6):489–509.
18. Molmen-Hansen HE, Stolen T, Tjonna AE, Aamot IL, Ekeberg IS, Tyldum GA, et al. Aerobic interval training reduces blood pressure and improves myocardial function in hypertensive patients. Eur J Prev Cardiol. 2012;19(2):151–60.
19. Tremblay A, Simoneau JA, Bouchard C. Impact of exercise intensity on body fatness and skeletal muscle metabolism. Metabolism. 1994;43(7):814–8.
20. Trapp EG, Chisholm DJ, Freund J, Boutcher SH. The effects of high-intensity intermittent exercise training on fat loss and fasting insulin levels of young women. Int J Obesity (2005). 2008;32(4):684–91.
21. Boutcher SH. High-intensity intermittent exercise and fat loss. J Obes. 2011;2011:868305.
22. Arseneau E, Mekary S, Leger LA. VO2 requirements of boxing exercises. J Strength Cond Res. 2011;25(2):348–59.
23. Alberti KG, Zimmet P, Shaw J. Metabolic syndrome–a new world-wide definition. A consensus statement from the International Diabetes Federation. Diabet Med. 2006;23(5):469–80.
24. Ainsworth B, Haskell W, Whitt M, Irwin M, Swartz A, Strath S, et al. Compendium of physical activities: an update of activity codes and MET intensities. Med Sci Sports Exer. 2000;32(9, Suppl):S498–516.
25. Stewart A, Marfell-Jones M, Olds T, de Ridder H. International standards for anthropometric assessment. In: Lower Hutt NZ, editor. 2011.
26. Norton K, Olds T, Commission AS. Anthropometrica: A Textbook of Body Measurement for Sports and Health Courses. Sydney: UNSW Press; 1996.
27. Thompson W, Gordon N, Pescatello L. ACSM's Guidelines for Exercise Testing and Prescription. Philadelphia: Wolters Kluwer/Lippincott Williams & Wilkins; 2010.
28. Wilkinson IB, Fuchs SA, Jansen IM, Spratt JC, Murray GD, Cockcroft JR, et al. Reproducibility of pulse wave velocity and augmentation index measured by pulse wave analysis. J Hypertens. 1998;16(12 Pt 2):2079–84.
29. Edwards DG, Lang JT. Augmentation index and systolic load are lower in competitive endurance athletes. Am J Hypertens. 2005;18(5):679–83.
30. Goldberg MJ, Boutcher SH, Boutcher YN. The effect of 4 weeks of aerobic exercise on vascular and baroreflex function of young men with a family history of hypertension. J Hum Hypertens. 2012;26(11):644–9.
31. Mustata S, Chan C, Lai V, Miller JA. Impact of an exercise program on arterial stiffness and insulin resistance in hemodialysis patients. J Am Soc Nephrol. 2004;15(10):2713–8.
32. Plotnikoff RC, Courneya KS, Trinh L, Karunamuni N, Sigal RJ. Aerobic physical activity and resistance training: an application of the theory of planned behavior among adults with type 2 diabetes in a random, national sample of Canadians. Int J Behav Nutr Phy. 2008;5(1):61-61.
33. Stewart A, Hays R, Je W. The MOS short-form general health survey: reliability and validity in a patient population. Med Care. 1988;26:724.
34. Hermand D, Mullet E, Rompteaux L. Societal risk perception among children, adolescents, adults, and elderly people. J Adult Dev. 1999;6(2):137–43.
35. Kaur G, Smyth RL, Williamson P. Developing a survey of barriers and facilitators to recruitment in randomized controlled trials. Trials. 2012;13(1):218.
36. Jacobs EJ, Newton CC, Wang Y, McCullough ML, Campbell PT, Thun MJ, et al. WAist circumference and all-cause mortality in a large us cohort. Arch Intern Med. 2010;170(15):1293–301.
37. Gonzalez A, Hartge P, Cerhan JR, Flint AJ, Hannan L, MacInnis RJ, et al. Body-mass index and mortality among 1.46 million white adults. N Engl J Med. 2010;23:2211–9.
38. Gómez-Ambrosi J, Silva C, Galofré JC, Escalada J, Santos S, Gil MJ, et al. Body adiposity and type 2 diabetes: increased risk with a high body fat percentage even having a normal BMI. Obesity. 2011;19(7):1439–44.

39. Stevens J, Truesdale KP, McClain JE, Cai J. The definition of weight maintenance. Int J Obesity (2005). 2006;30(3):391–9.
40. Terada T, Friesen A, Chahal BS, Bell GJ, McCargar LJ, Boule NG. Feasibility and preliminary efficacy of high intensity interval training in type 2 diabetes. Diabetes Res Clin Pract. 2013;99(2):120–9.
41. Keating SE, Machan EA, O'Connor HT, Gerofi JA, Sainsbury A, Caterson ID, et al. Continuous exercise but not high intensity interval training improves fat distribution in overweight adults. J Obes. 2014;2014:834865.
42. Helgerud J, Hoydal K, Wang E, Karlsen T, Berg P, Bjerkaas M, et al. Aerobic high-intensity intervals improve VO2max more than moderate training. Med Sci Sports Exerc. 2007;39(4):665–71.
43. Weston KS, Wisløff U, Coombes JS. High-intensity interval training in patients with lifestyle-induced cardiometabolic disease: a systematic review and meta-analysis. Br J Sports Med. 2013;48(16):1227–34.
44. Dogra S, Spencer MD, Paterson DH. Higher cardiorespiratory fitness in older trained women is due to preserved stroke volume. J Sports Sci Med. 2012;11(4):745.
45. McEniery CM, Wallace S, Mackenzie IS, McDonnell B, Newby DE, Cockcroft JR, et al. Endothelial function is associated with pulse pressure, pulse wave velocity, and augmentation index in healthy humans. Hypertension. 2006;48(4):602–8.
46. Tinken TM, Thijssen DH, Hopkins N, Dawson EA, Cable NT, Green DJ. Shear stress mediates endothelial adaptations to exercise training in humans. Hypertension. 2010;55(2):312–8.
47. Cash SW, Beresford SA, Henderson JA, McTiernan A, Xiao L, Wang CY, et al. Dietary and physical activity behaviours related to obesity-specific quality of life and work productivity: baseline results from a worksite trial. British J Nutri. 2012;108(6):1134–42.

11

Aerobic exercise modulates intracortical inhibition and facilitation in a nonexercised upper limb muscle

Amaya M Singh, Robin E Duncan, Jason L Neva and W Richard Staines*

Abstract

Background: Despite growing interest in the relationship between exercise and short-term neural plasticity, the effects of exercise on motor cortical (M1) excitability are not well studied. Acute, lower-limb aerobic exercise may potentially modulate M1 excitability in working muscles, but the effects on muscles not involved in the exercise are unknown. Here we examined the excitability changes in an upper limb muscle representation following a single session of lower body aerobic exercise. Investigating the response to exercise in a non-exercised muscle may help to determine the clinical usefulness of lower-body exercise interventions for upper limb neurorehabilitation.

Methods: In this study, transcranial magnetic stimulation was used to assess input–output curves, short-interval intracortical inhibition (SICI), long-interval intracortical inhibition (LICI) and intracortical facilitation (ICF) in the extensor carpi radialis muscle in twelve healthy individuals following a single session of moderate stationary biking. Additionally, we examined whether the presence of a common polymorphism of the brain-derived neurotrophic factor (BDNF) gene would affect the response of these measures to exercise.

Results: We observed significant increases in ICF and decreases in SICI following exercise. No changes in LICI were detected, and no differences were observed in input–output curves following exercise, or between BDNF groups.

Conclusions: The current results demonstrate that the modulation of intracortical excitability following aerobic exercise is not limited to those muscles involved in the exercise, and that while exercise does not directly modulate the excitability of motor neurons, it may facilitate the induction of experience-dependent plasticity via a decrease in intracortical inhibition and increase in intracortical facilitation. These findings indicate that exercise may create favourable conditions for adaptive plasticity in M1 and may be an effective adjunct to traditional training or rehabilitation methods.

Keywords: Aerobic exercise, Primary motor cortex, Transcranial magnetic stimulation, Intracortical inhibition, Intracortical facilitation

Background

The benefits of exercise on brain function have been widely documented. However, little is known about the direct effects of exercise on motor cortical excitability. In clinical settings, aerobic exercise is commonly prescribed to improve cardiovascular function following brain injury and can successfully improve aerobic capacity in neurological patient populations [1-4]. In addition to secondary cardiovascular disease prevention and improved quality of life, emerging evidence suggests exercise may also promote beneficial cortical adaptations. Plasticity in the motor cortex is among the primary goals of rehabilitation programs following brain injury, and much attention has been focused on the ability of exercise to act as a potential primer for subsequent task-specific changes in cortical excitability associated with learning-based rehabilitation. However, the mechanisms underlying such modulation are not yet known. While chronic physical activity is associated with increased metabolic capacity and increased angiogenesis in the primary motor cortex (M1) [5,6], little is known about how aerobic exercise

* Correspondence: rstaines@uwaterloo.ca
Department of Kinesiology, University of Waterloo, 200 University Avenue West, Waterloo, ON N2L 3G1, Canada

modulates cortical excitability, and the effects of an acute bout of aerobic exercise on the motor cortex are unclear.

Recently, pedaling exercise has been shown to decrease intracortical inhibition in the leg region of M1 [7], which suggest that such an intervention may be effective in increasing excitability. However, in clinical settings, spasticity and muscle weakness are seen frequently in the upper limbs, particularly following a stroke. Up to 85% of stroke patients present with hemiparesis of the upper limbs [8,9], and thus the upper limb musculature is often the focus of rehabilitation. Yet, the majority of clinical aerobic exercise interventions, such as walking, running and cycling, predominantly involve the lower limbs. Pedaling exercise is frequently used in rehabilitation settings for patients who exhibit gait disturbances, or who present with balance or stability issues. Recent evidence indicates that acute cycling modulates intracortical inhibition in the cortical representations of active muscles; however, it is not known if this response is limited to muscles involved in the exercise or if such responses can be observed in nonexercised limbs. Here, we use transcranial magnetic stimulation (TMS) to probe both the excitability of descending tracts of nonexercised muscles following exercise and the intracortical inhibitory and facilitatory networks within M1. We assessed the effect of aerobic exercise on corticospinal excitability by using single pulses to generate a stimulus–response (S-R) curve at varying intensities. Three paired-pulse paradigms were used to probe the effect of exercise on the intracortical networks within M1: short-interval intracortical inhibition (SICI), long-interval intracortical inhibition (LICI) and intracortical facilitation (ICF).

The primary aim of this study was to investigate the effects of a brief session of lower-limb aerobic exercise on the cortical excitability of an upper-limb muscle representation. In addition, we investigated whether the presence of a common single nucleotide polymorphism (a valine-to-methionine substitution at codon 66, or Val66Met) of the brain-derived neurotrophic factor (BDNF) gene would impact the cortical response to exercise. BDNF is a growth factor secreted by the brain that is critical for the growth and survival of neurons and plays a key role in the development of long-term potentiation (LTP). The Val66Met polymorphism is associated with decreased activity-dependent BDNF release and has been linked to diminished motor cortical plasticity, with Met carriers displaying decreased task-related M1 activation [10], reduced responses to the induction of experience-dependent plasticity [11], and impaired synaptic transmission [12]. Thus, we examined whether genetic variability in the BDNF gene would affect the response of M1 to aerobic exercise. We found that while the input–output curve and LICI were not significantly affected by exercise, lower-limb exercise induced a significant decrease in SICI and increase in ICF in a non-exercised muscle. None of the above measures were significantly affected by the presence of the BDNF polymorphism. These findings may have important implications for the use of aerobic exercise in treating upper limb motor deficits.

Methods

Participants

Twelve young, healthy, moderately active individuals were recruited (7 males; 1 left-handed, 11 right-handed; average age = 28 years). All participants had prior experience with TMS. Informed consent was obtained from all participants prior to undergoing the experimental protocol and they were screened for any contraindications to TMS using a standard screening form. All experimental procedures received clearance from the University Of Waterloo Office Of Research Ethics.

Exercise protocol

Heart rate (HR) and rate of perceived exertion (RPE) were collected at rest prior to exercise. During exercise, heart rate was monitored using a wrist-mounted heart rate monitor. Participants were instructed to work at 65-70% of their age-predicted maximal heart rate [average = 125-135 beats per minute (bpm)]. After a brief warm-up to elevate HR into the target zone, participants performed 20 minutes of continuous stationary biking on a recumbent bicycle in an isolated room. The duration and intensity were intended to mimic a standard aerobic workout. HR was carefully monitored and maintained throughout the session. Participants were seated comfortably with their feet strapped to the pedals and their backs against the backrest. RPE was verbally reported using the modified Borg scale every five minutes, and HR was continuously monitored throughout the exercise period. Instructions were given to work at a moderate intensity (RPE of 3–4), and participants could adjust either the pedaling resistance or the rate of pedaling to maintain the target heart rate. All participants reported intensity rates in the moderate range, with no individual exceeding an RPE of 4. The experimenters remained with the participant throughout the exercise and ensured that arms were resting comfortably by their sides and not gripping the handlebars during the session. The arms, and particularly the forearms, remained stationary during pedaling exercise. Participants were given free access to water. Immediately following exercise completion, participants returned to the TMS testing room for the collection of post-exercise measures. Post 1 occurred immediately following exercise and lasted approximately 10 minutes. Participants then rested in an upright chair in a quiet room for the remainder of the rest period. Post 2 was collected 30 minutes following exercise completion. In all cases, heart rate had returned to resting or near-resting levels (within 5 bpm) by the 30 minute mark post-exercise.

BDNF genotyping

The brain-derived neurotrophic factor (BDNF) Val66Met polymorphism (rs6265) was genotyped from saliva samples by qPCR on an ABI7500 using a TaqMan SNP genotyping assay (Applied Biosystems) with 10 ng of saliva genomic DNA isolated by standard procedures from anonymized samples. Random duplicate analyses showed 100% concordance with runs.

TMS protocol

Focal TMS was performed using a MagPro × 100 stimulator (Medtronic, Minneapolis, MN, USA) and a 'figure of eight' coil (MCF-B65; 70 mm). BrainSight Neuronavigation (Rogue Research, Canada) was used to guide the placement of the coil to the target motor region using a template MRI for all participants. Anatomical co-registration was performed prior to baseline collection and subsequent coil positioning was tracked using reflective markers affixed to custom-fitted glasses. The coil was placed at a 45° angle to the mid-sagittal line to induce a posterior to anterior current in the underlying neural tissue. EMG recordings of motor-evoked potentials (MEPs) were obtained using surface electrodes placed over the right extensor carpi radialis muscle (ECR). Raw EMG signals were recorded and stored in a customized Labview (National Instruments, Austin, TX, USA) program for offline analysis. The motor hotspot of the right ECR muscle was identified as the left M1 location that consistently elicited a maximal MEP in the resting muscle, as assessed by EMG amplitude, while producing a visible muscle twitch. The resting motor threshold (RMT) was determined by the stimulation intensity required to elicit a peak-to-peak MEP amplitude of >50 μV on 5 out of 10 trials. After localization of the hotspot, a stimulus–response curve was generated by assessing the cortical response to single-pulse TMS at a range of intensities. Ten single pulses were delivered with a minimum of 2-second intervals at stimulus intensities of 100%, 110%, 120%, 130%, and 140% of RMT. Three paired-pulse measures were also assessed using the following parameters for the conditioning stimulus (CS), test stimulus (TS) and inter-stimulus interval (ISI): a) SICI (CS = 80% and TS = 120% of RMT, 2.5 ms ISI); b) LICI (CS = 120% and TS = 120% of RMT, 100 ms ISI); and c) ICF (CS = 80% and TS = 120% of RMT, 12 ms ISI). Ten pairs of stimuli were delivered in each paired-pulse protocol with an ISI of 2 seconds between stimulus pairs. Thus, the following four measures were randomized across participants but the order remained consistent throughout each individual experiment: i) S-R curve, ii) SICI, iii) LICI, and iv) ICF. Measures were collected just prior to exercise, immediately following exercise, and again 30 minutes following exercise completion.

Statistical analysis

In all paired-pulse measures, the degree of inhibition or excitation was normalized to the single pulse amplitude at 120% RMT for each timepoint. Participants in whom intracortical inhibition could not be induced pre-exercise using standard protocols were excluded from the corresponding analysis. For SICI and ICF, the average amplitude elicited by the conditioned stimulus was expressed as a percentage of the average unconditioned MEP amplitude at 120%. For LICI, the amplitude of the MEP evoked by the test pulse was expressed as a percentage of the conditioning stimulus amplitude, and the average of 20 trials was taken. For the S-R curves, 10 MEPs were averaged at each intensity and the average values were compared. To assess changes in resting single-pulse excitability within the S-R curves, a two-way repeated measures ANOVA was conducted with time (pre, post 1 and post 2) and stimulus intensity (100%, 110%, 120%, 130% and 140% RMT) as factors. Paired-pulse measures were analyzed using three separate one-way repeated measures ANOVAs for SICI, LICI and ICF data using time as the main factor. Post hoc testing was performed using Tukey's HSD. To test the effect of the BDNF polymorphism, subjects were divided into Met carriers ($n = 6$) or non-Met carriers ($n = 6$). A mixed 2 × 3 × 5 ANOVA was conducted to assess differences in S-R curves between Met carriers and non-Met carriers using stimulus intensity and time as the within-subjects factors and genotype as the between-subjects factor. The response to paired-pulse measures within each group was assessed using separate two-way mixed ANOVAs for SICI, LICI, and ICF, with time as the within-subjects factor and genotype as the between-subjects factor. Significant main effects in the ANOVA were followed with post hoc tests using Tukey's HSD. The significance level for all tests was set at $p < 0.05$.

Results

Although EMG was not collected continuously during the exercise session, offline testing was conducted to monitor upper limb muscle activity during an identical biking task. There was no detectable muscle activity in right ECR, flexor carpi radialis (FCR), or first dorsal interosseous (FDI) during biking. For all measures, pre-exercise responses were taken as baseline values. Figure 1 displays the S-R curves, with the average MEP amplitude evoked in response to varying stimulus intensities at each timepoint. Not surprisingly, a two-way repeated

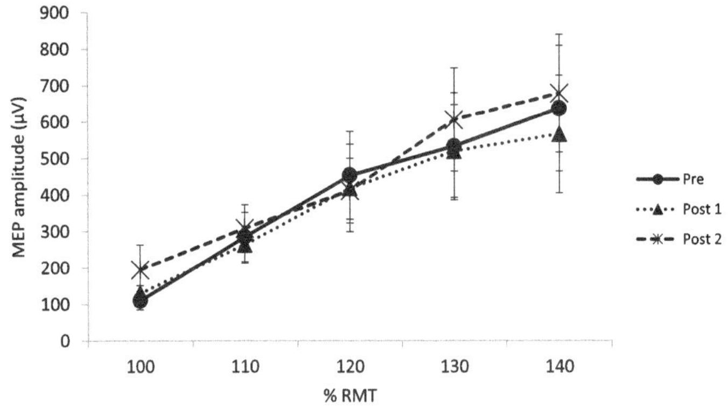

Figure 1 Recruitment curves before and after exercise. Stimulus–response curves pre- and post-exercise in response to stimulation at increasing percentages of RMT (n = 12). Bars represent SEM. (* = p < 0.05).

measures ANOVA showed a significant main effect of intensity ($F_{4, 44} = 9.70$, $p < 0.001$, Figure 1). Post-hoc testing using Tukey's HSD revealed that MEP amplitude differed significantly between 100% RMT and 120%, 130% and 140% RMT. In addition, evoked responses at 110% differed significantly from those at 130% and 140%. There was no main effect of timepoint relative to exercise ($F_{2, 22} = 1.59$, $p = 0.23$) and no interaction between intensity and timepoint ($F_{8, 88} = 1.11$, $p = 0.36$).

Average paired-pulse responses across all subjects are shown in Figures 2, 3 and 4. The above-noted exclusion criteria resulted in one participant being removed from the SICI analysis and one participant from the LICI analysis. Figure 2a displays the consistency of SICI induction across each timepoint. Results of a one-way repeated measures ANOVA showed that following exercise, SICI was significantly decreased ($F_{2, 20} = 4.30$, $p = 0.028$, Figure 2b). Prior to exercise, SICI induced an average (±standard error) of 53.8 ± 8.8% inhibition of the unconditioned stimulus. Immediately after exercise (post 1), SICI levels decreased to 21.8 ± 18.5% and remained at 19.4 ± 15.1% 30 minutes following exercise (post 2). Post-hoc testing using Tukey's HSD revealed a significant decrease in SICI from pre to post 2. Results from the LICI analysis demonstrate a similar trend (Figure 3): pre-exercise levels of LICI showed 54.2 ± 9.6% inhibition of test stimulus amplitude. Following exercise, this decreased to 25.0 ± 20.3% and increased slightly to 36.3 ± 21.5% at post 2; however, these differences were not statistically significant ($F_{2, 20} = 1.36$, $p = 0.28$, Figure 3b). Correspondingly, a one-way repeated measures ANOVA of ICF revealed that following exercise, ICF was significantly elevated ($F_{2, 22} = 5.29$, $p = 0.013$, Figure 4b). Baseline values showed a 140.1 ± 11.2% increase relative to unconditioned stimulus amplitudes. At post 1, ICF values increased to 224.8 ± 31.1% of unconditioned test pulses. ICF levels remained elevated at post 2, with an average of 193.7 ± 23.6% facilitation. Post-hoc testing revealed significant differences between pre and post 1, and while ICF levels remained elevated at post 2 relative to pre, this difference was not statistically significant.

Results from BDNF genotyping indicated that six of twelve subjects were Met carriers (two homozygous and four heterozygous). Results from a 2 × 3 × 5 mixed ANOVA performed on S-R curves indicated no significant

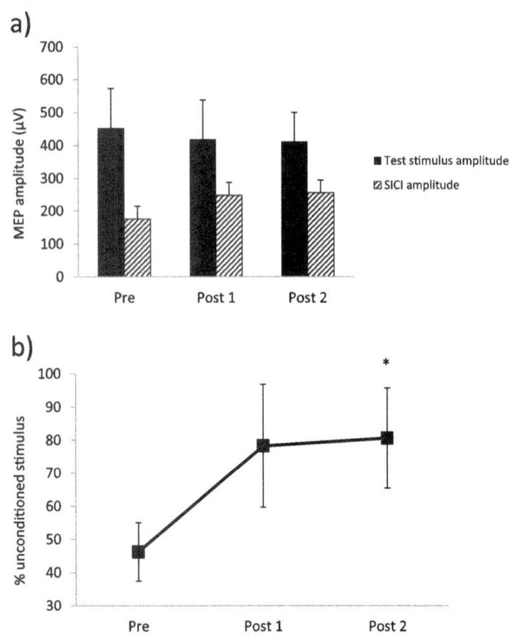

Figure 2 Modulation of SICI following exercise. (a) Induction of SICI across all participants (n = 11) at each timepoint and **(b)** % of test stimulus amplitude. Unconditioned single pulse amplitudes at 120% RMT are compared to conditioned stimulus amplitudes. Bars represent SEM. Asterisks indicate values significantly different from pre-exercise (p < 0.05).

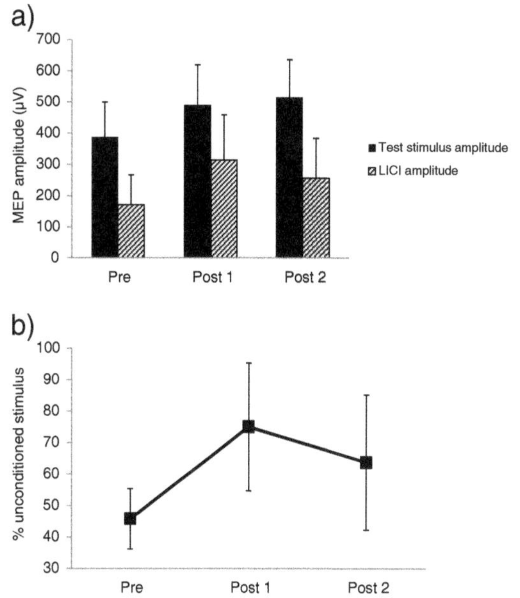

Figure 3 Modulation of LICI following exercise. Induction of LICI across all participants (n = 11) at each timepoint **(a)** and % of test stimulus amplitude **(b)**. Unconditioned single pulse amplitudes at 120% RMT are compared to conditioned stimulus amplitudes. Bars represent SEM.

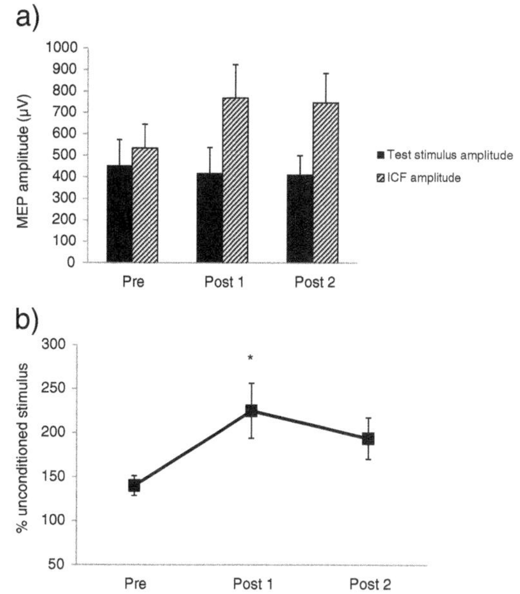

Figure 4 Modulation of ICF following exercise. Induction of ICF across all participants (n = 12) at each timepoint **(a)** and % facilitation of test stimulus **(b)**. Unconditioned single pulse amplitudes at 120% RMT are compared to conditioned stimulus amplitudes. Bars represent SEM. Asterisks indicate values significantly different from pre-exercise (p < 0.05).

differences between Met carriers and Val/Val subjects in single-pulse excitability at any timepoint or any stimulus intensity ($F_{1,\ 7} = 0.14$, $p = 0.71$, Figure 5).

Results from separate two-way mixed ANOVAs revealed no main effect of BDNF for SICI ($F_{1,\ 9} = 2.71$, $p = 0.13$), LICI ($F_{1,\ 9} = 2.66$, $p = 0.14$), or ICF ($F_{1,\ 10} = 0.00035$, $p = 0.95$), and no BDNF × time interaction for SICI ($F_{2,\ 18} = 0.3$, $p = 0.74$), LICI ($F_{2,\ 18} = 1.3$, $p = 0.30$), or ICF ($F_{2,\ 20} = 0.5$, $p = 0.62$) (Figure 6).

Discussion

The aim of this study was to test whether the modulation of the cortical excitability of a specific muscle representation in M1 following aerobic exercise is dependent on the involvement of that muscle in the exercise itself. Specifically, we sought to investigate whether aerobic exercise involving the lower limbs could modulate upper limb motor cortical excitability and also to determine the time course of this modulation and potential mechanisms that contribute to it. Thus, both S-R curves and paired-pulse measures of SICI, LICI and ICF were used to probe the excitability changes in a wrist extensor muscle following a single session of stationary biking. Immediately after exercise completion, there was a significant decrease in short-interval intracortical inhibition and a significant increase in intracortical facilitation. Immediately after exercise completion, there was a significant increase in intracortical facilitation, and a significant suppression of SICI was evident at 30 minutes post-exercise. While LICI displayed a similar trend to SICI, in this case the decrease in inhibition was not statistically significant. In contrast, the S-R curves indicate that the resting motor threshold was not modulated by exercise. There were no significant differences observed in MEP amplitudes pre- and post-exercise at any intensity. Thus, resting motor thresholds of inactive muscles appear unchanged by exercise. However, the current results indicate that aerobic activity using the lower limbs causes an immediate and sustained modulation of intracortical facilitation and inhibition of an upper limb muscle. Such excitability changes are a necessary precursor to the relatively more permanent changes in synaptic strength seen in the processes of long-term potentiation (LTP) and long-term depression (LTD). It is likely that the altered excitability state of these interneuronal pools will render them more receptive to strategies aimed at inducing plasticity, such as skilled motor training or targeted rehabilitation, when they are preceded by an exercise session. Furthermore, interventions that directly target the mechanisms of LTP/LTD, such as repetitive theta-burst stimulation (TBS), may benefit from the addition of exercise. It should be noted, however, that the benefits of such interventions will not necessarily be additive. The emerging principles of homeostatic metaplasticity suggest that

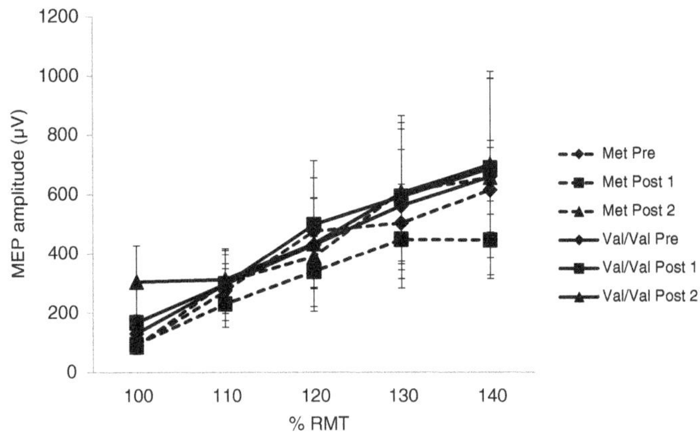

Figure 5 Effect of BDNF genotype on recruitment curves. Group differences between Met carriers (n = 6) and non-Met carriers (n = 6) in S-R curve outputs at each timepoint. Bars represent SEM.

the probability of LTP induction depends on prior synaptic activity and that when LTP has been recently induced, subsequent facilitatory interventions will be suppressed or even reversed in order to maintain a balance between LTP and LTD [13-15].

As indicated, previous research has demonstrated a decrease in SICI in exercising muscles [7]. The current results extend this finding to non-exercised muscles and indicate that such changes are not a direct consequence of preceding muscle activity. These results are in line with the findings of Takahashi et al. [16], who report that lower limb resistance exercise influences cortical excitability in nonexercised hand muscles. Takahashi and colleagues [16] propose several potential mechanisms for their findings, including facilitatory cortical pathways between synergistic arm and leg representations, and a spread of cortical excitability from active muscles to non-active muscles in proximal M1 areas. Neither of these possibilities can be ruled out here. However, the observed changes were seen at the motor hotspot of the ECR and not on the periphery of the representation, which would indicate a modulation of the ECR representation itself. Furthermore, the lack of an effect on single-pulse amplitude after exercise argues against a spread of excitability from active muscle representations. Nor do the current results address the contribution of spinal circuits. Although decreases in H-reflex amplitude following prolonged aerobic exercise have been reported in lower limb muscles [17], upper limb muscles are unaffected, indicating that such changes do not represent a generalized decrease in spinal excitability but rather are specific to those muscles involved in locomotion [18]. Additionally, one would expect a change in spinal networks to be reflected in the single pulse excitability. In contrast, emerging evidence suggests that aerobic exercise is uniquely suited to cause a more generalized increase in intracortical excitability following exercise [19-23]. Indeed, a model of a more widespread neural effect of exercise is well-supported. Chronic physical activity is associated with increased activation of regions as diverse as the superior parietal cortex and the dentate gyrus [19], and can modulate everything from pain perception [20] to mood [21]. Further, it is clear that lower limb aerobic exercise can affect vascular functioning in upper limb muscles [22]. Indeed, a single bout of moderate intensity stationary biking can induce a 20% increase in global cerebral blood flow (CBF) [23]. Yet, it has been hypothesized that with limited metabolic resources, exercise may upregulate those regions involved with maintaining exercise [24] which, it is assumed, includes movement-related cortical regions such as M1. Such a global response could be mediated by the supplementary motor area or the prefrontal cortex, both of which have shown increased activity with exercise [25-27].

Role of GABA and clinical significance

The mechanisms that may underlie a more widespread response to exercise are not entirely clear; however, there is strong evidence that exercise can modulate neurotransmission. Acute aerobic exercise has been shown to upregulate the activity and/or release of serotonin (5HT) [28,29], dopamine (DA) [28,30,31], and norepinephrine (NE) [31,32], all of which can modulate the excitability of M1 neurons [33-36]. Exercise-induced increases in blood lactate have shown corresponding increases in M1 excitability [37], while increased uptake of the trophic factor insulin-like growth factor 1 (IGF-1) appears to mediate an increase in neuronal sensitivity and firing rates post-exercise [38]. Both the time course of the exercise-induced changes in excitability and the

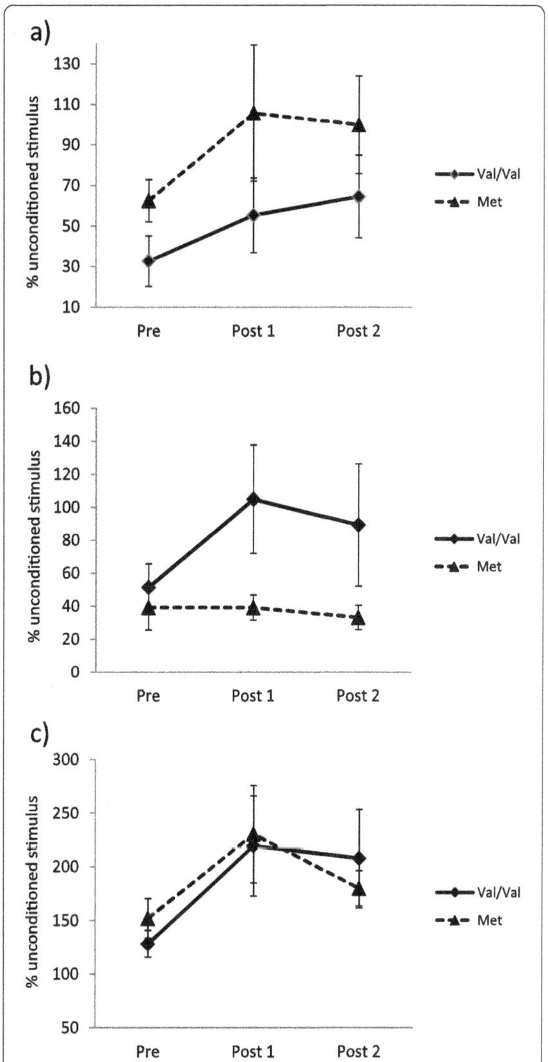

Figure 6 Effect of BDNF genotype on intracortical inhibition and facilitation. Group differences between **a)** Met carriers (n = 6) and non-Met carriers (n = 5) for SICI; **b)** Met carriers (n = 5) and non-Met carriers (n = 6) for LICI, and **c)** Met carriers (n = 6) and non-Met carriers (n = 6) for ICF. Bars represent SEM.

optimal exercise parameters for stimulating the release of neurotrophic factors remain under investigation. While the potential contribution of such excitatory neurotransmitters cannot be discounted here, the current results point to modulations in GABA (γ-aminobutyric acid) as a primary outcome of exercise. GABA is the principal inhibitory neurotransmitter in the CNS and exerts its effects via multiple receptors, particularly in cortical inhibitory networks. SICI is thought to be mediated by $GABA_A$ receptors [39], which are ligand-gated chloride channels, while LICI is believed to activate $GABA_B$ receptors [40], which are coupled to G-protein complexes that activate downstream K^+ ion channels. Although the cortical mechanisms of ICF are not fully understood, it appears to be mediated by glutamatergic interneurons, and possibly NMDA receptors [41,42]. While both LICI and SICI directly affect the excitability of corticospinal neurons, there are also interactions between them, as LICI appears to reduce SICI, likely via GABA-mediated inhibition of GABA-release [39,43]. The current results indicate that SICI is more sensitive to the effects of aerobic exercise than LICI. This is perhaps not surprising given that there appears to be little correlation between SICI and LICI measures [40,43]. Indeed, it has been suggested that $GABA_A$ and $GABA_B$ receptors may differ in their activation thresholds, with $GABA_A$ receptors requiring greater levels of exposure to the neurotransmitter [44]. Another potential reason for this disconnect is the variation in test stimulus intensities, in that SICI and ICF both employ a subthreshold conditioning pulse that is assumed to activate intracortical connections, while LICI requires two suprathreshold pulses, and may therefore be activating a different pool of neurons.

Such intracortical networks are critical to the modulation of cortical output and are implicated in cortical plasticity and reorganization [45]. The release of GABA at inhibitory synapses directly modulates the excitability of pyramidal cells and the current results suggest this process may be sensitive to exercise. There is limited information available on GABA levels immediately following exercise; however, a downregulation of GABA signalling on baroreceptor neurons is thought to contribute to post-exercise hypotension [46]. Further, mRNA levels of a key $GABA_A$ receptor subunit are reduced after only 3 days of exercise training [47]. Meeusen et al. [31] report up to a 76% increase in striatal GABA levels following 60 minutes of treadmill running, although their data did not reach statistical significance. There are considerable clinical implications of an exercise-induced modulation of GABA activity. Decreases in GABA are critical for motor learning and M1 plasticity [48,49]. Indeed, excessive inhibition is a key cause of post-stroke motor impairment [50-52]. GABA blockade removes tonic inhibition and promotes plasticity [53], and indeed, a decrease in GABA levels is key to functional recovery after stroke [53-55]. It is clear that motor reorganization following a brain injury is dependent on functional plasticity. As GABA levels were not directly measured in this study, we cannot determine whether exercise results in changes in GABA release, uptake, or activity, or alters the sensitivity of $GABA_A$ receptors. However, these results indicate that there is a reduction in short-interval intracortical inhibition following aerobic exercise, which is likely mediated by exercise-induced changes in $GABA_A$ activity.

Our results, taken together with previously observed increases in excitatory neurotransmission, indicate that the net effect of exercise appears to be a decrease in M1 inhibition that may facilitate the induction of plasticity. In the current study, these effects are seen immediately after exercise and persist at 30 minutes after exercise completion. Thus, it is possible that the intracortical network changes seen here are a necessary precursor for cortical plasticity, and that exercise creates the conditions under which more permanent plastic changes may occur. The current results indicate that in non-active muscles, exercise alone does not directly affect the resting motor threshold of pyramidal cells, but instead modulates the balance of inhibitory and excitatory inputs to these cells. This is supported by the findings of Smith et al. [23], who despite observing a global increase in CBF following exercise, did not see an observable modulation in M1 until a subsequent motor task was performed. In addition, McDonnell et al. report no changes in MEP amplitude in the FDI muscle following cycling exercise, but instead demonstrate that the effects of theta-burst stimulation (TBS) are potentiated when preceded by exercise [56]. Thus, while exercise may not modulate CST excitability in and of itself, it can potentially create favourable conditions for the induction of cortical plasticity with subsequent motor training. Indeed, aerobic exercise training has been shown to improve motor arm function after stroke [57,58], and the combination of exercise and skilled motor training improves motor recovery to a greater extent than training alone [59].

Thus, in this context, it is perhaps not surprising that the paired-pulse measures here do not correlate with the single-pulse data, in which we observed a decrease in SICI and an increase in ICF, but no concomitant increases in single-pulse MEP amplitude. This would seem to indicate that there is not a direct correlational relationship between these two measures. Previous studies have reported a similar disconnect between single and paired-pulse measures of CST excitability [33,43,60]. Indeed, Ilic et al. [33] propose that single and paired-pulse measures may reflect substantially different mechanisms. The final corticospinal output reflects the summation of all inhibitory and excitatory inputs to the descending neuron, and can be influenced by many factors, both cortical and subcortical. The paired-pulse measures taken here reflect the activity of particular cortical interneuron pools whose activity may be modulated by exercise, but which are only one of a multitude of inputs on the descending motor neuron.

BDNF

As a neurotrophic factor, the relationship between acute exercise and BDNF is not clear. Although increases in levels of serum BDNF have been reported following acute aerobic exercise [61-65], BDNF is known to exert its effects primarily over longer time frames and is correlated with the induction of LTP and postsynaptic modification [66]. Thus, it is unlikely that BDNF levels significantly influenced the response to exercise seen here.

Although not the principal aim of this study, we were interested in exploring the relationship between a relatively common single nucleotide polymorphism of the BDNF gene and exercise-related changes in cortical excitability. The valine-to-methionine substitution at codon 66 of the BDNF gene occurs in approximately 30% of the population [67] and is associated with decreased activity-dependent BDNF release and impaired synaptic and cortical plasticity [10,11,68]. Here, as in the majority of the literature, Val/Met and Met/Met individuals were grouped together and compared to Val/Val subjects. There was no difference between the groups in the S-R curves before or at either time point following exercise. Nor was there any interaction between BDNF and time, indicating that genotype did not influence the response to exercise. Previous studies investigating the response to facilitatory intermittent TBS have reported impairments [68,69] or no difference [70,71] in Met carriers, but methodological differences prevent direct comparisons of these studies. While the current sample size is smaller than in the above studies, a key difference is their use of a technique known to induce LTP-like plasticity. The neurological response to exercise is not well-understood, and as such it is not clear how such changes relate to the mechanisms underlying LTP. In the current study, two interesting trends are evident, in that Met carriers, on average, display a complete abolition of SICI following exercise (Figure 6a). Secondly, Met carriers appear to be more resistant to the modulation of LICI following exercise (Figure 6b). Indeed, the lack of response in this group is likely the reason the overall group effect for LICI failed to reach significance. While preliminary, these trends suggest modulations in $GABA_B$ receptor activity or sensitivity may contribute to the impaired short-term plasticity frequently observed in Met carriers, and warrants further investigation with a larger subject pool. Our aim was to investigate whether Met carriers would still display these exercise-induced effects, and these results suggest that Met carriers display no impairment in the response to exercise-induced modulations in SICI and ICF.

Conclusions

The present results suggest that lower-body focused aerobic activity can modulate cortical excitability in an upper limb muscle and that at the cortical level, exercise may prime the motor cortex for the induction of plasticity. While these findings have potential clinical utility, further research will be required to determine how the relationship between exercise and cortical excitability may be altered by disruptions to the balance of cortical inhibition and facilitation following a brain injury, and how the response to exercise is affected by characteristics such as the location, severity and type of brain injury. However, the current findings support the use of aerobic training as an adjunct to traditional rehabilitation methods. A potential limitation of this study is that EMG data was not collected during the exercise session. Although a lack of upper limb activity was confirmed with offline EMG, there nevertheless remains the slight possibility of upper limb muscle activation during the biking session. A second limitation of this study is the investigation of only one upper limb muscle. However, given that changes in upper limb excitability following lower body aerobic exercise are not well-studied, our goal was to create a comprehensive profile of excitability changes that would be sensitive to modulations in both motor neurons and interneurons. This, combined with the time-sensitive nature of the post-exercise measures, made it difficult to test additional muscles. The generalizability of our findings across the upper limb is an interesting direction for future studies.

Competing interests

The authors declare they have no competing interests.

Authors' contributions

AMS carried out the study and data analysis and drafted the manuscript. RD carried out the genetic analysis and assisted with manuscript preparation. JLN assisted with the study design, data collection, and data analysis. WRS helped to conceive the study, wrote the collection and analysis programs, and critically revised the manuscript. All authors read and approved the final manuscript.

Acknowledgements

The authors thank Philip Marvyn and Ashley Patterson for technical assistance with genotyping. This work was supported by a research grant to WRS from the Natural Sciences and Engineering Research Council of Canada (NSERC).

References

1. Bergen JL, Toole T, Elliott RG, Wallace B, Robinson K, Maitland CG: **Aerobic exercise intervention improves aerobic capacity and movement initiation in Parkinson's disease patients.** *NeuroRehabilitation* 2002, **17**:161–168.
2. Pang MY, Eng JJ, Dawson AS, Gylfadóttir S: **The use of aerobic exercise training in improving aerobic capacity in individuals with stroke: a meta-analysis.** *Clin Rehabil* 2006, **20**:97–111.
3. Mossberg KA, Orlander EE, Norcross JL: **Cardiorespiratory capacity after weight-supported treadmill training in patients with traumatic brain injury.** *Phys Ther* 2008, **88**:77–87.
4. Mackay-Lyons M, McDonald A, Matheson J, Eskes G, Klus M-A: **Dual effects of body-weight supported treadmill training on cardiovascular fitness and walking ability early after stroke: a randomized controlled trial.** *Neurorehabil Neural Repair* 2013, **27**:644–653.
5. McCloskey DP, Adamo DS, Anderson BJ: **Exercise increases metabolic capacity in the motor cortex and striatum, but not in the hippocampus.** *Brain Res* 2001, **891**:168–175.
6. Kleim JA, Cooper NR, VandenBerg PM: **Exercise induces angiogenesis but does not alter movement representations within rat motor cortex.** *Brain Res* 2002, **934**:1–6.
7. Yamaguchi T, Fujiwara T, Liu W, Liu M: **Effects of pedaling exercise on the intracortical inhibition of cortical leg area.** *Exp Brain Res* 2012, **218**:401–406.
8. Feys HM, De Weerdt WJ, Selz BE, Cox Steck GA, Spichiger R, Vereeck LE, Putman KD, Van Hoydonck GA: **Effect of a Therapeutic Intervention for the Hemiplegic Upper Limb in the Acute Phase After Stroke: A Single-Blind, Randomized, Controlled Multicenter Trial.** *Stroke* 1998, **29**:785–792.
9. Wade DT, Langton-Hewer R, Wood VA, Skilbeck CE, Ismail HM: **The hemiplegic arm after stroke: measurement and recovery.** *J Neurol Neurosurg Psychiatry* 1983, **46**:521–524.
10. McHughen SA, Rodriguez PF, Kleim JA, Kleim ED, Marchal Crespo L, Procaccio V, Cramer SC: **BDNF val66met polymorphism influences motor system function in the human brain.** *Cereb Cortex* 2010, **20**:1254–1262.
11. Kleim JA, Chan S, Pringle E, Schallert K, Procaccio V, Jimenez R, Cramer SC: **BDNF val66met polymorphism is associated with modified experience-dependent plasticity in human motor cortex.** *Nat Neurosci* 2006, **9**:735–737.
12. Pattwell SS, Bath KG, Perez-Castro R, Lee FS, Chao MV, Ninan I: **The BDNF Val66Met polymorphism impairs synaptic transmission and plasticity in the infralimbic medial prefrontal cortex.** *J Neurosci* 2012, **32**:2410–2421.
13. Abraham WC, Bear MF: **Metaplasticity: the plasticity of synaptic plasticity.** *Trends Neurosci* 1996, **19**:126–130.
14. Müller JFM, Orekhov Y, Liu Y, Ziemann U: **Homeostatic plasticity in human motor cortex demonstrated by two consecutive sessions of paired associative stimulation.** *Eur J Neurosci* 2007, **25**:3461–3468.
15. Murakami T, Müller-Dahlhaus F, Lu M-K, Ziemann U: **Homeostatic metaplasticity of corticospinal excitatory and intracortical inhibitory neural circuits in human motor cortex.** *J Physiol* 2012, **590**(Pt 22):5765–5781.
16. Takahashi K, Maruyama A, Hirakoba K, Maeda M, Etoh S, Kawahira K, Rothwell JC: **Fatiguing intermittent lower limb exercise influences corticospinal and corticocortical excitability in the nonexercised upper limb.** *Brain Stimul* 2011, **4**:90–96.
17. Racinais S, Girard O, Micallef JP, Perrey S: **Failed excitability of spinal motoneurons induced by prolonged running exercise.** *J Neurophysiol* 2007, **97**:596–603.
18. Motl RW, Dishman RK: **Acute leg-cycling exercise attenuates the H-reflex recorded in soleus but not flexor carpi radialis.** *Muscle Nerve* 2003, **28**:609–614.
19. Hillman CH, Erickson KI, Kramer AF: **Be smart, exercise your heart: exercise effects on brain and cognition.** *Nat Rev Neurosci* 2008, **9**:58–65.
20. Naugle KM, Fillingim RB, Riley JL: **A meta-analytic review of the hypoalgesic effects of exercise.** *J Pain* 2012, **13**:1139–1150.
21. Schneider S, Askew CD, Diehl J, Mierau A, Kleinert J, Abel T, Carnahan H, Strüder HK: **EEG activity and mood in health orientated runners after different exercise intensities.** *Physiol Behav* 2009, **96**:709–716.
22. Green DJ, Maiorana AJ, Cable NT: **Point: exercise training does induce vascular adaptations beyond the active muscle beds.** *J Appl Physiol* 2008, **105**:1002–1004. discussion 1007.
23. Smith JC, Paulson ES, Cook DB, Verber MD, Tian Q: **Detecting changes in human cerebral blood flow after acute exercise using arterial spin labeling: implications for fMRI.** *J Neurosci Methods* 2010, **191**:258–262.
24. Dietrich A: **Transient hypofrontality as a mechanism for the psychological effects of exercise.** *Psychiatry Res* 2006, **145**:79–83.
25. Christensen LOD, Johannsen P, Sinkjaer T, Petersen N, Pyndt HS, Nielsen JB: **Cerebral activation during bicycle movements in man.** *Exp Brain Res* 2000, **135**:66–72.
26. Fukuyama H, Ouchi Y, Matsuzaki S, Nagahama Y, Yamauchi H, Ogawa M, Kimura J, Shibasaki H: **Brain functional activity during gait in normal subjects: a SPECT study.** *Neurosci Lett* 1997, **228**:183–186.
27. Yanagisawa H, Dan I, Tsuzuki D, Kato M, Okamoto M, Kyutoku Y, Soya H: **Acute moderate exercise elicits increased dorsolateral prefrontal activation and improves cognitive performance with Stroop test.** *Neuroimage* 2010, **50**:1702–1710.
28. Kitaoka R, Fujikawa T, Miyaki T, Matsumura S, Fushiki T, Inoue K: **Increased noradrenergic activity in the ventromedial hypothalamus during treadmill running in rats.** *J Nutr Sci Vitaminol (Tokyo)* 2010, **56**:185–190.
29. Gomez-Merino D, Béquet F, Berthelot M, Chennaoui M, Guezennec CY: **Site-dependent effects of an acute intensive exercise on extracellular 5-HT and 5-HIAA levels in rat brain.** *Neurosci Lett* 2001, **301**:143–146.
30. Goekint M, Bos I, Heyman E, Meeusen R, Michotte Y, Sarre S: **Acute running stimulates hippocampal dopaminergic neurotransmission in rats, but has**

no influence on brain-derived neurotrophic factor. *J Appl Physiol* 2012, **112**:535–541.

31. Meeusen R, Smolders I, Sarre S, de Meirleir K, Keizer H, Serneels M, Ebinger G, Michotte Y: **Endurance training effects on neurotransmitter release in rat striatum: an in vivo microdialysis study.** *Acta Physiol Scand* 1997, **159**:335–341.
32. Zouhal H, Jacob C, Delamarche P, Gratas-Delamarche A: **Catecholamines and the effects of exercise, training and gender.** *Sport Med* 2008, **38**:401–423.
33. Ilic TV, Korchounov A, Ziemann U: **Complex modulation of human motor cortex excitability by the specific serotonin re-uptake inhibitor sertraline.** *Neurosci Lett* 2002, **319**:116–120.
34. Herwig U, Bräuer K, Connemann B, Spitzer M, Schönfeldt-Lecuona C: **Intracortical excitability is modulated by a norepinephrine-reuptake inhibitor as measured with paired-pulse transcranial magnetic stimulation.** *Psychopharmacology (Berl)* 2002, **164**:228–232.
35. Plewnia C, Hoppe J, Hiemke C, Bartels M, Cohen LG, Gerloff C: **Enhancement of human cortico-motoneuronal excitability by the selective norepinephrine reuptake inhibitor reboxetine.** *Neurosci Lett* 2002, **330**:231–234.
36. Molina-Luna K, Pekanovic A, Röhrich S, Hertler B, Schubring-Giese M, Rioult-Pedotti M-S, Luft AR: **Dopamine in motor cortex is necessary for skill learning and synaptic plasticity.** *PLoS One* 2009, **4**:e7082.
37. Coco M, Alagona G, Rapisarda G, Costanzo E, Calogero RA, Perciavalle V, Perciavalle V: **Elevated blood lactate is associated with increased motor cortex excitability.** *Somatosens Mot Res* 2010, **27**:1–8.
38. Carro E, Nunez A, Busiguina S, Torres-Aleman I: **Circulating Insulin-Like Growth Factor I Mediates Effects of Exercise on the Brain.** *J Neurosci* 2000, **20**:2926–2933.
39. Chen R: **Interactions between inhibitory and excitatory circuits in the human motor cortex.** *Exp Brain Res* 2004, **154**:1–10.
40. McDonnell MN, Orekhov Y, Ziemann U: **The role of GABA (B) receptors in intracortical inhibition in the human motor cortex.** *Exp Brain Res* 2006, **173**:86–93.
41. Liepert J, Schwenkreis P, Tegenthoff M, Malin J-P: **The glutamate antagonist Riluzole suppresses intracortical facilitation.** *J Neural Transm* 1997, **104**:1207–1214.
42. Ziemann U, Chen R, Cohen LG, Hallett M: **Dextromethorphan decreases the excitability of the human motor cortex.** *Neurology* 1998, **51**:1320–1324.
43. Sanger TD, Garg RR, Chen R: **Interactions between two different inhibitory systems in the human motor cortex.** *J Physiol* 2001, **530**(Pt 2):307–317.
44. Otis TS, Mody I: **Differential activation of GABAA and GABAB receptors by spontaneously released transmitter.** *J Neurophysiol* 1992, **67**:227–235.
45. Chen R, Corwell B, Yaseen Z, Hallett M, Cohen LG: **Mechanisms of Cortical Reorganization in Lower-Limb Amputees.** *J Neurosci* 1998, **18**:3443–3450.
46. Chen C-Y, Bechtold AG, Tabor J, Bonham AC: **Exercise reduces GABA synaptic input onto nucleus tractus solitarii baroreceptor second-order neurons via NK1 receptor internalization in spontaneously hypertensive rats.** *J Neurosci* 2009, **29**:2754–2761.
47. Molteni R, Ying Z, Gomez-Pinilla F: **Differential effects of acute and chronic exercise on plasticity-related genes in the rat hippocampus revealed by microarray.** *Eur J Neurosci* 2002, **16**:1107–1116.
48. Floyer-Lea A, Wylezinska M, Kincses T, Matthews PM: **Rapid modulation of GABA concentration in human sensorimotor cortex during motor learning.** *J Neurophysiol* 2006, **95**:1639–1644.
49. Stagg CJ, Bachtiar V, Johansen-Berg H: **The role of GABA in human motor learning.** *Curr Biol* 2011, **21**:480–484.
50. Classen J: **The motor syndrome associated with exaggerated inhibition within the primary motor cortex of patients with hemiparetic.** *Brain* 1997, **120**:605–619.
51. Honaga K, Fujiwara T, Tsuji T, Hase K, Ushiba J, Liu M: **State of intracortical inhibitory interneuron activity in patients with chronic stroke.** *Clin Neurophysiol* 2013, **124**:364–370.
52. Takeuchi N, Tada T, Toshima M, Ikoma K: **Correlation of motor function with transcallosal and intracortical inhibition after stroke.** *J Rehabil Med* 2010, **42**:962–966.
53. Clarkson AN, Huang BS, Macisaac SE, Mody I, Carmichael ST: **Reducing excessive GABA-mediated tonic inhibition promotes functional recovery after stroke.** *Nature* 2010, **468**:305–309.
54. Lazar RM: **Reemergence of Stroke Deficits With Midazolam Challenge.** *Stroke* 2002, **33**:283–285.
55. Clarkson AN: **Perisynaptic GABA Receptors The Overzealous Protector.** *Adv Pharmacol Sci* 2012, **2012**:708428.
56. McDonnell MN, Buckley JD, Opie GM, Ridding MC, Semmler JG: **A single bout of aerobic exercise promotes motor cortical neuroplasticity.** *J Appl Physiol* 2013, **114**:1174–1182.
57. Potempa K, Lopez M, Braun LT, Szidon JP, Fogg L, Tincknell T: **Physiological outcomes of aerobic exercise training in hemiparetic stroke patients.** *Stroke* 1995, **26**:101–105.
58. Quaney BM, Boyd LA, McDowd JM, Zahner LH, He J, Mayo MS, Macko RF: **Aerobic exercise improves cognition and motor function poststroke.** *Neurorehabil Neural Repair* 2009, **23**:879–885.
59. Ploughman M, Attwood Z, White N, Doré JJE, Corbett D: **Endurance exercise facilitates relearning of forelimb motor skill after focal ischemia.** *Eur J Neurosci* 2007, **25**:3453–3460.
60. Roy FD: **Suppression of EMG activity by subthreshold paired-pulse transcranial magnetic stimulation to the leg motor cortex.** *Exp Brain Res* 2009, **193**:477–482.
61. Gold SM, Schulz K-H, Hartmann S, Mladek M, Lang UE, Hellweg R, Reer R, Braumann K-M, Heesen C: **Basal serum levels and reactivity of nerve growth factor and brain-derived neurotrophic factor to standardized acute exercise in multiple sclerosis and controls.** *J Neuroimmunol* 2003, **138**:99–105.
62. Rojas Vega S, Strüder HK, Wahrmann BV, Schmidt A, Bloch W, Hollmann W: **Acute BDNF and cortisol response to low intensity exercise and following ramp incremental exercise to exhaustion in humans.** *Brain Res* 2006, **21**:59–65.
63. Ferris LT, Williams JS, Shen C-L: **The effect of acute exercise on serum brain-derived neurotrophic factor levels and cognitive function.** *Med Sci Sports Exerc* 2007, **39**:728–734.
64. Rasmussen P, Brassard P, Adser H, Pedersen MV, Leick L, Hart E, Secher NH, Pedersen BK, Pilegaard H: **Evidence for a release of brain-derived neurotrophic factor from the brain during exercise.** *Exp Physiol* 2009, **94**:1062–1069.
65. Griffin ÉW, Mullally S, Foley C, Warmington SA, O'Mara SM, Kelly AM: **Aerobic exercise improves hippocampal function and increases BDNF in the serum of young adult males.** *Physiol Behav* 2011, **104**:934–941.
66. Kovalchuk Y, Hanse E, Kafitz KW, Konnerth A: **Postsynaptic Induction of BDNF-Mediated Long-Term Potentiation.** *Science* 2002, **295**:1729–1734.
67. Shimizu E, Hashimoto K, Iyo M: **Ethnic difference of the BDNF 196G/A (val66met) polymorphism frequencies: the possibility to explain ethnic mental traits.** *Am J Med Genet B Neuropsychiatr Genet* 2004, **126B**:122–123.
68. Cheeran B, Talelli P, Mori F, Koch G, Suppa A, Edwards M, Houlden H, Bhatia K, Greenwood R, Rothwell JC: **A common polymorphism in the brain-derived neurotrophic factor gene (BDNF) modulates human cortical plasticity and the response to rTMS.** *J Physiol* 2008, **586**(Pt 23):5717–5725.
69. Antal A, Chaieb L, Moliadze V, Monte-Silva K, Poreisz C, Thirugnanasambandam N, Nitsche MA, Shoukier M, Ludwig H, Paulus W: **Brain-derived neurotrophic factor (BDNF) gene polymorphisms shape cortical plasticity in humans.** *Brain Stimul* 2010, **3**:230–237. 3.
70. Li Voti P, Conte A, Suppa A, Iezzi E, Bologna M, Aniello MS, Defazio G, Rothwell JC, Berardelli A: **Correlation between cortical plasticity, motor learning and BDNF genotype in healthy subjects.** *Exp Brain Res* 2011, **212**:91–99.
71. Mastroeni C, Bergmann TO, Rizzo V, Ritter C, Klein C, Pohlmann I, Brueggemann N, Quartarone A, Siebner HR: **Brain-derived neurotrophic factor–a major player in stimulation-induced homeostatic metaplasticity of human motor cortex?** *PLoS One* 2013, **8**:e57957.

12

Development of the Brazilian Portuguese version of the Achilles Tendon Total Rupture Score (ATRS BrP): a cross-cultural adaptation with reliability and construct validity evaluation

Roberto Zambelli[1], Rafael Z. Pinto[2,3], João Murilo Brandão Magalhães[1], Fernando Araujo Silva Lopes[1], Rodrigo Simões Castilho[1], Daniel Baumfeld[4], Thiago Ribeiro Teles dos Santos[5] and Nicola Maffulli[6,7*]

Abstract

Background: There is a need for a patient-relevant instrument to evaluate outcome after treatment in patients with a total Achilles tendon rupture. The purpose of this study was to undertake a cross-cultural adaptation of the Achilles Tendon Total Rupture Score (ATRS) into Brazilian Portuguese, determining the test-retest reliability and construct validity of the instrument.

Methods: A five-step approach was used in the cross-cultural adaptation process: initial translation (two bilingual Brazilian translators), synthesis of translation, back-translation (two native English language translators), consensus version and evaluation (expert committee), and testing phase. A total of 46 patients were recruited to evaluate the test-retest reproducibility and construct validity of the Brazilian Portuguese version of the ATRS. Test-retest reproducibility was performed by assessing each participant on two separate occasions. The construct validity was determined by the correlation index between the ATRS and the Orthopedic American Foot and Ankle Society (AOFAS) questionnaires.

Results: The final version of the Brazilian Portuguese ATRS had the same number of questions as the original ATRS. For the reliability analysis, an $ICC_{(2,1)}$ of 0.93 (95 % CI: 0.88 to 0.96) with SEM of 1.56 points and MDC of 4.32 was observed, indicating excellent reliability. The construct validity showed excellent correlation with $R = 0.76$ (95 % CI: 0.52 to 0.89, $P < 0.001$).

Conclusion: The ATRS was successfully cross-culturally validated into Brazilian Portuguese. This version was a reliable and valid measure of function in patients who suffered complete rupture of the Achilles Tendon.

Keywords: Achilles Tendon Total Rupture Score (ATRS), Complete rupture of the Achilles Tendon, Functional questionnaires, Cross-cultural adaptation

* Correspondence: n.maffulli@qmul.ac.uk
[6]Department of Musculoskeletal Disorders, University of Salerno School of Medicine and Surgery, Salerno, Italy
[7]Centre for Sports and Exercise Medicine, Queen Mary University, Mile End Hospital, London, UK
Full list of author information is available at the end of the article

Background

The use of patient-reported questionnaires to estimate functional capacity, pain and limitation in activities of daily living is an important outcome measure to monitor treatment progress in clinical and research settings [1]. The Knee Injury and Osteoarthritis Outcome Score (KOOS) [2] and the Foot and Ankle Outcome Score (FAOS) [3] are examples of patient-reported questionnaires widely used to assess perceived activity limitations in patients with osteoarthritis of the knee and patients with ankle ligament injury respectively. With increasing number of publications from different countries, cross-cultural adaptation of patient-reported questionnaires is essential when the aim is to compare the results of interventions across different populations [4, 5].

Ruptures of the Achilles tendon are relatively common in adults, especially in individuals aged 30–50 years. Men are three to four times more likely to sustain an injury than women [6–8]. The incidence has been reported to vary between 9.9 to 37.3 cases per 100,000 people [6, 9]. The recent increase in incidence has been associated with increased participation in high demand competitive and recreational sports, aging population, lack of fitness and performing strenuous physical activities [10–12]. Another explanation may be the increasing incidence of metabolic and other chronic diseases, which are associated with acute Achilles tendon ruptures [13].

An important tool for evaluation of patients who have suffered a complete rupture of the Achilles tendon is the Achilles Tendon Total Rupture Score (ATRS). The ATRS is a valid questionnaire with high reproducibility and sensitivity for measuring outcome after treatment in patients with total Achilles tendon rupture [14]. The ATRS was originally developed in Swedish, and has been translated and cross-culturally adapted into several languages, including Danish [15], and British English [16, 17].

To facilitate comparison among studies at an international level, cross-cultural adaptation of this questionnaire for the Brazilian population is warranted. The aim of this study was to perform the translation and cross-cultural adaptation of the Achilles Tendon Total Rupture Score (ATRS) into Brazilian Portuguese, and to determine its reproducibility and validity.

Methods

Design

This is a cross sectional study approved by the Ethics and Research Committee of our institution (Hospital Mater Dei, Belo Horizonte, Minas Gerais, Brazil). Patients from three tertiary hospitals were included into this study. All were examined for the purposes of the present study in our centre (Orthopedic Department, Hospital Mater Dei, Belo Horizonte, Minas Gerais, Brazil). All patients gave written informed consent to participate in this study.

Translation

The ATRS is a self-reported questionnaire composed of ten items that reflect the opinion of patients regarding their symptoms, limitations in daily activities and physical activities after a complete rupture of the Achilles tendon. At the end of each question, the patient is given a scale from 0 to 10, where 0 corresponds to more symptoms and greater limitations of physical activity, and 10 indicates no symptoms and limitations. The final score is obtained by the sum of the responses for each item. The ATRS total score ranges from 0 to 100, with higher scores equal to less symptoms and limitations [10] (Additional file 1).

The cross-cultural adaptation of the ATRS was divided into 5 phases: initial translation (two bilingual Brazilian translators), synthesis of translation, back-translation (two native English language translators), consensus version and evaluation (expert committee), and testing phase [4] (Fig. 1). The first phase was the initial translation of the ATRS into the Brazilian-Portuguese, by two Brazilian bilingual translators, who produced two distinct versions, T1 version and T2. Only one of the translators had prior knowledge of the content of questionnaire [18].

The second stage was the synthesis of the translation, where the T1 and T2 versions were discussed with both translators, thus producing a single translation, the T1-2 version.

In the third phase, two bilingual translators, whose native language was English, translated separately the T1-2 version back into English, which results in the BT1 and BT2 versions. These two translators had no previous contact with the original questionnaire. This new translation into English allowed us to identify possible translation errors and grammatical inconsistencies, and was compared with the original version [19, 20].

The fourth phase consisted of the evaluation of all reports by an expert committee, which was composed by the authors of this work. The purpose of this phase was to review all translations to obtain a single version. For that purpose, the semantic equivalence, with regard to the meanings of words, with attention to idioms and colloquialisms, experimental equivalence, meaning to match activities of daily living in different countries and cultures and conceptual equivalence, ensuring the words have the same definition, were evaluated.

The final phase was the testing phase, where the final version of the Brazilian-Portuguese version of the ATRS was administered to 46 patients who suffered a total rupture of the Achilles tendon between the years 2007 and 2012 in 3 private hospitals in MG, Brazil. After answering the questionnaire, patients were asked about the

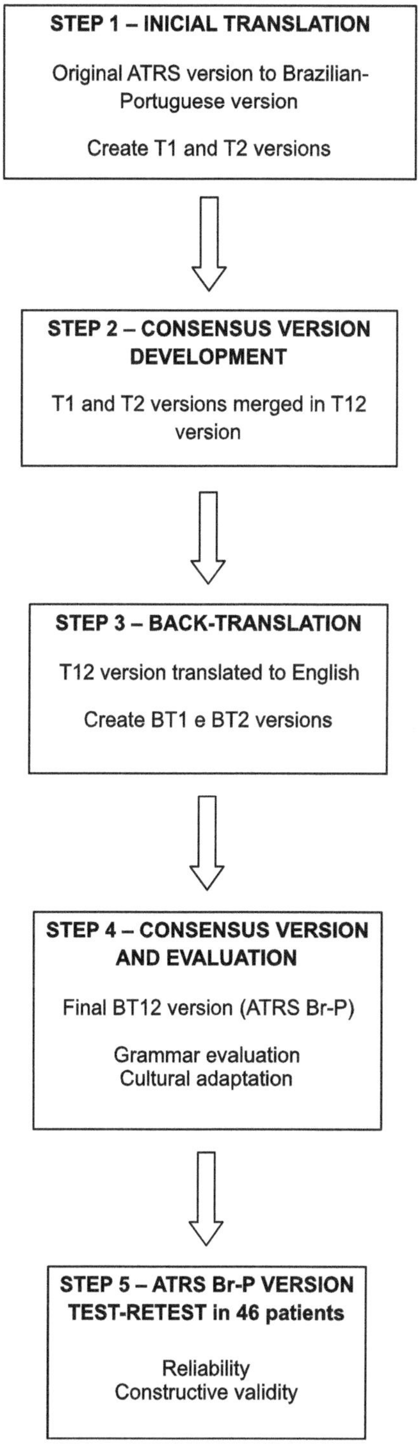

Fig. 1 Five-step approach used to translate the Achilles Tendon Total Rupture Score (ATRS)

difficulty of interpreting the questions or any other limitation in understanding the questionnaire.

Test-retest reproducibility

This test-retest reproducibility of the Brazilian Portuguese version of the ATRS was conducted with a minimum interval of one week and a maximum interval of two months for each patient. The coefficient of Intra-Class Correlation (ICC) type 2,1 was used to determine the reproducibility of ATRS. The strength of agreement was classified using the following benchmarks: poor reproducibility for values below 0.40, good reproducibility for values between 0.40 and 0.75, and excellent reproducibility for those values above 0.75 [21]. We also calculated the standard error of the measurement (SEM) and the minimal detectable change (MDC) as additional measures. The SEM and MDC were calculated as follows: $SEM = s\sqrt{1 - ICC}$ (where s is the standard deviation of the baseline) [21] and $MDC = 1.96 \times \sqrt{2} \times SEM$, respectively [14, 22]. The SEM reflects the error of the instrument; and the MDC reflects the smallest within-person change in a score that, with $p < 0.05$, can be interpreted as a "real" change, above the measurement error.

Validity

The construct validity, which is the ability of the instrument to measure an abstract concept, [21] in this case, functional limitation, was determined by the Pearson coefficient between the ATRS and Orthopedic American Foot and Ankle Society (AOFAS) questionnaire for the hindfoot. The AOFAS questionnaire, already translated into Portuguese, was developed to evaluate the different anatomic regions of the foot, including the ankle and hindfoot. The questionnaire consists of nine items, divided into three categories: pain (40 points), functional aspects (50 points) and alignment (10 points), totaling 100 points [23]. In the analysis of construct validity, the Pearson correlation coefficient was calculated and its 95 % confidence interval estimated using bootstrapping (1000 samples). Pearson correlation coeficient were interpreted as follow: values between 0.00 and 0.25 indicate little or no correlation, between 0.25 and 0.50 indicate low correlation, between 0.50 and 0.75 a moderate correlation, above 0.75 indicate excellent correlation [24].

To characterize the sample, the mean (range) for age, median (interquartile range) for time of assessment after surgery, and frequency for gender and limb affected were calculated. Mean and standard deviation as well as median and interquartile range were reported for ATRS data. Sample size calculation followed the proposed method by Walter et al. [25] for reliability studies. Based on an expected ICC of 0.85, two measures per participant on two separate days and accepting at least moderate reliability coefficient (ICC = 0.7), a total of 46 participants was required. Wilcoxon paired test was used to compare test-retest data since the score presents in ordinal data. Independent t test and Chi square test were used to compare groups for age, gender and ATRS variables, respectively. IBM SPSS (IBM Corporation, Somers, NY) software 18.0 version was used for all statistical analyses.

Results

Forty-six patients with complete rupture of the Achilles Tendon were recruited. This group of patients was composed of 39 men (84.7 %) and 7 women (15.3 %), with the left lower limb being slightly more frequently affected (52 %). The average age of participants was 49 (range: 26–63) years. The median (interquatile range) time of assessment was 32.5 (26) months after the surgery.

During the process of translation and cultural adaptation of the ATRS, none of the patients assessed had doubts while answering the questionnaire, considering it self-explanatory, easy to understand and adapted to activities of daily living. No question was modified after the formal testing of the questionnaire, and the T1-2 version was considered the final version in Brazilian Portuguese of ATRS (Additional file 2).

From the total population sample, we analyzed data from 41 individuals undergoing test-retest after suffering total rupture of the Achilles Tendon. Five patients did not undergo the retest session, because we could not contact them or because they refused to answer the questionnaire again. For the reproducibility analysis, an $ICC_{(2,1)}$ of 0.93 (95 % CI: 0.88 to 0.96) with SEM of 1.56 points and MDC of 4.32 was observed, indicating excellent reproducibility (Table 1).

Figure 2 shows the results for construct validity of the Brazilian-Portuguese version of the ATRS using the AOFAS score of 46 patients for the study as a reference. Using the Pearson correlation coefficient, we obtained an excellent correlation with $r = 0.76$ (95 % CI: 0.52 to 0.89), ($P < 0.001$).

Discussion

The most important finding of the present study is that, during the process of cross-cultural adaptation to Brazilian-Portuguese of the ATRS, no significant changes in any of the questions were needed. Patients were able to interpret all questions and understand the functional activities included in the questionnaire. The Brazilian-Portuguese version of the ATRS showed to be a reliable and valid tool to be used in the Brazilian population.

Table 1 Test-retest reproducibility– Portuguese-Brazilian version of Achilles Tendon Total Rupture Score (ATRS)

ATRS ($n = 41$)	First session	Second session	Wilcoxon paired test (p-value)	$ICC_{(2,1)}$ (95 % CI)
Mean (median)	94.3 (96)	93.8 (95)	0.2	0.93 (0.88 to 0.96)
SD (IQR)	5.9 (9.0)	6.1 (9.5)		

SD standard deviation, *IQR* interquartile range, *ICC* intraclasscorrelation coeficiente, *CI* confidence interval

The reproducibility index found in this study is similar to the original version of the ATRS (ICC = 0.98), [10] the Danish version (ICC = 0.91), [15] and the British English version (ICC = 0.98) [16]. The MDC of 4.3 reported in this study was smaller than the one reported among the British English population [16] (MDC = 6.8), meaning that, to detect true change in the Brazilian population, clinicians should expect a difference of at least 4.3 between different time points.

The construct validity analysis showed an excellent correlation between the ATRS and the AOFAS with a Pearson coefficient of 0.76 (95 % CI: 0.52 to 0.89). Other questionnaires culturally adapted into Brazilian Portuguese have shown similar results for the analysis of construct validity. For instance, a study investigating the psychometric properties of the Brazilian Portuguese version of the Foot Health Status Questionnaire (FHSQ) found that five out of eight domains on the FHSQ were significantly correlated with Health Assessment Questionnaire and Numeric Rating Scale [19]. Similarly, the Brazilian Portuguese version of the American Orthopedic Foot and Ankle Society (AOFAS) Ankle-hindfoot scale showed moderate correlation with pain ($r = 0.64$, $p < 0.01$) and functional capacity ($r = 0.67$, $p < 0.01$) domains [23].

The present study has some limitations. Firstly, the time between the test and retest sessions was not the same for all patients. Patients were assessed with a minimum interval of one week or a maximum interval of two months. Some would argue that long intervals could have had a negative impact on the reproducibility index. However, the excellent reproducibility found in this study could be explained by the fact that the majority of patients were assessed at least one year after the surgery. At this point in time, patients might be less prone to change as improvements in functional level are expected, in most cases, in the early stages after surgery. Secondly, the only two psychometric properties investigated were reproducibility and construct validity. Future studies investigating other properties such as responsiveness and internal consistency are needed to study these properties in our Brazilian population.

Conclusion

The cultural adaptation of the ATRS into Brazilian Portuguese showed that the new version is easy to apply, self-explanatory and with good ability to assess the functional limitations of patients who suffered a complete rupture of the Achilles tendon. This version will allow Brazilian clinicians to reliably compare the results of their

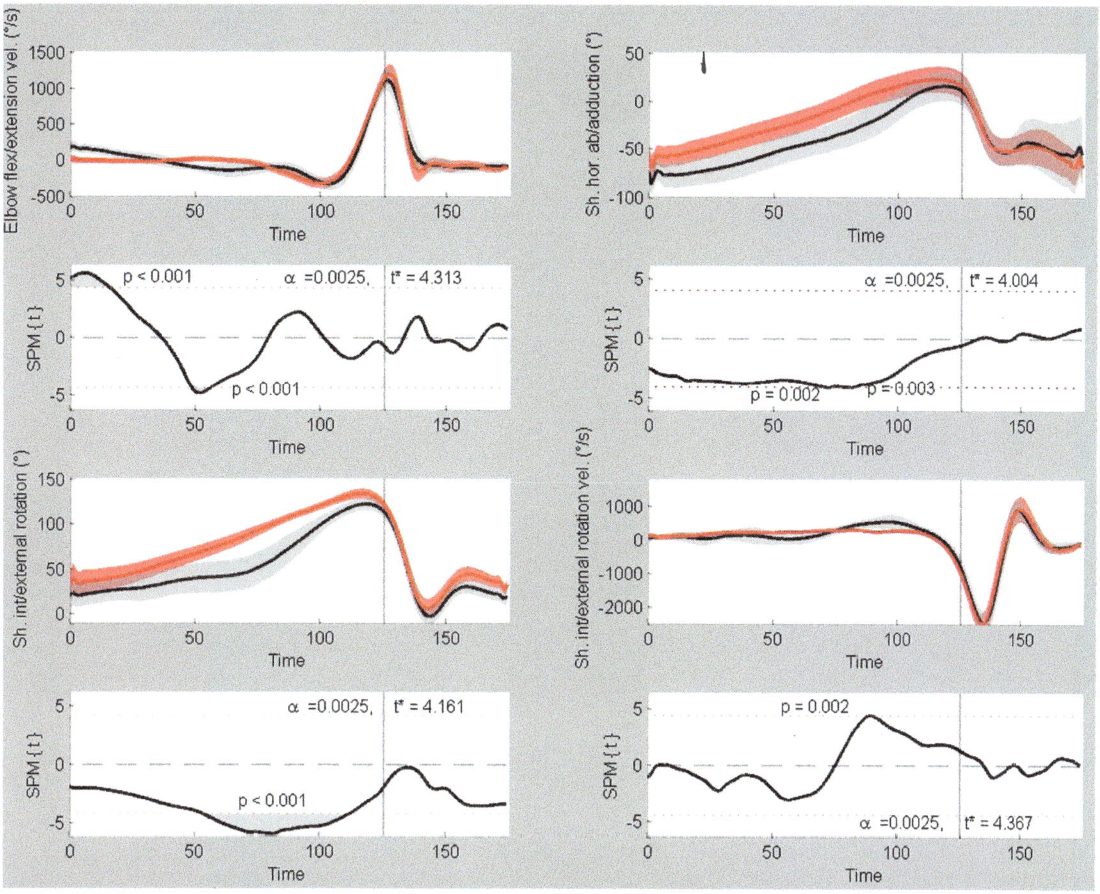

Fig. 4 Shoulder and elbow kinematics. Mean ± SD time series with their respective SPM{t} fields below them for elbow flexion(−)/extension(+) velocity (upper left figure), shoulder horizontal ab(−)/adduction(+) (upper right figure), shoulder internal(−)/external(+) rotation (lower left figure) and shoulder internal(−)/external(+) rotation velocity (lower right figure). Black = male, red = female

could be caused by the differences in body seize. It is possible that the different throwing patterns are the result of specific optimization strategies under the constraints of anthropometric features. Nevertheless, the observed differences can suggest important kinematic features to explain the throwing mechanics and can later be used to design intervention studies. This is not to say that the mean male throwing pattern was better than the female throwing pattern and that athletes should try to imitate a 'role model pattern'. If these throwing kinematics are in fact influenced by the anthropometric profile, gender-specific guidelines for coordination- and strength training might be in order.

The trunk endo/exorotation velocity time series revealed an interesting gender difference. The higher exorotation velocity in the preparation phase, which was absent for female players, could be a strategy to apply a pre-stretch on the oblique abdominal muscles leading to a more explosive trunk endorotation. Trunk endorotation velocity was indeed higher for male players, but did not reach statistical significance. This result can be compared with the results of Wagner et al. [18] who found significant and positive correlations between ball release speeds and maximal trunk endorotation velocity ($r = 0.78$) and maximal trunk exorotation angle ($r = 0.65$). A second gender difference for trunk kinematics was found in trunk flexion/extension velocity during the acceleration phase. The female players exhibited a higher trunk flexion velocity and their timing (onset and maximal velocity) was earlier. Male players reached their peak trunk flexion velocity nearly at ball release, whereas the female players were already accelerating towards trunk extension (countermotion movement).

Elbow angular velocity showed two significant clusters in the preparation phase. Many studies illustrated the importance of maximal elbow extension velocity and

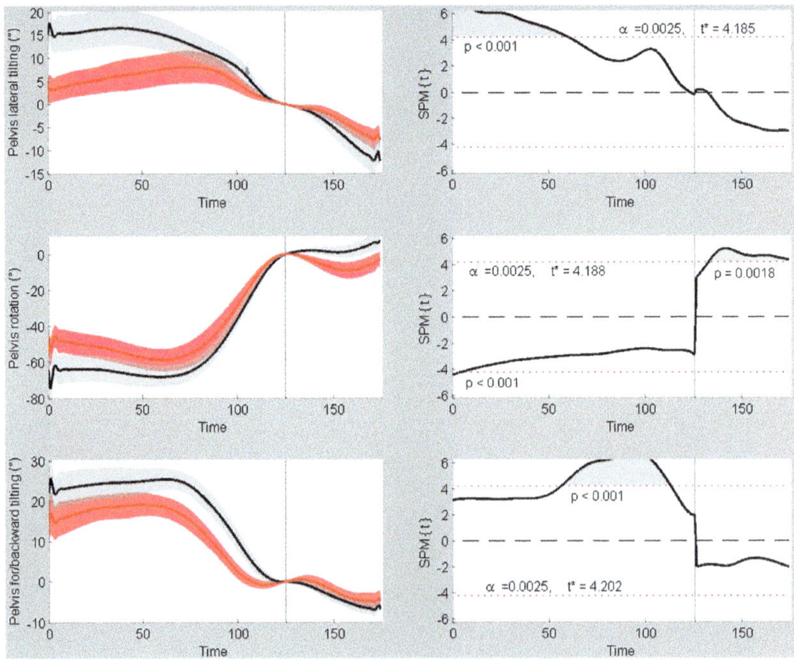

Fig. 5 Pelvis kinematics (angles). Mean ± SD time series with their respective SPM{t} fields beside them for pelvis left(−)/right(+) tilting (upper figure), pelvis outward(−)/inward(+) rotation (middle figure) and pelvis forward(−)/backward(+) tilting (lower figure). Black = male, red = female

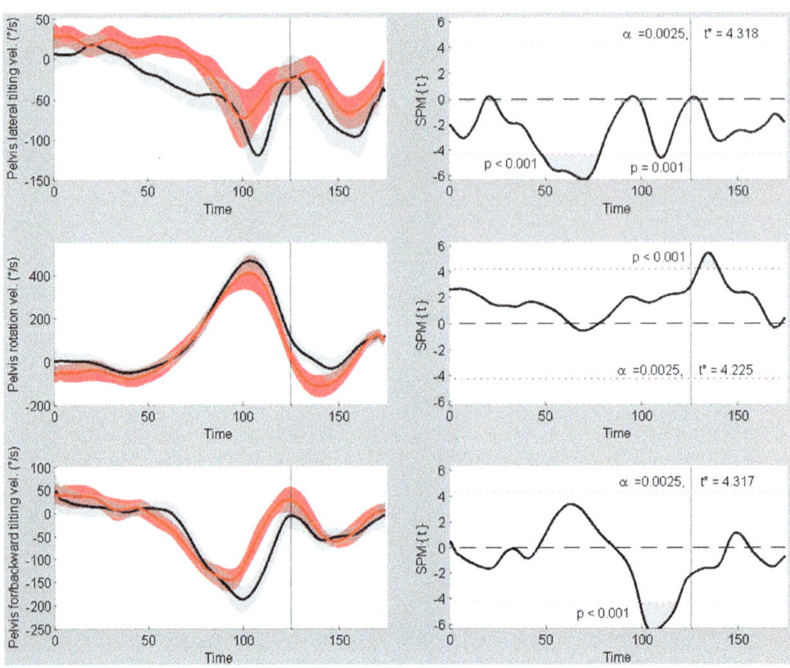

Fig. 6 Pelvis kinematics (angular velocities). Mean ± SD time series with their respective SPM{t} fields beside them for pelvis left(−)/right(+) tilting velocity (upper figure), pelvis outward(−)/inward(+) rotation velocity (middle figure) and pelvis forward(−)/backward(+) tilting velocity (lower figure). Black = male, red = female

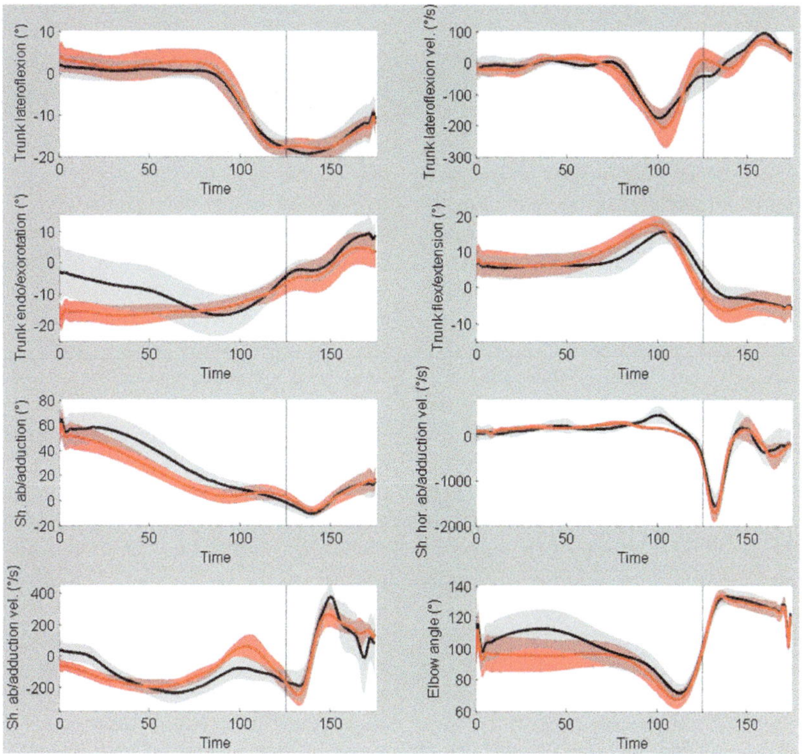

Fig. 7 Other kinematic variables. Mean ± SD time series for trunk left(−)/right(+) tilting, trunk left(−)/right(+) tilting velocity, trunk endo(+)/exorotation (−), trunk flexion(−)/extension(+), shoulder ab(+)/adduction(−), shoulder horizontal ab(+)/adduction(−) velocity, shoulder ab(−)/adduction(+) velocity and elbow flexion/extension(full extension = 180°)

elbow extension velocity at ball release [18, 23], but in this study, we were unable to find differences in elbow extension velocity in the acceleration phase. Another variable that is frequently reported in literature to be associated with higher ball release speeds is maximal shoulder endorotation velocity (or velocity at ball release) [18, 23, 26]. We found a difference between the two shoulder rotation velocity curves, but not during the maximal values or around ball release. Figure 4 shows that right before the onset of shoulder endorotation velocity, the male players had a short-term and small-in-magnitude exorotation velocity. This whip-like motion in the throwing shoulder did not lead to higher shoulder endorotation velocities however and thus could not have contributed to ball release speed.

Male players had higher shoulder horizontal abduction angles during the cocking phase, which gives a larger pre-stretch on the Pectoralis Major - and anterior Deltoid muscle fibers. This potential energy created by decelerating the horizontal shoulder abduction motion can be used to accelerate the ball. In shoulder rotation, we see that female players having higher exorotation angles during the cocking phase (pre-stretch on Pectoralis Major and Subscapularis muscles), indicating the difference in the arm cocking maneuver.

All angles and angular velocities describing the pelvis motion reached a significant gender difference at a given point during the time series. Inter-individual differences in approach angle were spatially normalized by expressing all pelvis angles in function of its orientation at ball release (=0°). Pelvis lateral tilting to the right (counter-motion tilt) was higher for male players during the preparation phase. Right thereafter, a significant cluster of pelvis leftward tilting velocity (higher for male players) was present. Also around the peak pelvis left tilt velocity, a significant cluster indicated higher values for male players and this peak was located much closer to ball release than for female players. Pelvis rotation showed a significant gender difference after ball release speed, indicating that female players, after ball release, did not exhibit a follow through pelvis rotation. Their pelvis started to rotate backward in exorotation. This is probably because of the lower pelvis rotation velocity during the acceleration phase (although this was not significant). Van den Tillaar & Ettema [26] found a correlation (r = 0.84) between timing of maximal pelvis rotation angle (countermotion angle) and ball release speed, this was confirmed by Wagner et al. [18], r = 0.64. We could not find a difference at this location in time with our sample. Wagner et al. [18] also found a high correlation (r = 0.72) between ball release speed and maximal pelvis internal rotation velocity. Male players had higher pelvis backward tilting angles and higher pelvis forward tilting velocities than female players. The onset of forward pelvis tilting appears to occur around the same time, but the maximal forward pelvis tilting velocity for males occurs closer to ball release. The fact that all pelvis kinematics were significantly different, suggests, that this is a very important segment within the chain of motion. The pelvis serves as a connection between the motion of the legs and the motion of the trunk. A stable, but fast rotating pelvis is necessary for the trunk, the pelvis is used as a base whereon the trunk can start its rotation. Saeterbakken et al. [27] examined the effect of core-stability training on throwing velocity in female team-handball players and found an increased velocity after 6 weeks. They proposed that a stronger and more stable lumbopelvic-hip complex may contribute to higher rotational velocity in multi-segmental movements. However, they did not measure the kinematics of the pelvis (and trunk) motions. This would be a very interesting topic and can give more insights into the actual role of the pelvis.

From the previous discussion, it is clear that male and females throwers differ in generating momentum and transferring it from the ground through the kinematic chain towards the throwing arm and finally to the ball (we did not study the kinematics of the final joint, the wrist). Male team-handball players showed more activity in the transverse plane (pelvis and trunk rotation and shoulder horizontal abduction) whereas female team-handball players showed more activity in the sagittal plane (trunk flexion). An important aspect in the transfer of momentum is proximal-to-distal sequencing [8–10]. An analysis with SPM offers many advantages (no data reduction and thus no directed hypothesis testing and an easier graphical way to communicate results of 1D time series), but a clear distinction within a cluster, of differences in magnitudes or timing would need post-hoc scalar tests. The team-handball specific proximal-to-distal sequence as indicated by maximal joint velocities (starting with pelvis rotation, followed by trunk rotation, trunk flexion, elbow extension, shoulder horizontal adduction and shoulder internal rotation) was also observed in our data as illustrated in Fig. 8. Most gender differences were observed in the early and late preparation phases of the throw. This period is probably the most important, because in this phase, the build-up of momentum from the pelvis and trunk (with their large masses) is maximal. At the end of the preparation phase, the reversal of the torques working on the pelvis and trunk will create a torque on the shoulder [28] and the transfer of momentum to the throwing arm will occur. Even more gender differences might be apparent in the standing throw with run-up, but did we not detect them. We have set our significance threshold at a fairly conservative level (Bonferroni correction; indicating 20 independent variables, which is of course not the case). This needs to be taken into account when interpreting the results, because within a kinematic chain, all variables have a time-varying covariance and are thus not independent. Further research needs to be done to determine these interrelations between variables.

The standing throw with run-up that was analyzed in this study is the second most popular throwing technique (14–18 %) in team-handball [29], but it is the throwing technique which produces the highest ball release speed [18]. In future studies, this gender difference should be confirmed in the jump shot which is the most popular throwing technique in team-handball games [29]. An additional limitation of this study is the low sample size, only 10 players from each gender participated. In future studies, this number should be higher to extrapolate to a larger population. This study was situated within a deterministic framework [11] where we studied differences in kinematic time series and ball release speed. Future studies are needed to assess see if these differences are caused by the anthropometric profile and if they can be used to increase throwing speed. The relationships among all variables are not taken into account and are not studied in one statistical test. Multivariate techniques in SPM can be a solution to this problem and will be a very interesting research area in the future. Also other techniques in the field of mechanics such as Induced Acceleration Analysis [30] and in the field of pattern recognition such as Neural Networks [31, 32] could give further insights into throwing mechanics and coordination in team-handball and other overhead throwing sports.

Conclusions

We can conclude that, in contrast to previous research [4], gender differences in throwing kinematics are present. The exact nature of the role of kinematics in the relation between anthropometric profile and ball speed still remains unclear. Differences were found in the orientation and velocities of pelvis, trunk, shoulder and elbow kinematic time series. We could say that male players showed more activity in the transverse plane while female players showed more activity in the sagital plane. Based on our results, the motion of the pelvis may be serving as a more important segment than was previously stated. As stated by Wagner et al. [12],

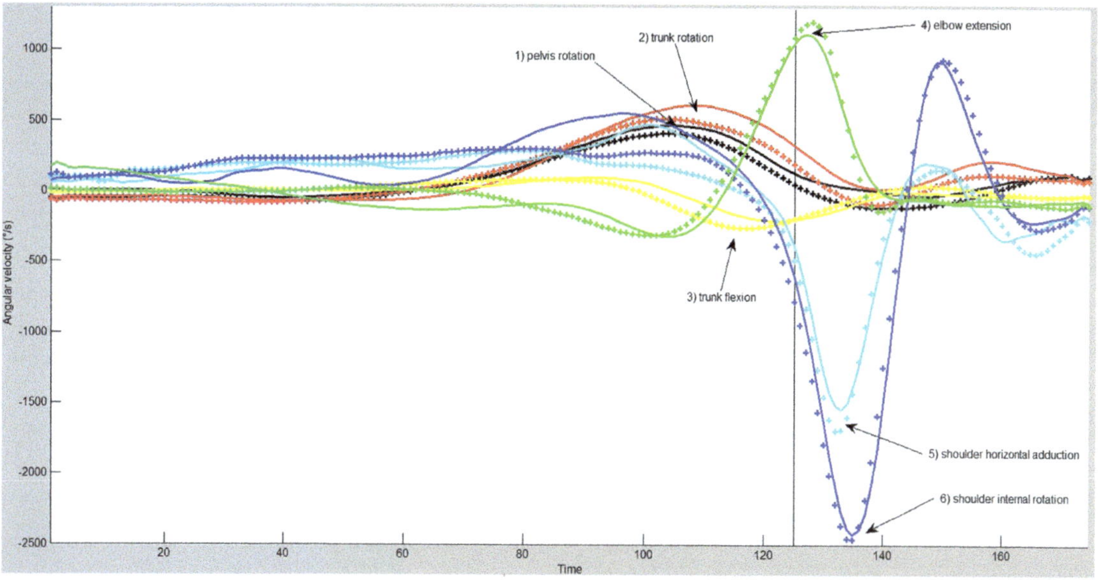

Fig. 8 Proximal-to-distal sequencing in male (---) and female (+++) team-handball throwing in terms of angular velocity profiles. The sequence of the maximal angular velocities follows the typical team-handball proximal-to-distal sequence of pelvis rotation, trunk rotation, trunk flexion, elbow extension, shoulder horizontal adduction and shoulder internal rotation

coaches can easily observe the motions of pelvis and trunk because these are the largest segments and rotate at a relatively lower angular velocity. Coordination training (especially in youth training) should focus more on pelvis and trunk motions. Also, future research should examine the effect of different types of training such as core-stability/core-strength training and differential training on pelvis- and trunk kinematics to establish a causal link between differences in throwing pattern and differences in ball release speed.

Statistical Parametric Mapping clearly offers an advantage for sports biomechanics, because it allows us to use the entire data-sets and thus, more differences may be observed that would slip past researchers if they would extract only minima/maxima.

Competing interests

The authors report no competing interests.

Authors' contributions

RC and JPB performed the measurements and coordinated the study. BS and JB prepared the raw data in VICON Nexus and Mathcad software. BS performed the statistical analysis with help from MG. BS drafted the first version of the manuscript and all authors were involved in reviewing for substantive and grammatical adjustments and approved the final manuscript.

Acknowledgements

The authors wish to thank all players that participated in this study and the help of the following students in performing the measurements: Dominique Senn, Miryam Leyrer, Kenny Bosmans, Martina Buël and Judith Odermatt.

Author details

[1]Department Biomechanics, Vrije Universiteit Brussel, Brussels, Belgium. [2]Thim Van Der Laan University College, Landquart, Switzerland. [3]University of Antwerp, ICT-electronics, Antwerp, Belgium. [4]Department Health Sciences, University of Applied Sciences and Arts of Southern Switzerland, Landquart, Switzerland.

References

1. International Handball Federation. 2014. https://en.wikipedia.org/wiki/Handball. Accessed 20 Dec 2014
2. Jöris HJJ, Edwards van Muyen AJ, van Ingen Schenau GJ, Kemper HCG. Force, velocity and energy flow during the overarm throw in female handball players. J Biomech. 1985;18:409–14.
3. van den Tillaar R, Ettema G. Effect of body size and gender in overarm throwing performance. Eur J Appl Physiology. 2004;91:413–8.
4. van den Tillaar R, Cabri JMH. Gender differences in the kinematics and ball velocity of overarm throwing in elite team handball players. J Sports Sci. 2012;30:807–13.
5. van den Tillaar R, Ettema G. Influence of instruction on velocity and accuracy of overarm throwing. Percept Mot Skills. 2003;96:423–34.
6. van den Tillaar R, Ettema G. A comparison between novices and experts of the velocity-accuracy trade-off in overarm throwing. Percept Mot Skills. 2006;103:503–14.
7. Wagner H, Finkenzeller T, Würth S, von Duvillard SP. Individual and team performance in team-handball: A review. J Sports Sci Med. 2014;13:808–16.
8. Fradet L, Botcazou M, Durocher C, Cretual A, Multon F, Prioux J, et al. Do handball throws always exhibit a proximal-to-distal segmental sequence? J Sports Sci. 2004;22:439–47.
9. van den Tillaar R, Ettema G. Is there a proximal-to-distal sequence in overarm throwing in team handball? J of Sports Sci. 2009;27:949–55.
10. Wagner H, Pfusterschmied J, von Duvillard SP, Müller E. Skill-dependent proximal-to-distal sequence in team-handball throwing. J Sports Sci. 2012;30:21–9.

11. Chow JW, Knudson DV. Use of deterministic models in sports and exercise biomechanics research. Sports Biomech. 2011;10:219–33.
12. Wagner H, Buchecker M, von Duvillard SP, Müller E. Kinematic description of elite vs. low level players in team-handball jump throw. J Sports Sci Med. 2010;9:15–23.
13. Ohnjec K, Antekolović L, Gruić I. Comparison of kinematic parameters of jump shot performance by female handball players of different ages. Acta Kinesiologica. 2010;4:33–40.
14. Wagner H, Pfusterschmied J, Tilp M, Landlinger J, von Duvillard SP, Müller E. Upper-body kinematics in team-handball throw, tennis serve, and volleyball spike. Scand J Med Sci Sports. 2014;24:345–54.
15. van den Tillaar R, Ettema G. A comparison of overarm throwing with the dominant and non-dominant arm in experienced team-handball players. Perceptual Motor Skills. 2009;109:315–26.
16. van den Tillaar R, Ettema G. A Comparison of Kinematics Between Overarm Throwing With 20 % Underweight, Regular, and 20 % Overweight Balls. J Appl Biomech. 2011;27:252–7.
17. Wagner H, Buchecker M, von Duvillard SP, Müller E. Kinematic comparison of team-handball throwing with two different arm positions. Int J Sports Physiology and Performance. 2010;5:469–83.
18. Wagner H, Pfusterschmied J, von Duvillard SP, Müller E. Performance and kinematics of various throwing techniques in team-handball. J Sports Sci Med. 2011;10:73–80.
19. van den Tillaar R, Zondag A, Cabri JMH. Comparing performance and kinematics of throwing with a circular and whip-like wind up by experienced handball players. Scand J Med Sci Sports. 2013;23:e373–80. doi:10.1111/sms.
20. Friston KJ, Ashburner JT, Kiebel SJ, Nichols TE, Penny WD. Statistical Parametric Mapping: The analysis of functional brain images. Amsterdam: Elsevier/Academic Press; 2007.
21. Pataky TC, Robinson MA, Vanrenterghem J. Vector field statistical analysis of kinematic and force trajectories. J Biomech. 2013;46:2394–401.
22. Adler RJ, Taylor JE. Random Fields and Geometry. New York: Springer-Verslag; 2007.
23. van den Tillaar R, Ettema G. Force-velocity relationship and coordination patterns in overarm throwing. J Sports Sci Med. 2004;3:211–9.
24. Robertson G, Caldwell G, Hamill J, Kamen G, Whittlesey S. Research Methods in Biomechanics. 2nd ed. Leeds: Human Kinetic; 2014.
25. Pataky TC, Vanrenterghem J, Robinson MA. Two-way ANOVA for scalar trajectories with experimental evidence of non-phasic interactions. J Biomech 2014. doi:10.1016/j.jbiomech.2014.10.013.
26. van den Tillaar R, Ettema G. A Three-Dimensional Analysis of Overarm Throwing in Experienced Handball Players. J Appl Biomech. 2007;23:12–9.
27. Saeterbakken AH, van den Tillaar R, Seiler S. Effect of core-stability training on throwing velocity in female handball players. J Strength and Conditioning Res. 2011;25:712–8.
28. Herring RM, Chapman AE. Effects of changes in segmental values in timing of both torque and torque reversal in simulated throws. J Biomech. 1992;25:1173–84.
29. Wagner H, Kainrath S, Müller E. Koordinative und taktische Anforderungen beim Torwurf im Handball. Der Zusammenhang von Leistungsniveau, Qualität der Wurfbewegung und ausgewählten technisch-taktischen Parametern. Leistungssport. 2008;38:35–42.
30. Hirashima M, Yamanec K, Nakamura Y, Ohtsuki T. Kinetic chain of overarm throwing in terms of joint rotations revealed by induced acceleration analysis. J Biomech. 2008;41:2874–83.
31. Bauer HU, Schöllhorn W. Self-organizing maps for the analysis of complex movement patterns. Neural Process Lett. 1997;5:193–9.
32. Lamb PF, Bartlett RM, Robins A. Artificial neural networks for analyzing inter-limb coordination: The golf chip shot. Hum Mov Sci. 2011;30:1129–43.

16

Cutaneous stimulation of discrete regions of the sole during locomotion produces "sensory steering" of the foot

E Paul Zehr[1,7,8,9*], Tsuyoshi Nakajima[2], Trevor Barss[1,7,8], Taryn Klarner[1,7,8], Stefanie Miklosovic[1], Rinaldo A Mezzarane[3,4,6], Matthew Nurse[5] and Tomoyoshi Komiyama[6]

Abstract

Background: While the neural and mechanical effects of whole nerve cutaneous stimulation on human locomotion have been previously studied, there is less information about effects evoked by activation of discrete skin regions on the sole of the foot. Electrical stimulation of discrete foot regions evokes position-modulated patterns of cutaneous reflexes in muscles acting at the ankle during standing but data during walking are lacking. Here, non-noxious electrical stimulation was delivered to five discrete locations on the sole of the foot (heel, and medial and lateral sites on the midfoot and forefoot) during treadmill walking. EMG activity from muscles acting at the hip, knee and ankle were recorded along with movement at these three joints. Additionally, 3 force sensing resistors measuring continuous force changes were placed at the heel, and the medial and lateral aspects of the right foot sole. All data were sorted based on stimulus occurrence in twelve step-cycle phases, before being averaged together within a phase for subsequent analysis.

Methods: Non-noxious electrical stimulation was delivered to five discrete locations on the sole of the foot (heel, and medial and lateral sites on the midfoot and forefoot) during treadmill walking. EMG activity from muscles acting at the hip, knee and ankle were recorded along with movement at these three joints. Additionally, 3 force sensing resistors measuring continuous force changes were placed at the heel, and the medial and lateral aspects of the right foot sole. All data were sorted based on stimulus occurrence in twelve step-cycle phases, before being averaged together within a phase for subsequent analysis.

Results: The results demonstrate statistically significant dynamic changes in reflex amplitudes, kinematics and foot sole pressures that are site-specific and phase-dependent. The general trends demonstrate responses producing decreased underfoot pressure at the site of stimulation.

Conclusions: The responses to stimulation of discrete locations on the foot sole evoke a kind of "sensory steering" that may promote balance and maintenance of locomotion through the modulation of limb loading and foot placement. These results have implications for using sensory stimulation as a therapeutic modality during gait retraining (e.g. after stroke) as well as for footwear design and implementation of foot sole contact surfaces during gait.

* Correspondence: pzehr@uvic.ca
[1]Rehabilitation Neuroscience Laboratory, University Victoria, PO Box 3010 STN CSC, Victoria, BC V8W 3P1, Canada
[7]Human Discovery Science, International Collaboration on Repair Discoveries (ICORD), Vancouver, BC, Canada
Full list of author information is available at the end of the article

Background

Somatosensory feedback serves as a crucial means of communication between the environment and the central nervous system. There is a dynamic interaction between many different types of receptors in the lower limb including: nociceptors, muscle and skeletal mechanoreceptors, as well as cutaneous and subcutaneous mechanoreceptors [1,2]. Although all play relevant roles in locomotion, the activities of cutaneous and subcutaneous plantar reflex pathways are particularly important to ascertain in what way activation of cutaneous regions may differentially modulate pressure under the foot.

The role sensory feedback plays in sculpting human locomotion incorporates complex functional reflex modulation [3]. Reflexes have functional roles in locomotion that demonstrate context-dependent behavioural relevance. Reflex amplitudes (and thus the role of sensory input) are dependent upon task (standing vs. walking), stimulus intensity (nociceptive vs. non-nociceptive), and phase of movement (heel contact vs. stance to swing transition). The precise modulation of walking that is generated by cutaneous input from the foot depends upon the nerve that is stimulated [4,5]. Additionally, removal of the "normal" sensation from the skin of the foot alters muscle activation and gait mechanics [6]. Thus, cutaneous afferent feedback is suggested to assist in balance regulation and ensure proper foot placement during the stance phase [3,7,8].

There is a distinct nerve or location specificity of cutaneous reflexes. Activation of the foot dorsum, the lateral foot margin (sural nerve) and the plantar foot surface (tibial nerve) show differential responses [4,5,9-11]. In particular, receptors in the foot sole are the unseen sensory organs through which we perceive the ground during locomotion. Due to a high concentration of receptors including Meissner's corpuscles, Merkel disk receptors, Ruffini endings, and Pacinian corpuscles, the glaborous skin of the plantar foot is sensitive to tactile input throughout the step cycle.

With electrical stimulation of the tibial nerve at tactile intensities, enhanced ankle dorsiflexion occurs at the stance to swing transition while ankle plantar flexion can be enhanced at swing to stance transition [4,10,12]. Non-nociceptive stimulation of the sural nerve during stance enhances dorsiflexion and eversion at the ankle in order to restore balance when on uneven terrain at the lateral foot surface and near the heel [11].

While non-noxious cutaneous reflexes have been studied for the three main nerve trunks innervating the dorsal and plantar foot, only recently have attempts to isolate specific tactile effects from regions of the foot sole been made [13,14]. These studies were restricted to sitting and standing conditions, and limited to forefoot medial, forefoot lateral, and heel stimulation but clearly showed that cutaneous reflexes evoked by stimulation of discrete foot sole regions produced topographical organized reflexes in human ankle muscles [13,14].

Forefoot stimulation produced inhibitory responses in the soleus (Sol) and medial gastrocnemius (MG), but excitatory responses in tibialis anterior (TA) muscles. Following heel stimulation, an opposite effect was evoked [14]. Systemic stimulations from the fifth toe to the heel on the lateral margin of the plantar foot demonstrated that the border of this Sol and TA reflex reversal occurred roughly around the middle of the foot sole, providing greater resolution in the fine sculpting of motor output than previously revealed by sural or tibial nerve stimulation.

It was also observed that stimulation at the lateral forefoot and heel evoked excitatory responses in peroneus longus (PL), but following medial forefoot stimulation an inhibitory response was evoked [13,14]. These results suggest tactile stimulation mimics a destabilization of posture and thus modulates PL responses to counteract uneven terrain through stabilization of the ankle joint [13,14].

An overarching principle in neuroscience, however, is that neural function is exquisitely task-dependent. As such we cannot predict with surety the pattern of reflexes evoked by foot sole stimulation during locomotion from data obtained during standing or sitting. The purpose of the current study was to examine cutaneous reflexes evoked by distinct plantar foot regions during locomotion. Additionally, we simultaneously look to determine the neuromechanical role of specific regions from the foot sole in shaping locomotor output and to initiate the process of developing a more detailed topographical view of the neuromechanical effects of cutaneous input from the foot during walking.

There were thus two main hypotheses tested in this study. Firstly, we hypothesized that stimulation at discrete skin locations on the foot sole would evoke topographically discrete cutaneous reflexes during walking. Secondly, we hypothesized that neural responses evoked in the form of cutaneous reflexes would have mechanical correlates detected as changes in force under the foot and kinematics of the stimulated leg.

Methods

Participants

Fourteen neurologically intact volunteers (8 females and 6 males) participated in the study. Participants were 30.3 ± 10 years old, with an average height of 174.4 ± 8.4 cm and weight of 73.7 ± 15.3 kg. Informed, written consent was obtained from all participants prior to the experiment under a protocol approved by the University of Victoria Human Research Ethics Committee and performed in accordance with the Declaration of Helsinki.

Experimental protocol

To improve procedural standardization and consistency, all participants were provided and fitted with the same make and model of running shoe with flexible foot sole (Nike Free 3.0 V4). The sipes (grid like horizontal cuts along rubber sole) enhanced flexibility, while the seamless upper and stretchy inner-sleeve provided a sock-like snug fit, both of which were useful in evaluating plantar cutaneous reflex effects during locomotion. The right shoe was then equipped with an insole containing five paired stimulating electrodes and three force sensing resistors (FSRs), as shown in Figure 1.

Participants walked on a motorized treadmill (Woodway USA, Waukesha, WI) at a self-selected, comfortable walking pace (2.1 ± 0.5 mph) that remained constant throughout the experiment. During each trial (average duration 315.6 ± 11.4 seconds), participants walked continuously while electrical stimulation was delivered to one of the five stimulation sites. In total, five separate trials were performed in order to obtain responses to stimuli for each regions stimulated. Prior to the experiment, the order of presentation for each of the five trials was randomized.

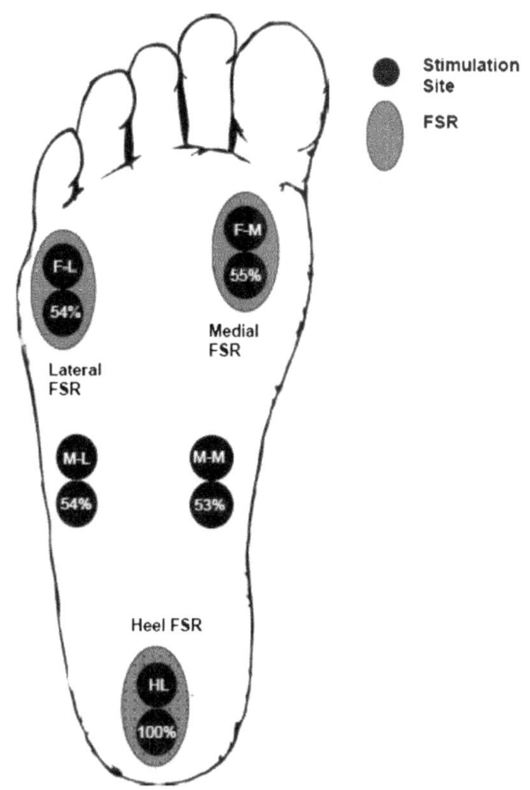

Figure 1 Cartoon schematic illustrating the positions of the paired stimulation electrodes (solid circles) for the 5 sites: HL (S1), M-M (S2), M-L (S3), F-M (S4), and F-L (S5). The position of the force-sensing resistors (FSRs) are shown as the hatched ovals at heel (F1), medial (F2), and lateral (F3) regions. Abbreviations: M-M = mid-foot medial, M-L = mid-foot lateral, F-M = forefoot medial, F-L = forefoot lateral.

Cutaneous stimulation

Transcutaneous electrical stimulation was delivered separately and in random order to five sites on the sole of the right foot. These sites were: calcaneous (HL); medial aspect of the transverse arch of the foot (M-M); proximal end of the fifth metatarsal (M-L); head of the first metatarsal (F-M); and, distal end of the fifth metatarsal (F-L) (Figure 1).

Stimulation was provided by a Digitimer Constant Current High Voltage Stimulator (Model DS7AH) with trains of 5 × 1.0 ms pulses at 300 Hz. Stimulation to the bottom of the foot was delivered via paired surface electrodes (cathode distal) (Narco Bio-systems INC, Houston, TX) placed within the insole of the right shoe to minimize undesired sensation, discomfort, and movement of the electrodes. Holes were cut and bevelled at the locations indicated in Figure 2. Figure 2a shows the relative position of the 5 stimulus sites on one of the sock liners. Figures 2b and c show the medial and lateral profiles, respectively, for the sock liner when viewed from the side. The plastic electrodes were then inserted through these holes and adhered with tape to provide a flush fit against the bottom of the sock liner. Two sided tape (cut with appropriate holes for each electrode) was then affixed over each electrode site and attached tightly to the foot sole.

Next, the electrodes were filled with electrode gel (Parker Laboratories, INC, Orange, NJ) to improve electrical conduction with the skin surface of the bare foot of each Participant. During each trial, a total of 160 randomly-timed stimulations (1–3 seconds) were delivered throughout the step cycle.

Stimulation intensity

Immediately prior to each trial, perceptual threshold (PT) was determined for each stimulation site. PT was defined as the stimulus intensity found to evoke detectable tactile sensation at the lowest intensity possible. Participants remained standing, while stimulation intensities were gradually decreased by the researchers until the participant could barely discern the stimulus (identified as PT). The stimulation intensity delivered to the sole of the foot was set to approximately three times PT. The actual stimulator output needed to reach PT was the same at all sites except for the heel where it was ~ twice as high. (The actual percentage of stimulator output needed to achieve PT in all sites with HL as the reference is shown within the lower circles for stimulation sites in Figure 1). The stimulation intensity of 3 × PT was chosen in order to evoke a non-noxious cutaneous sensation

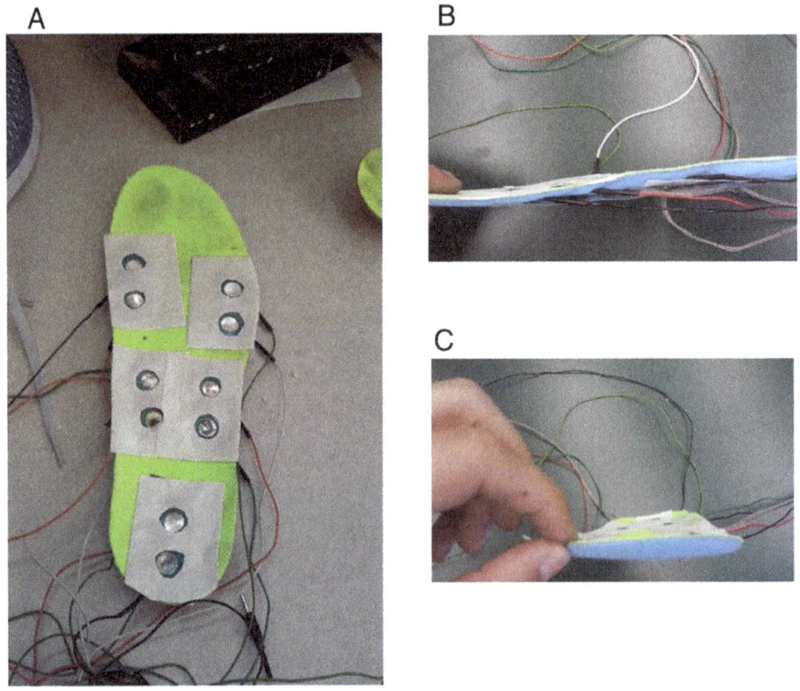

Figure 2 Photographs showing the configuration of the stimulating electrode array in the sock liner. A. the electrode pairs cut-out from the sock liner and overlaid with 2 sided tape; and profile of the integrated sock liner with electrode pairs and FSRs shown from the medial side **(B)** and from the front **(C)**.

during each trial by activating cutaneous afferents immediately under the electrodes and to provide the same relative activation at all stimulation sites.

Electromyography

Once the skin was cleaned with alcohol wipes, disposable surface electrodes were placed on the skin over muscles in the upper and lower leg and shoulder. All EMG recordings were ipsilateral to the site of stimulation (right side). Muscles recorded from included TA, MG, PL, vastus lateralis (VL), biceps femoris (BF), gracilis (GR), gluteus medius (GM) and posterior deltoid (PD). Ground electrodes were placed over electrically neutral tissue. EMG signals were amplified at 5000 times and filtered from 100–300 Hz (Grass P511, Astro-Med Grass Inc.).

Mechanical measures: force sensing resistors and goniometry

Force sensing resistors (FSRs) were firmly attached to the insole of the participant's right shoe. The forces produced at the foot-insole interface during the step cycle were recorded by three custom-made FSRs located at anatomically distinct landmarks: calcaneous (heel), head of the first metatarsal (medial), and distal end of the fifth metatarsal (lateral) (Refer to Figure 1). These signals were also used to establish step cycle parameters (such as heel contact and stance to swing transition) based on methods previously described [4]. Throughout the experiment, force signals were pre-amplified, and sent directly to the computer system. FSR signals from both unperturbed steps, serving as the control, and perturbed steps were recorded in volts and saved for later analysis.

Angular positions of the hip (flexion/extension), knee (flexion/extension), and ankle (inversion/eversion and dorsi/plantarflexion) were measured with electrogoniometers (Biometrics Ltd., Gwent, UK).

Data analysis

As with our other similar studies ([4,15-17]), all EMG, kinetic and kinematic data were sampled at 1000 Hz with a 12 bit A/D converter connected to a PC running custom-written LabVIEW (National Instruments Corp., Austin, Texas, USA) acquisition software and stored on hard disk for off-line analysis. Offline data were analysed using custom written software MATLAB (MathWorks, Inc., Natick, MA, USA). Custom-written software programs were used to separate the step cycle into 12 separate phases, beginning with heel contact and ending with the subsequent heel contact at the swing to stance transition. Using the FSR data, all responses for all data for each stimulus condition occurring in the same phase of the step cycle (n = ~10–20 responses per phase; See Figure 3 for schematic illustration of the phases of walking) were aligned to stimulus delivery and averaged together. Assignment to phase of step cycle was based on the time of the stimulation delivery in the data sweep. Averages from the same phase of walking during unstimulated cycles ("control" EMG n = ~50–60 per phase) were then subtracted from each of the corresponding 12 averages after stimulation yielding subtracted traces of reflex EMG, and stimulation induced changes in kinematic and kinetics. For evaluation of reflex effects the subtracted data traces were analyzed in all instances.

Cutaneous reflexes were determined as the average cumulative reflex activity occurring 150 ms after stimulation (ACRE150). This "net reflex" has been shown to be well correlated with kinematic responses in the legs [4,11,12,18] and arms [19]. This measure involved calculating a subtracted reflex (see above) then cumulatively summing the signal over a post-stimulus period of 150 ms. The summed value was then divided by the time interval of integration to measure an overall reflex effect. Net reflex values were normalized to peak control EMG amplitude.

Mechanical data were low pass filtered at 20 Hz using a dual-pass third order Butterworth filter. Stimulated data were subtracted from unstimulated data to yield a reflex trace. Mechanical reflex changes were analyzed within a 140–220 ms window post stimulus [4,19]. Responses were considered significant if they exceeded a 2-SD band of the mean value of the subtracted prestimulus level of the ongoing mechanical parameter at each phase.

Statistics

All statistical analyses were completed using SPSS version 18 (Chicago, IL). In all instances, analysis was conducted on averaged data from each part of the step cycle for each Participant. Each data set was analyzed separately, as was each phase of walking, in order to determine if the site of stimulation at a specific location on the foot sole and during a particular part of the step cycle had a discernible effect.

To test our first hypothesis that stimulation at discrete locations on the foot sole would evoke topographically distinct cutaneous reflexes, the initial approach for all data was to conduct 12 omnibus 12 (Phase) × 5 (Sites of stimulation) repeated measures ANOVAs. Note that all significant differences indicated on the figures also showed a significant 1× 5 ANOVA main effect. Fisher's LSD post hoc tests were used to determine site specific differences.

Based on the critical function of somatosensory feedback particularly at transition points and less stable phases of walking [3] we predicted enhanced effects from stimulation sites at early stance (phase 1; see Figure 3), late stance (phase 6), the swing transition (phase 7), early swing (phase 8), late swing (phase 11), and the stance transition (phase 12). Thus, using an approach applied in prior work [16,20], we subsequently performed planned comparisons between stimulation sites at these phases (also noted with asterisks on Figure 3). On all data figures across phases of walking, these phases are identified with black borders around the plots.

All statistical tests were 2-tailed and significance was accepted at $p < 0.05$. Thus, all data described in the following text or shown in the accompanying figures and described as "significant" or indicated with an * were determined as a main effect or interaction from the Omnibus and from the RM ANOVA and tested with Fisher's LSD post hoc test at the level of $p < 0.05$.

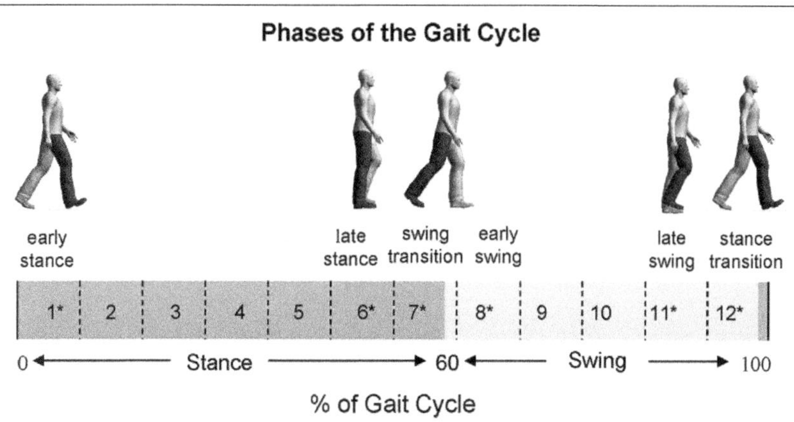

Figure 3 Schematic illustration of the walking cycle along with phase numbering for analysis and highlights of specifically targeted parts of stepping.

Results

Cutaneous reflexes

To view any evoked reflexes in all muscles studied we present the phase-independently averaged data in Figure 4. The data traces represented are averages across all Participants from all stimuli given across the entire step cycle for each Participant. This process reveals strong reflex effects but can obscure phase-modulation and other subtleties. This figure is useful, though, for representing the general trends in the evoked responses.

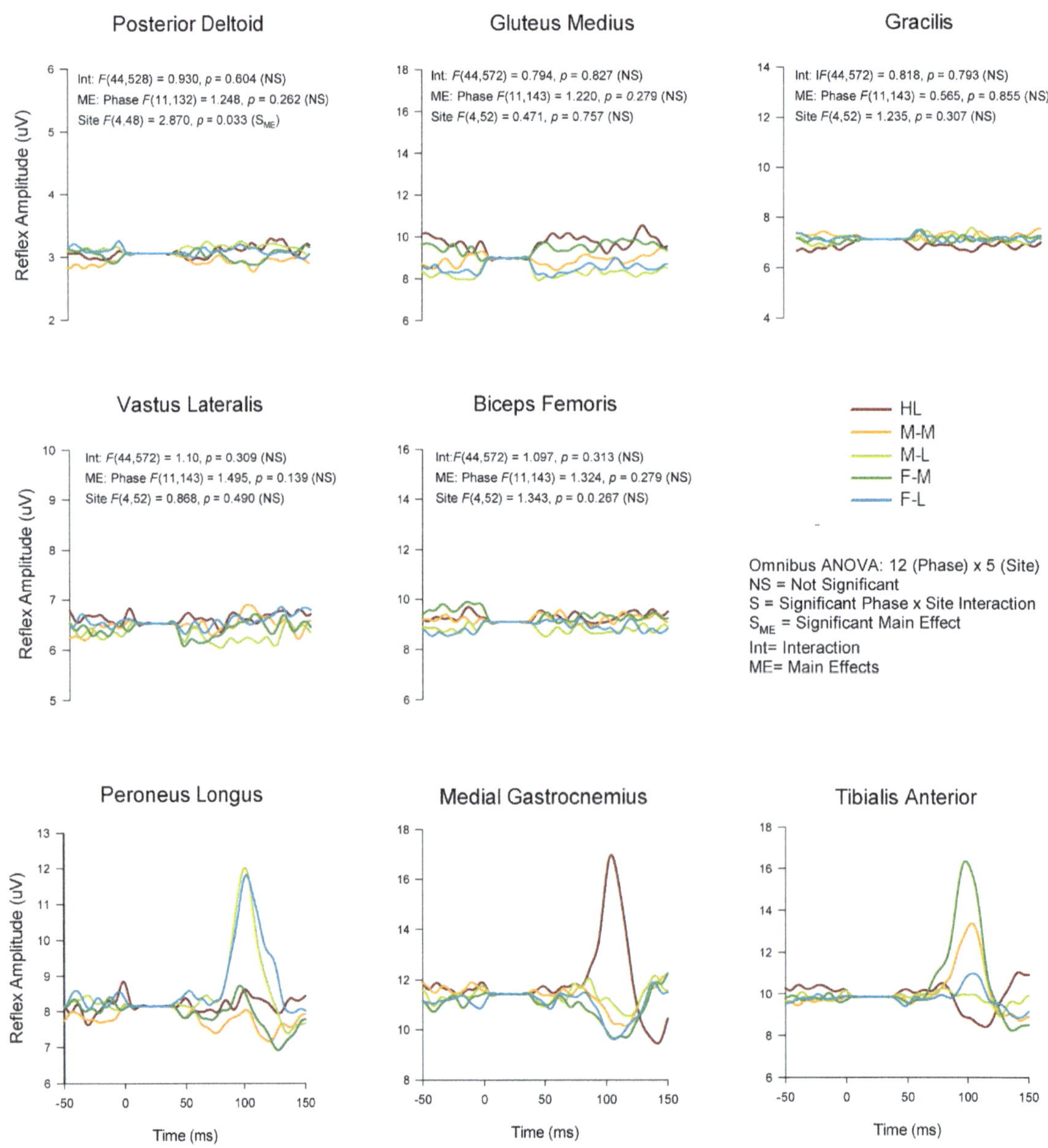

Figure 4 Grand average reflex traces taken across the entire walking cycle for all 5 stimulation conditions across all participants in all 8 muscles. Note that presentation of the data in this format shows nothing about phase-modulation since all stimulation irrespective of phase are averaged together. This presentation emphasizes the major trends in the reflexes but can obscure details such as phase-modulation. Abbreviations: HL (heel), M-M (midfoot medial), M-L (midfoot lateral), F-M (forefoot medial), F-L (forefoot lateral). The stimulus artefact beginning at time 0 has been blanked out and replaced by a flat line. The outcomes from interaction terms in the omnibus ANOVA are listed in the panel for those muscles not subjected to further analysis.

When looking at specific phases of walking, differences in evoked cutaneous reflexes were found extensively across the walking cycle in lower leg muscles PL, MG, and TA. In the other muscles examined, differences based upon site of stimulation were not typically observed. Taking into account PD, BF, VL, and GM, only 2 phases of walking (one in VL, one in PD; out of a possible 48 phases across muscles) showed a main effect for stimulation site. Thus these data are not discussed further below and the focus remains on the 3 lower leg muscles acting predominately at the ankle.

On Figure 4 are also shown the results of main effects and interaction terms from the omnibus ANOVA for each that did not show site-specific effects. The data shown in Figure 4 clearly illustrate that the main outcomes of regional foot sole stimulation emerged in PL, MG, and TA muscles (statistical details found on subsequent figures).

Grand averages taken across all participants for each stimulation condition for PL, MG, and TA muscles are shown in Figure 5 row A for Phase 1 (early stance) and for Phase 9 (swing) in row B. Three main observations are demonstrated in this Figure. First, comparison across stimulation conditions within a muscle show the site-dependence of the reflexes. For example, reflexes in MG at Phase 1 show clear antagonism with facilitation in the HL condition and suppression for F-L (see arrows). Similarly, reflexes at Phase 9 for PL muscle in the F-M and MF Med show opposite effects as do HL and F-M for TA muscle (again see arrows on Figure). Second, comparison across muscles within a stimulation condition show that the reflex effects are differentially specified to muscle. For example, compare responses for F-M in PL (facilitation), MG (no effect) and TA (facilitation) for F-M at Phase 9. Third, comparison within a muscle and stimulation site across phases shows clear phase dependence. For example, compare F-M in PL muscle from Phase 1 (suppression) to phase 9 (facilitation).

Characteristics evident in the reflex traces are illustrated in the quantified PL net reflexes shown in Figure 6. As indicated on the figure, PL reflexes showed a significant main effect for phase and site and a phase × site interaction. Site-dependence can be assessed in several ways including statistical differences across stimulation condition and sign of the evoked responses. In PL muscle, functional dorsiflexor and ankle invertor, significant site-dependence of foot sole stimulation was found in 5 of the 12 step cycle phases: four during stance (phases 1,3–5) and one during swing (phase 9). During stance, a key observation is that F-M and F-L were always (phases 1,3,4 &5) significantly different from each other and M-M and M-L differed from each other in mid-stance (phases 3 and 4). During swing (phase 9) the distal sites (M-L, F-M, F-L) differed from more proximal sites (HL & M-M).

Additionally, when considering the sign of the responses, there were clear site-dependent effects that can be seen in the Figure. Notably, facilitation was evoked in PL for all 12 phases of the step cycle when stimulation was applied to the lateral region of the foot (M-L and F-L). Heel stimulation produced facilitation in 7 phases and suppression in 5 whereas the opposite distribution was found at M-M with 5 phases with facilitation and 7 with suppression. F-M had 4 phases with facilitation and 8 with suppression.

MG muscle, is a strong plantarflexor and ankle evertor. Within the Achilles tendon, the fibers of the MG make their way to the lateral portion of the calcaneus as originally described by Parsons in 1894 [21] and discussed in Zehr et al. (1998) [11]. As shown on Figure 7, for reflexes in MG there was a significant main effect for phase and stimulation site, but no significant interaction. Phase 1 (early stance) showed significant differences between nerve stimulation sites. A main observation for MG muscle was that the HL site typically differed from at least one other stimulation site, particularly during stance.

As for the sign of the evoked responses, the most notable effect was 11 phases with facilitation for HL and only one with suppression. The medial sites showed mostly suppression (M-M = 9 and F-M = 7). There were similar effects for the lateral sites with F-L (n = 8) and F-M (n = 7) showing largely suppression.

In TA muscle (see Figure 8), functional dorsiflexor and ankle invertor, cutaneous reflexes showed significant main effects for phase and site and a significant phase × site interaction. Five of the step cycle phases showed significant differences across nerve stimulation sites. Three were during swing (8, 9 & 11), and 2 included the transition to stance (phase 12) and early stance (phase 1) itself. A main observation during swing phases 8, 9 and 11 was that F-M significantly differed from most other sites except M-M. Stimulation at the medial sites of M-M ad F-M produced facilitation of TA muscle at swing to stance transition (Phase 12).

In terms of the sign of the responses, for the medial stimulation sites, facilitation dominated (M-M = 12 and F-M = 12) all the phases of walking. Mixed results were seen at the HL (n = 6) and M-L (n = 6) and F-L had 8 phases with facilitation.

Kinetics

Heel FSR

Statistical analysis of heel FSR data revealed main effects for phase and site and a significant phase × site interaction. Data from the heel FSR along with results from the statistical tests are plotted in Figure 9. During stance HL stimulation tended to produce reduction in force at the heel FSR. At the stance transition (phase 12) both

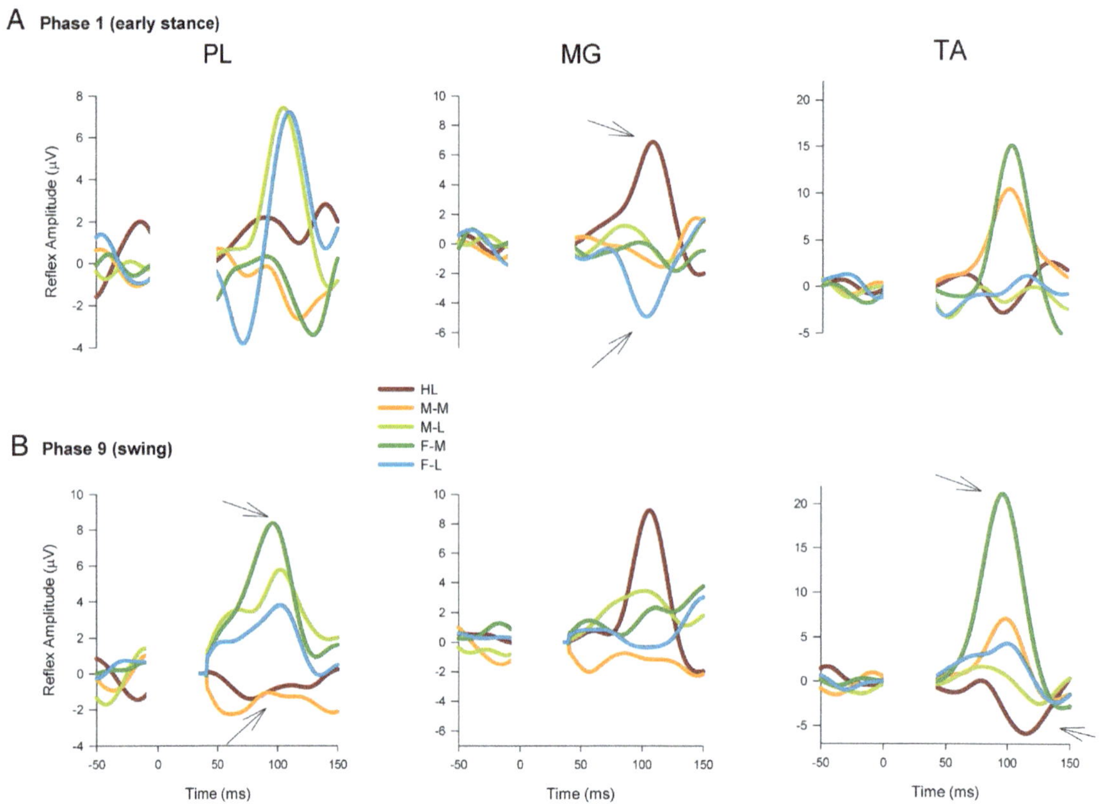

Figure 5 Grand average reflex traces for all 5 stimulation conditions across all Participants (n = 16) in PL, MG, and TA muscles at specific walking phases. A) early stance (phase 1), and **B)** swing (phase 9). Abbreviations: PL = peroneus longus, MG = medial gastrocnemius, TA = tibialis anterior. Other abbreviations as in Figure 4. Note that the stimulus artefact has been removed from all traces and replaced by a flat line extending from time 0 to ~50 ms post-stimulation.

forefoot sites and the M-L were significantly increased compared with HL stimulation.

Medial FSR

Statistical analysis of medial FSR data revealed main effects for phase and site and a significant phase × site interaction. Data from the medial FSR along with summary results from the statistical tests are plotted in Figure 10. Medial FSR showed site dependence at early (phase 1) and late stance (phase 6). Generally, lateral stimulation sites (M-L & F-L) tended to produce increases in force detected at the medial FSR during stance.

Lateral FSR

Statistical analysis of lateral FSR data revealed no main effects for phase and site nor a significant phase × interaction. Data from the lateral FSR along with results from the statistical tests are plotted in Figure 11. Generally, medial stimulation sites M-M (phases 1 & 6) and F-M (phase 6) tended to produce reduced forces at the lateral FSR. The lateral FSR showed site dependence at early stance (phase 1) where medial stimulation at site M-M (reduction) and HL (increase) showed opposite effects at the lateral FSR.

Kinematics

As with the EMG data for the upper leg, there were no differences across stimulation conditions for knee or hip kinematics and these data are not plotted.

Ankle inversion and eversion

Ankle kinematics for inversion-eversion showed significant main effects for phase and site and a significant phase × site interaction. Data for stimulus-induced changes in ankle inversion-eversion across the step cycle along with results from the statistical tests are plotted in Figure 12. Significant site-dependent changes in kinematics were detected at the ankle for inversion and eversion during stance (phase 2) and throughout swing (phases 9–11).

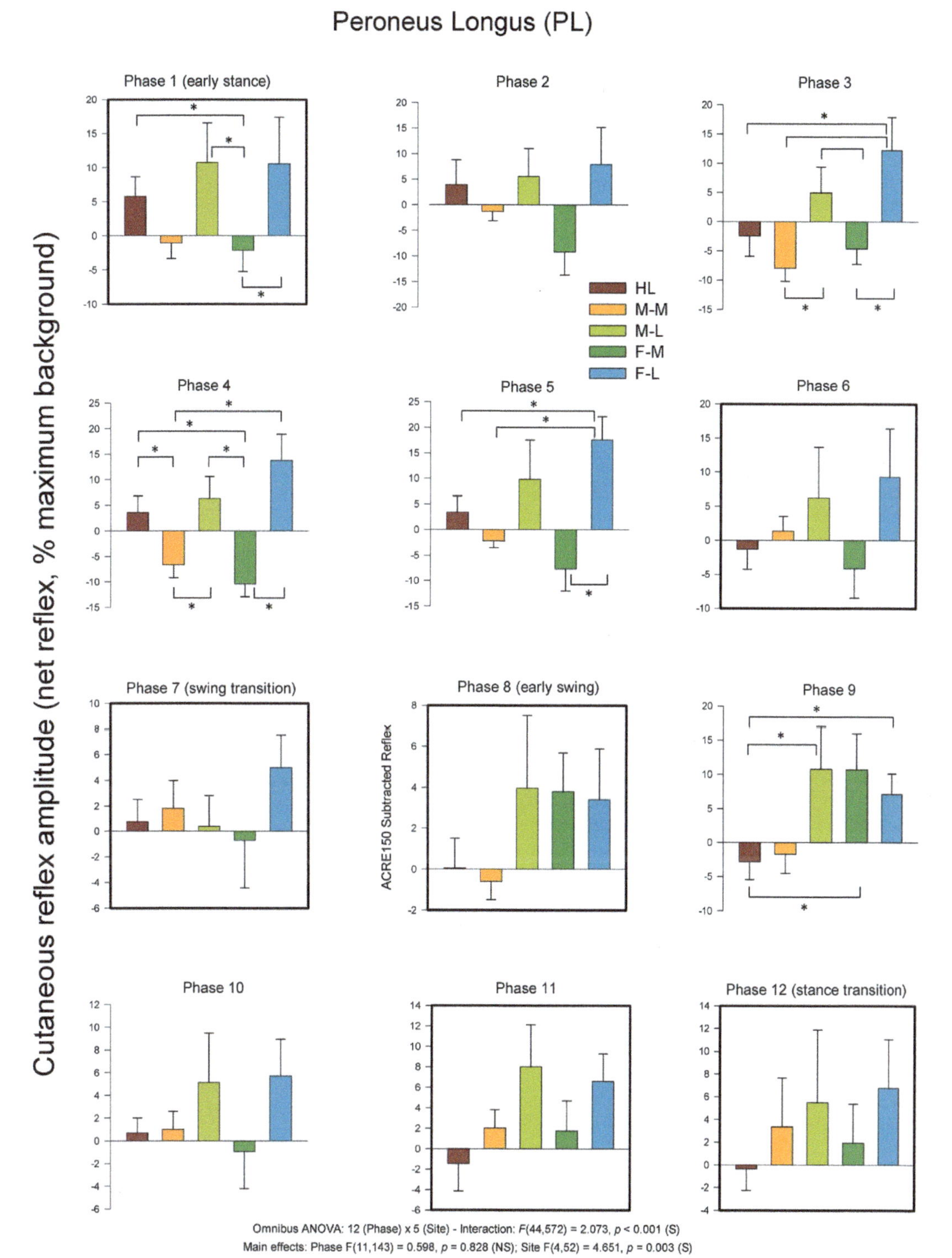

Figure 6 (See legend on next page.)

(See figure on previous page.)
Figure 6 Average quantified net ($ACRE_{150}$) cutaneous reflexes across all 12 phases of the step cycle for ankle plantarflexor and evertor muscle peroneus longus. Data are percentages normalized to maximum background EMG measured across all phases of walking. Negative values indicate overall suppression and positive values overall facilitation of muscle activity. There were significant main effects for phase and stimulus region as well as a phase × region interaction. Phases of walking analyzed with planned comparisons are indicated by black borders. *indicates statistical differences at $p < 0.05$ between stimulation conditions within a phase.

During stance, M-M stimulation reduced eversion and statistically differed from both HL and from M-L. During swing, a common feature for In/Ev was that FF Med differed from most other conditions. Stimulation at lateral sites (M-L and F-L) produced opposite responses (reduced inversion) to that seen with stimulation of medial sites (M-M and F-M; reduced eversion).

Ankle plantar and dorsiflexion
Statistical analysis of ankle plantar and dorsiflexion revealed main effects for phase and site and a significant phase × site interaction. Data for plantar and dorsiflexion along with summary results from the statistical tests are plotted in Figure 13. Significant site-dependent differences were seen throughout swing, at those phases were significant effects were also detected for ankle inversion/eversion (phases 9–11; Figure 13). During swing, a common feature for DF/PF was that FF Med differed from most other conditions. HL stimulation produced consistent reductions in dorsiflexion throughout swing and plantar and dorsiflexion during swing (phases 9–11).

Discussion
In this paper we examined the site and phase-dependency of gait adaptation in response to non-noxious cutaneous stimulation at five discrete sites on the plantar foot surface. We thus evaluated the topographic organisation and neuromechanical reflex effects from cutaneous afferents innervating the foot sole. Our results suggest that cutaneous inputs from discrete regions on the foot sole stabilize and enhance coupling between afferent feedback from the foot sole and neuromechanical function during locomotion. Stimulation evoked clear phase and location-specific reflexes in muscles acting at the ankle and the topographic distribution of responses produced changes in forces under the foot and ankle kinematics. As described for electrical stimulation of whole cutaneous nerves innervating the foot, mechanical changes in kinematics were mostly found during swing and kinetic changes in forces under the foot during stance [4,11].

Neuromechanical expression depends upon the phase of locomotion
Functional interpretations of the integrated neuromechanical responses are found below, organized within 4 functional phases of walking in which distinct responses occurred [3]: stance transition, stance, swing transition, and swing (see Figure 3).

Stance transition
The dominant site-specific features of stimulation applied at the swing to stance transition were effects on TA muscle activity and force detected at the heel FSR. At the transition to stance, HL stimulation led to unloading at the heel FSR. Functionally, non-noxious cutaneous input at the heel may have increased TA activity to facilitate eversion if needed to avoid scuffing or tripping, and initiate weight acceptance by the stance limb. As ground contact is expected from swing to stance, tactile input from heel stimulation was likely interpreted as enhanced ground contact initiation. These observations are supported by research on late swing tibial nerve stimulation (innervating the heel, midfoot medial, and forefoot medial foot sole), which evoked a form of placing reaction characterized by ankle plantarflexion [4].

Effects with stimulation of sites distal to the heel may be perceived as uneven terrain requiring increased loading of the heel to accommodate the stance limb and is consistent with previous research demonstrating that stance phase sural nerve stimulation during walking produced dorsiflexion and eversion to accommodate for what could be perceived as uneven terrain along the lateral foot margin and near the heel [11]. With regard to M-M and F-M effects, although previous literature reports plantarflexion following tibial stimulation, there has been evidence of reflex reversal in Sol and TA muscle activity at a plantar boundary existing approximately midfoot [14]. This boundary exists along the foot sole's lateral margin, but is likely mirrored along the medial margin. Heel stimulation during seated and standing isometric contractions respectively produced excitatory responses in Sol and inhibitory responses in TA, while forefoot medial and lateral stimulation resulted in the opposite effect [14]. This provides support for TA facilitation following F-M and F-L stimulation, but also for M-M stimulation given the reflex reversal boundary near the midfoot. M-M and F-M effects may thus simply reflect distinct reflexes that arise from activating the specific medial plantar branches of the tibial nerve.

At heel contact, stimulation delivered to the F-L site produced a significant increase in pressure at the Medial FSR, when compared to the decrease of force output with M-M stimulation. These effects may be the result

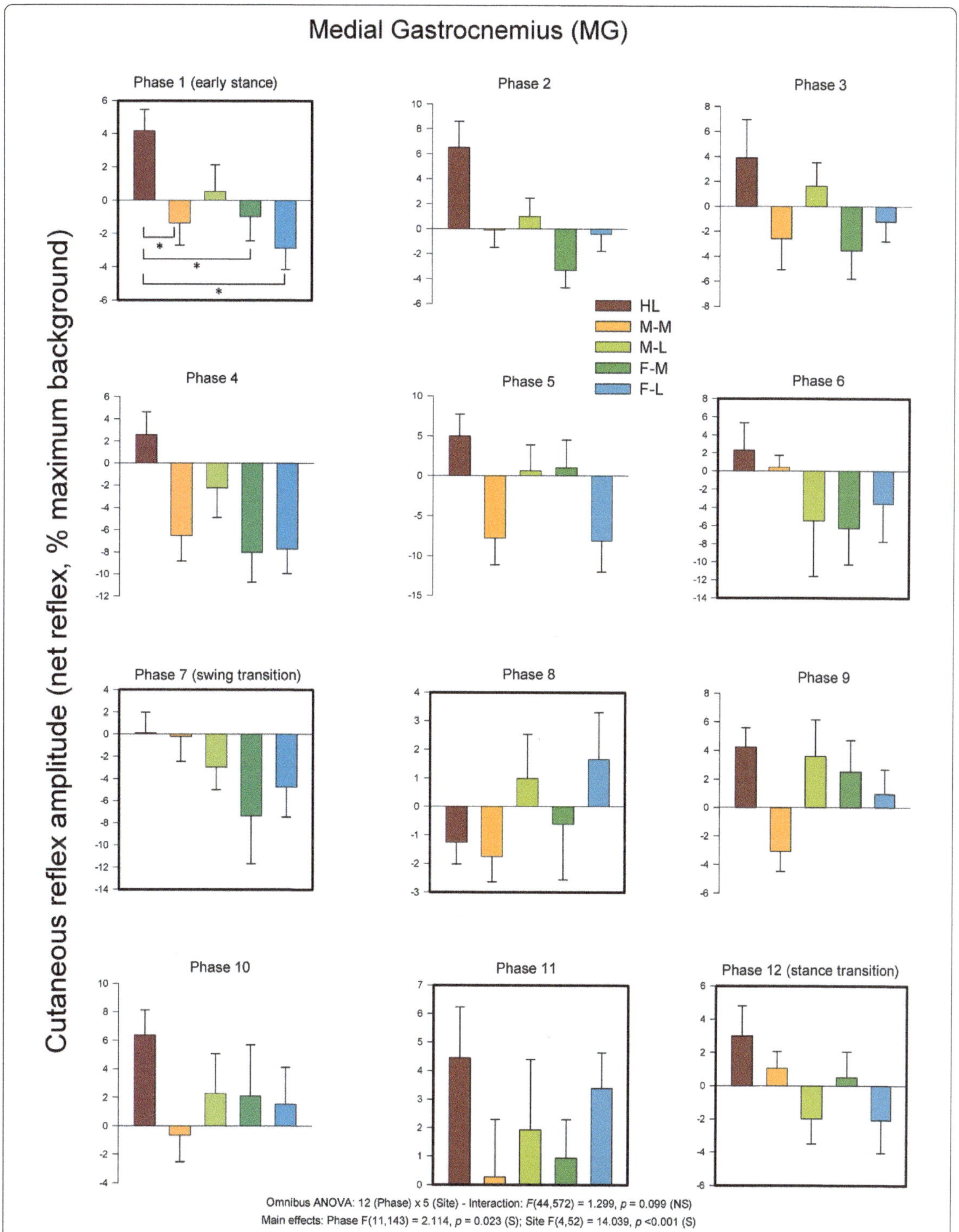

Figure 7 (See legend on next page.)

(See figure on previous page.)

Figure 7 Average quantified net ($ACRE_{150}$) cutaneous reflexes across all 12 phases of the step cycle for ankle plantarflexor and evertor muscle medial gastrocnemius. Data are percentages normalized to maximum background EMG detected across all phases of walking. Negative values indicate overall suppression and positive values overall facilitation of muscle activity. There were significant main effects for phase and stimulus region. Phases of walking analyzed with planned comparisons are indicated by black borders. *indicates statistical differences at $p < 0.05$ between stimulation conditions within a phase.

of balance restoration and ankle stabilization in response to the increased tactile input from opposing plantar margins. Nakajima et al., [14] provide supporting evidence for decreased medial loading following F-L stimulation as each stimulation along the lateral plantar border facilitated ankle eversion. This interpretation makes functional sense, given the widespread facilitation of PL at this phase.

Stance

The dominant effects of stimulation applied during early stance were changes in PL, MG, and TA muscle activity, forces in the medial and lateral FSRs, and ankle IN/EV. With regards to heel stimulation, as it has been shown that heel and tibial nerve stimulation produce plantarflexion, the increase in lateral loading may simply reflect a general increase in forefoot loading in response to what is perceived as uneven terrain [4]. This may be particularly evident during early stance as the lateral FSR is in contact with the ground at this phase. Additionally, inversion was typically produced by stimulation of all sites except the most medial midfoot site. During heel contact and early stance, tactile stimulation at the heel likely results in corrective changes due to an imbalance of pressure at the heel, thus altering motor output to promote readying of the stance limb for balanced weight support through an increase in forefoot pressure application. This would be reflected in the facilitation of TA (dorsiflexor and invertor) muscle found with medial stimulation and contrasted with facilitation of PL (dorsiflexor and evertor) muscle with lateral stimulation.

PL and MG muscles showed strong effects during stance along with changes in the force recorded from the medial FSR. Both M-L and F-L stimulation produced increased loading of the Medial aspect of the foot sole, indicating a shift in weight to ensure even loading of the foot in response to uneven terrain and thus improved balance. These effects are supported by Nakajima et al., [13,14]. The larger force output following M-L stimulation when compared to that of F-L may be indicative of greater forefoot stability during late stance when compared to the midfoot, as the body's centre of mass is directly over the forefoot region in this phase.

Swing transition

At the swing transition (phase 7) and into early swing (phase 8) we found modest effects of site-dependence. Generally, stimulation at lateral and distal sites (e.g. towards the forefoot) tended to enhance PL muscle activity and produce mixed results in MG muscle. TA muscle did show significant site dependence suggesting ankle plantar/dorsiflexion and inversion/eversion are main variables of control at this part of the step cycle. This was mirrored by forces under the heel FSR (generally increased from similar sites), as well as the medial and lateral FSR (generally reduced with stimulation). The overall impression is that regional plantar foot stimulation has a less specific regulatory role at the swing transition. This may be consistent with prior suggestion of general ground contact signalling (e.g. from distal tibial nerve) based upon whole cutaneous nerve stimulation [3-5].

Swing

During swing (phases 9–11), PL, MG, and TA muscles showed dominant site-specific effects that were associated with changes in ankle IN/EV and DF/PF. Forefoot stimulation generally resulted in facilitation of all 3 muscles that produced eversion from medial and proximal sites and inversion elsewhere. This functional effect on inversion and eversion was differentially specified along the width and length of the foot such that F-L was always different from M-L and F-M. A related differential was also seen in DF/PF at the ankle during swing where forefoot stimulation tended to produce a DF response and more proximal stimulation a compensation at the ankle towards PF. Interestingly, stimulation at HL consistently produced PF. Taken together these can be interpreted as finely tuned obstacle avoidance to guide the foot away from perturbations during swing phase as previously described for whole nerve stimulation [4,11].

Discrete activation of the sole produces "sensory steering" of foot motion during walking

The present observations support and extend to a locomotor context the earlier work of Nakajima and colleagues [13,14]. This earlier work in a postural context suggested a distinct organization of reflexes from the foot sole. The functional organization of the neural and mechanical responses evoked by stimulation of the foot sole are shown here to produce a kind of guided tuning—we suggest a "sensory steering"—of foot motion that accommodates to the perturbations mimicked by the electrical activation. A cartoon illustration of the general impressions from the synthesis of our data is shown in Figure 11. This illustration is not meant to be interpreted literally

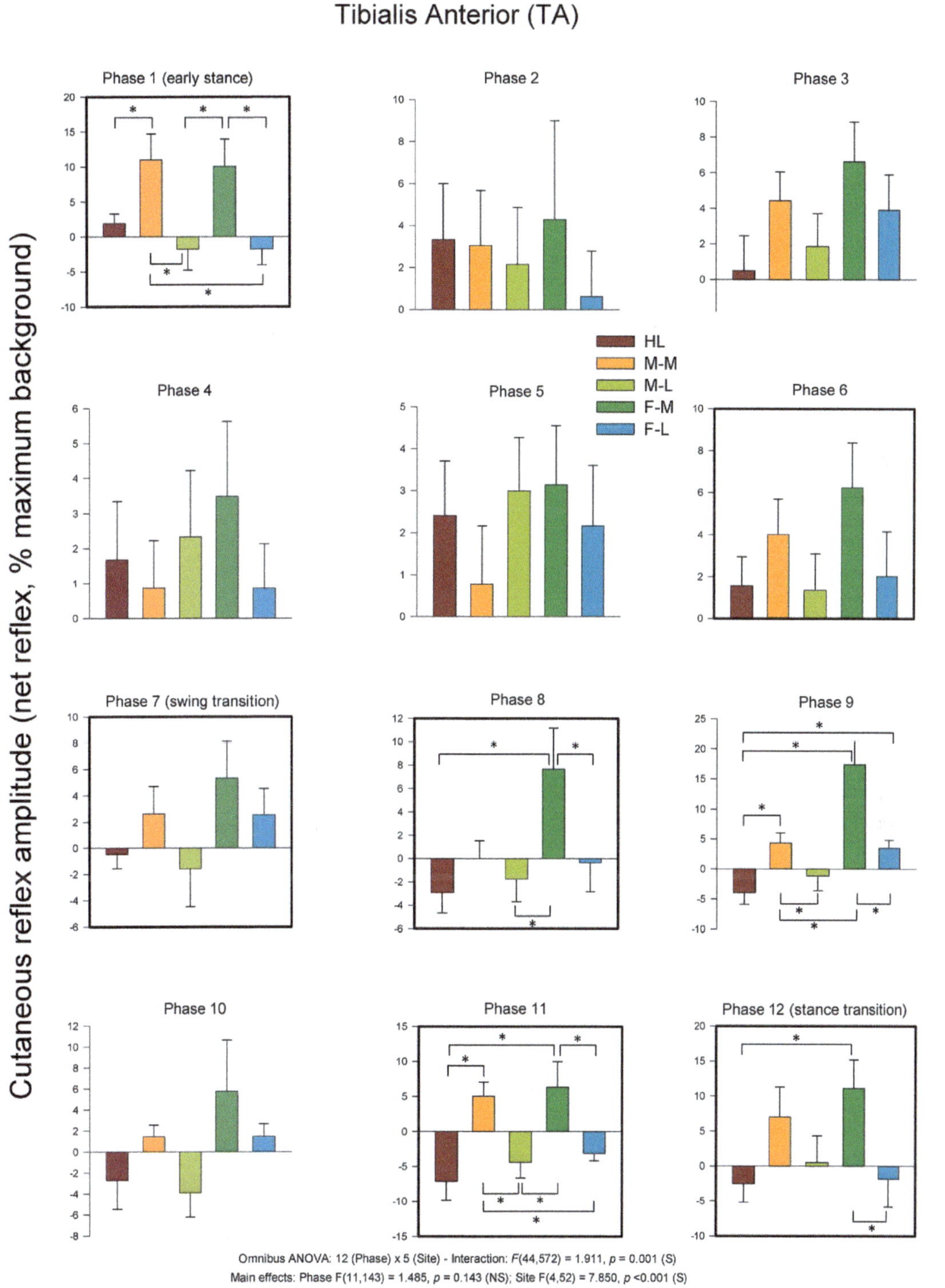

Figure 8 (See legend on next page.)

(See figure on previous page.)

Figure 8 Average quantified net ($ACRE_{150}$) cutaneous reflexes across all 12 phases of the step cycle for ankle dorsiflexor and invertor muscle tibialis anterior. Data are percentages normalized to maximum background EMG detected across all phases of walking. Negative values indicate overall suppression and positive values overall facilitation of muscle activity. There were significant main effects for phase and stimulus region as well as a phase x region interaction. Phases of walking analyzed with planned comparisons are indicated by black borders. *indicates statistical differences at $p < 0.05$ between stimulation conditions within a phase.

and also does not highlight any of the details of phase-dependency found in the figures above, but rather graphically shows the overall effects of stimulation.

The illustration in Figure 14 shows the general concept that activation under the foot sole produces a kind of tuned "sensory steering" response detected in EMG from the ankle muscles and manifesting itself mechanically by changes in ankle trajectory and pressure under the foot. The functional outcome of sensory steering is to guide foot trajectory away from or around the mimicked obstacle for foot placement. This overall interpretation is highly reminiscent of the earlier work of Arendt-Nielsen, Ole Andersen and colleagues who, in an elegant series of studies, showed a clear modular organization of nociceptive responses from the foot sole [22-26]. Our present results are consistent with a generally similar topographical and possibly modular organization of neuromechanical outcomes for both tactile and nociceptive sensory activation.

In any case, with our tactile stimulation intensities, generally the neuromechanical outcomes could be seen as movement medio-lateral (with activation at the lateral and medial sites; Figure 14A), proximal-distal (with activation at the heel or forefoot; Figure 14B), and on the diagonal axis of the foot (comparing forefoot medial and midfoot lateral; not illustrated) depending upon the site of stimulation.

Failure to observe differential effects of discrete stimulation in muscles distant from the ankle

In this study we observed distinct topographical effects of discrete foot sole stimulation only in the muscles acting predominately at the ankle (PL, MG, and TA). Muscles acting at the upper leg and hip (BF, VL, GM) and arm (PD) did not express this topography (see Figure 4). This was somewhat unexpected given the strong interlimb reflexes evoked in muscles across the body by cutaneous stimulation of the superficial peroneal [15,27] and sural [16] nerves. Interestingly, in static conditions Nakajima and colleagues also showed topographic effects in muscles acting at the ankle that were not observed in VL acting at the knee [14]. These observations could be a function of a difference in the quality of the perturbation represented by whole nerve versus discrete regional skin site stimulation. That is, discrete regional activation may represent smaller perturbations easily accommodated solely by responses controlling the ankle whereas whole nerve stimulation may be interpreted by the nervous system as a larger perturbation requiring more widespread responses across the body to avoid tripping and falling [3]. We await further research to clarify this issue.

Methodological considerations with foot region stimulation

It must be pointed out that there is likely a major difference in constancy of stimulation input using the methodology of foot region stimulation during walking applied here and other studies using whole nerve stimulation. During stance the full body weight of each Participant put more pressure on stimulating electrodes on the foot than during swing, a difference likely to be absent with nerve stimulation. To help offset this concern, we created the low profile electrode interface and used 2 sided adhesive to keep the insole interface on the foot. We were most concerned with the insole "dropping" away from the foot during swing but the use of the adhesive was effective in this regard. In order to attempt a quantification of this, we determined the stimulator output needed to produce sensation at PT at all 5 stimulation sites in 3 conditions: standing (to mimic stance phase), sitting with feet on ground (to mimic partial body loading), and unloaded with the stimulated foot held off the ground (to mimic swing phase). Using standing as the "reference" position we found that the conditions with less body loading (sitting and mimicked swing phase) required stimulator outputs that ranged between 5 and 17% higher to achieve PT. Thus, this could lead to an small underestimation of the effects of stimulation from the M-M, M-L, F-M, and F-L regions compared to HL, or viewed conversely and overestimation of the relative effects of stimulation applied to HL. Despite that, we do not think this is a major concern with interpretation of our data since the actual evoked responses were an order of magnitude larger than those that would be anticipated by small changes in stimulation input. Indeed responses during swing (representing an unloaded condition) could often exceed those evoked during stance (loaded condition) (See Figure 4 for Peroneus Longus, Medial Gastrocnemius, and Tibialis Anterior).

Conclusion

The results of this study further support suggestions that cutaneous nerves of the foot sole produce highly organised, topographic reflex effects in the lower limb of

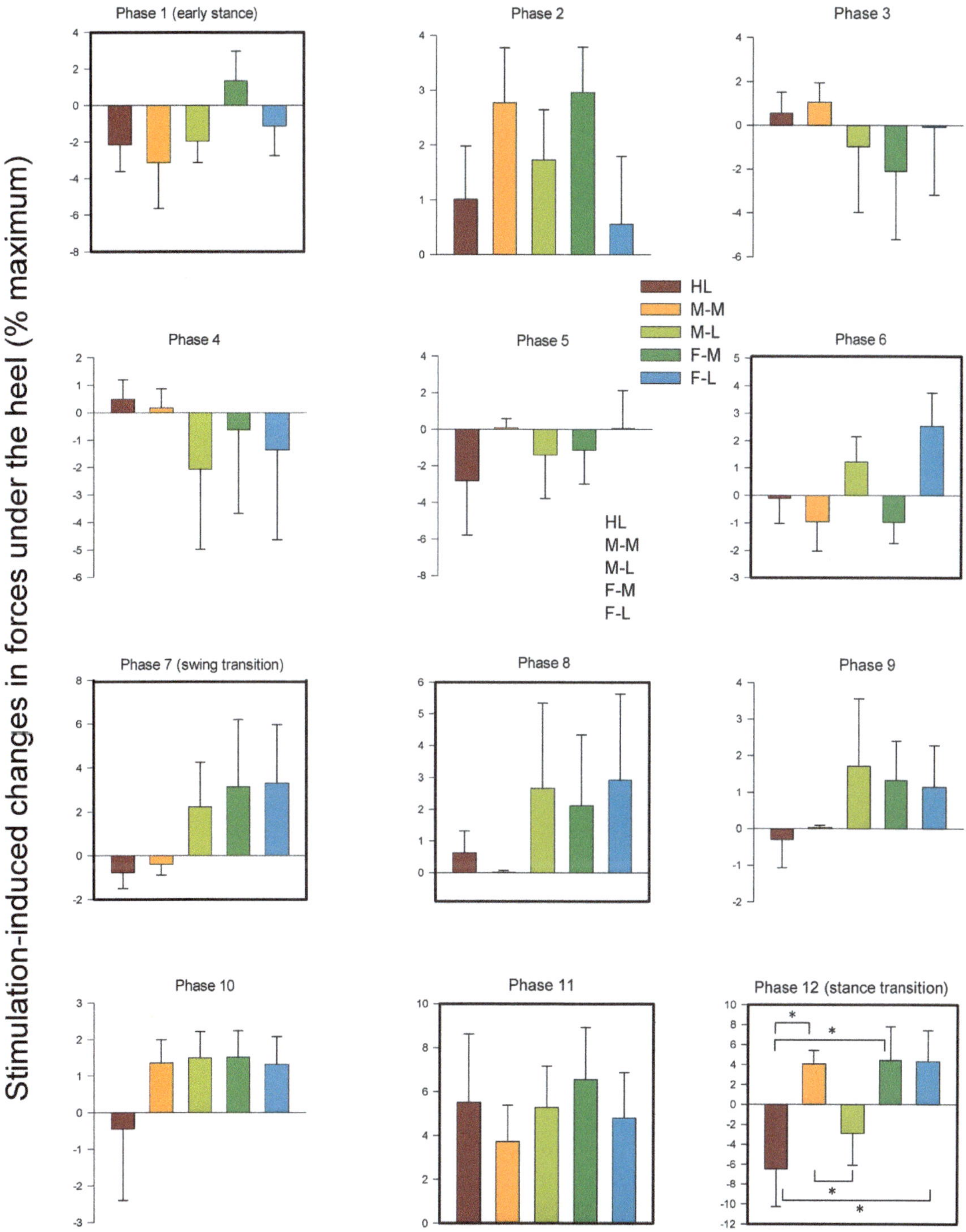

Omnibus ANOVA: 12 (Phase) x 5 (Site) - Interaction: $F(44,572) = 1.349$, $p = 0.070$ (NS)
Main Effects: Phase: $F(11,143) = 1.933$, $p = 0.040$ (S); Site: $F(4,52) = 3.543$, $p = 0.012$ (S)

Figure 9 Stimulation-induced average changes in forces under the foot detected by FSRs at the heel. Data are percentages normalized to maximum FSR load detected in the stance phase of walking. Phases of walking analyzed with planned comparisons are indicated by black borders. *indicates statistical differences at $p < 0.05$ between stimulation conditions within a phase.

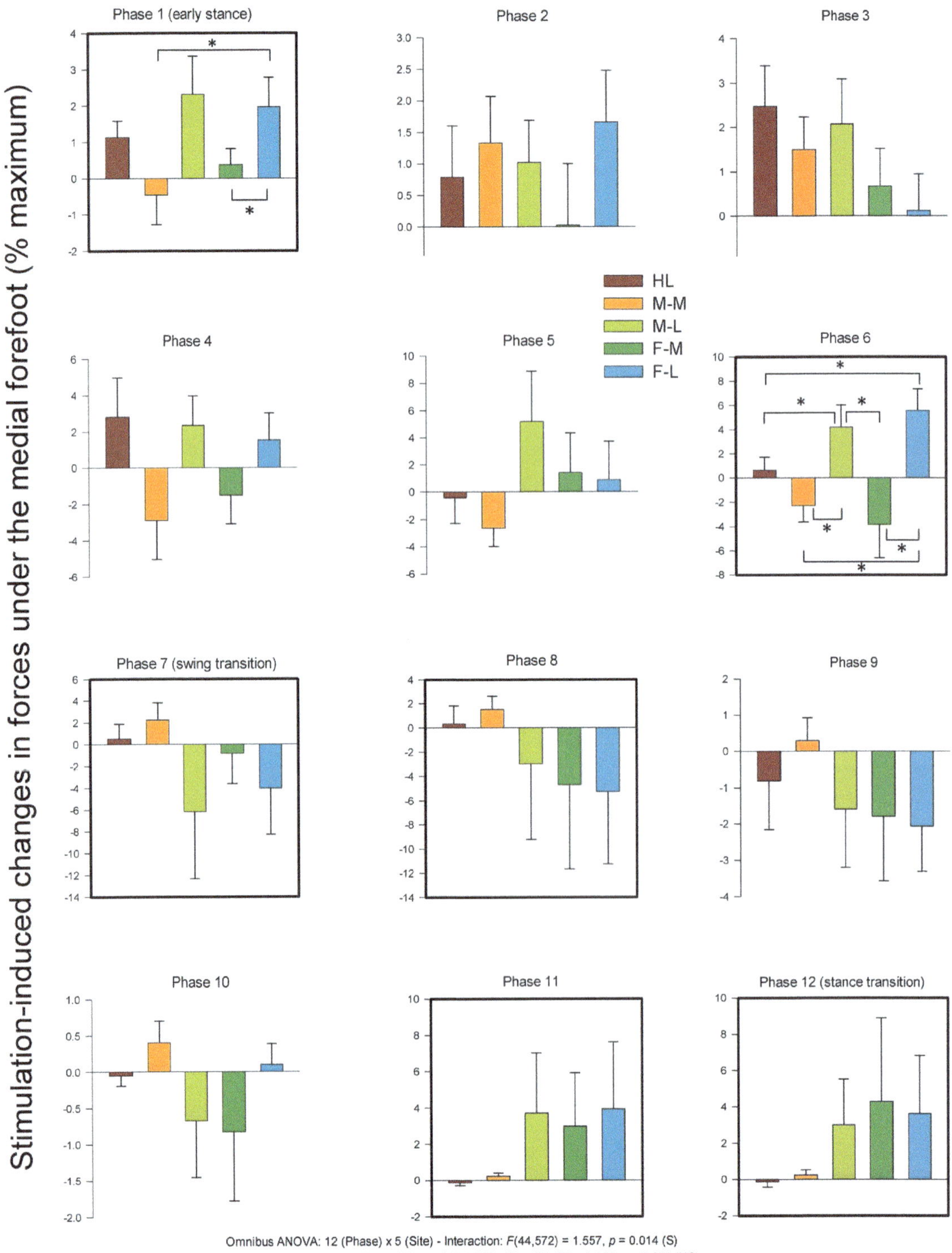

Figure 10 Stimulation-induced average changes in forces under the foot detected by FSRs at the medial foot. Data are percentages normalized to maximum FSR load detected in the stance phase of walking. Phases of walking analyzed with planned comparisons are indicated by black borders. *indicates statistical differences at $p < 0.05$ between stimulation conditions within a phase.

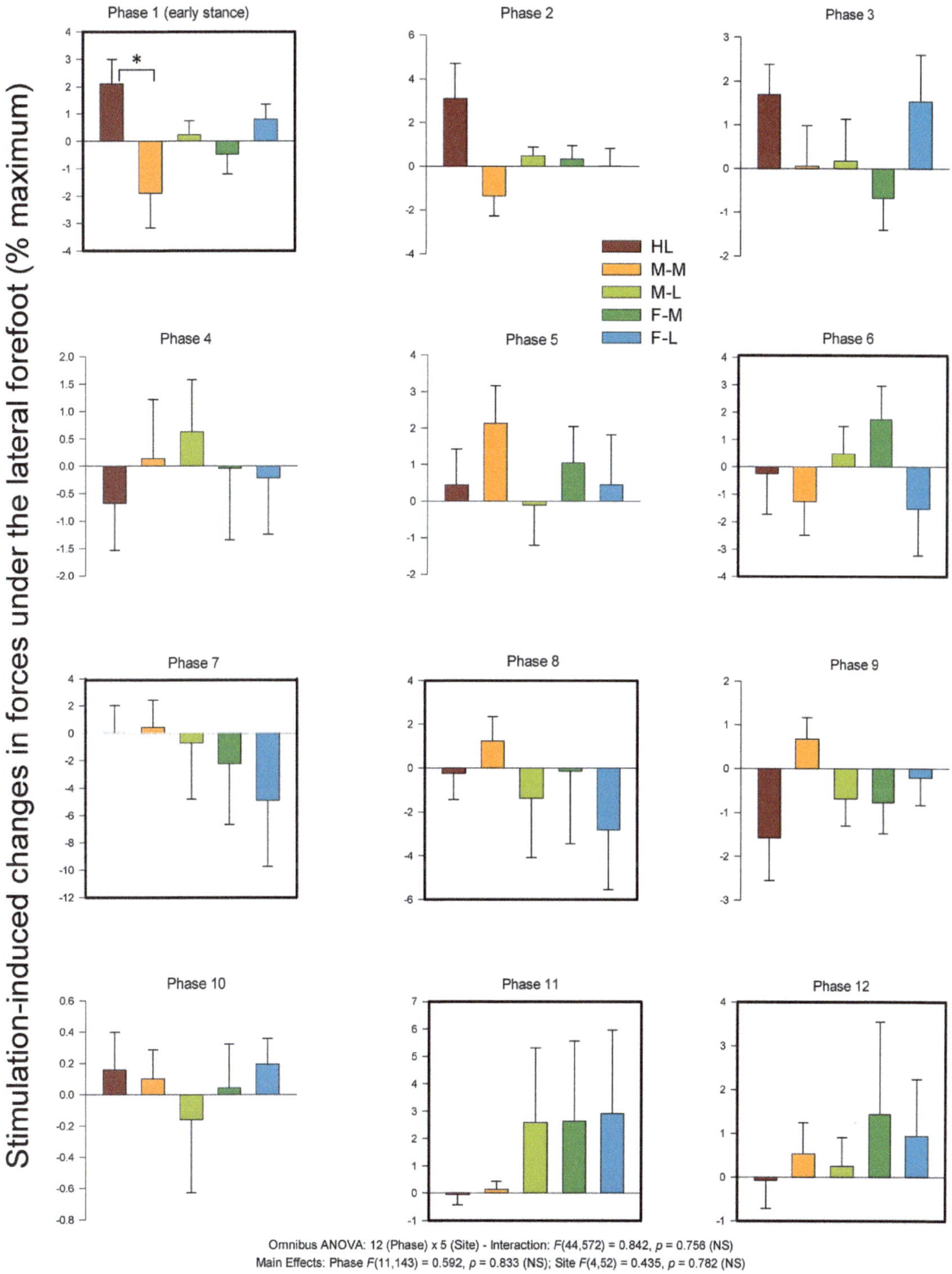

Figure 11 Stimulation-induced average changes in forces under the foot detected by FSRs at the lateral margin. Data are percentages normalized to maximum FSR load detected in the stance phase of walking. Phases of walking analyzed with planned comparisons are indicated by black borders. *indicates statistical differences at $p < 0.05$ between stimulation conditions within a phase.

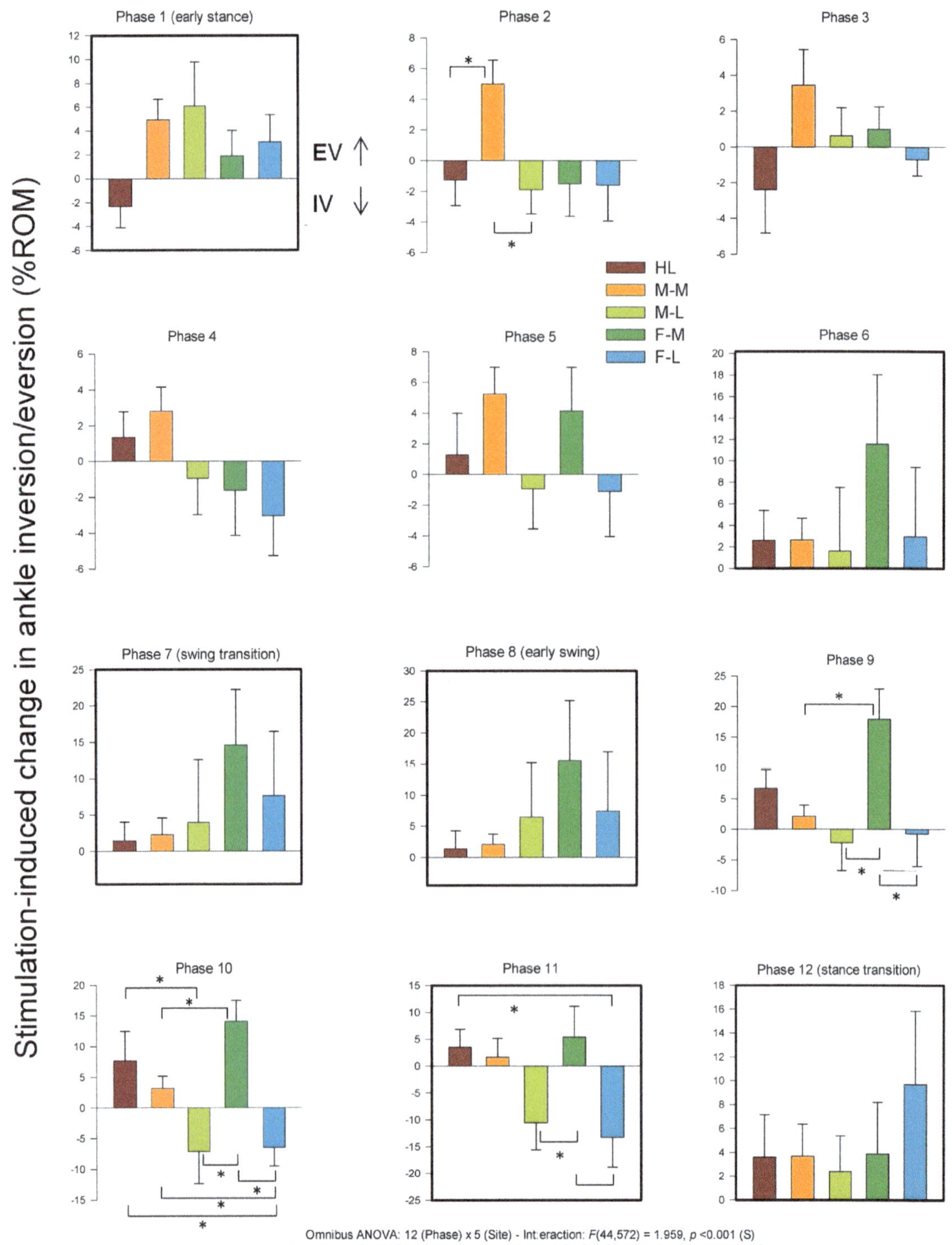

Figure 12 Stimulation-induced average changes in ankle joint kinematics for inversion/eversion (eversion = up). Data are percentages normalized to maximum range of motion across all phases of walking. Phases of walking analyzed with planned comparisons are indicated by black borders. *indicates statistical differences at $p < 0.05$ between stimulation conditions within a phase.

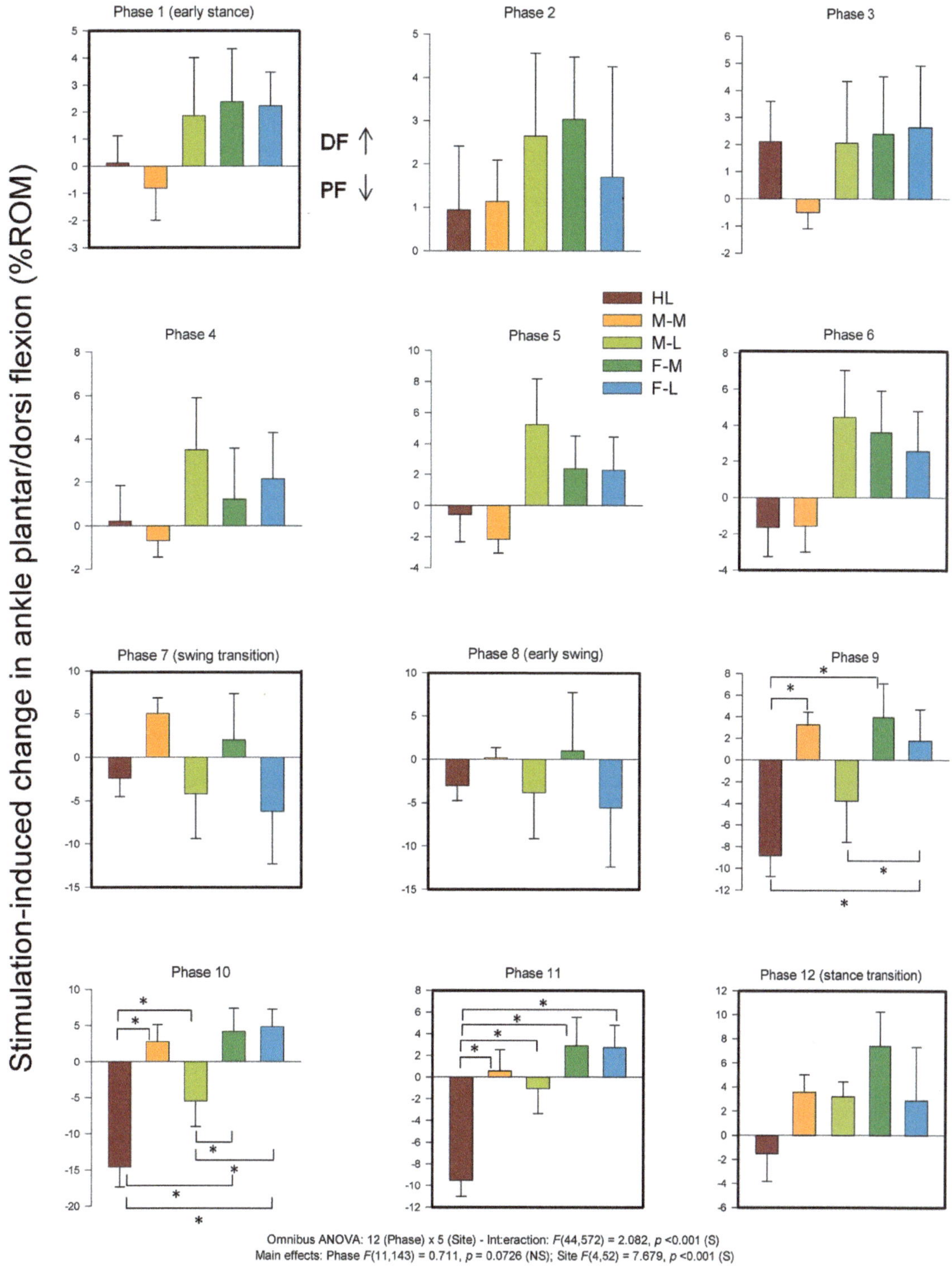

Figure 13 Stimulation-induced average changes in ankle joint kinematics for dorsiflexion and plantarflexion (dorsiflexion = up). Data are percentages normalized to maximum range of motion across all phases of walking. Phases of walking analyzed with planned comparisons are indicated by black borders. *indicates statistical differences at $p < 0.05$ between stimulation conditions within a phase.

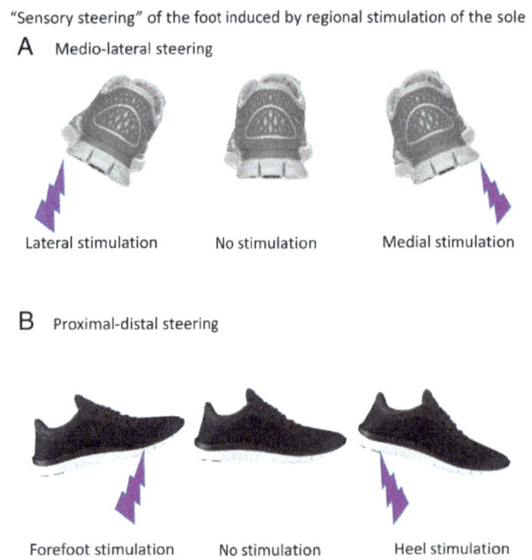

Figure 14 Cartoon schematic illustrating the overall neuromechanical outcomes ("sensory steering") found in the data. Medio-lateral steering around a longitudinal axis is shown in **(A)** and proximal-distal steering along a transverse axis is shown in **(B)**. "Sensory steering" is as shown in this schematic is not meant as a literal representation of the amplitude of the evoked evokes at each phase of walking. Rather it is a general distillation of the overall neuromechanical outcomes found in our data.

humans. Both site and phase dependence were observed in the kinetic responses, expressed as changes in force production at the foot sole, and offer additional evidence that non-noxious cutaneous perturbations applied to the bottom of the foot provide important tactile sensations for balance and maintenance of locomotion through the modulation of limb loading and foot placement [4,7,10]. While functional interpretation of cutaneous reflex effects on gait modulation have been determined for the dorsum of the foot [4,5,15] and with direct stimulation of tibial and sural nerve trunks [4,5], few studies have isolated cutaneous reflexes to specific regions of the foot sole [13,14]. The main findings of site and phase specificity do support previous literature and are important to providing further detail in our understanding of the topographical organisation of cutaneous reflexes.

This information is of importance to increase our understanding of how afferent feedback from specific cutaneous locations on the foot sole influences the mechanisms involved in locomotor output. This information may also have potential for rehabilitation strategies in impaired gait, such as in those arising after neurological damage. With a better understanding of how each receptive site on the plantar foot contributes to locomotion, researchers may be able to harness the effects of cutaneous reflexes to aid in enhancing functional modulation of gait following injury.

This study provides further evidence of site-specific and phase dependent gait modulation in response to non-noxious cutaneous stimulation at individual locations of the foot sole and could provide a better understanding of the behavioral relevancy, and potential rehabilitative use, of cutaneous input from specific regions on the plantar foot during locomotion.

Competing interests

A portion of the funding for this project was obtained from a research contract-for-hire from NIKE Inc. One author (EPZ) has worked in the capacity as consultant for NIKE Inc. and one author (MN) is the current Director of the NIKE Sport Research Laboratory. We further certify and declare that none of these competing interests had any impact on the analysis, interpretation of results, or conclusions derived within the MS.

Authors' contributions

EPZ conceived the experiment, directed the analysis, and wrote the MS. TN, RAM, MN, and TK contributed to the experimental design, analysis, and interpretation. TB, TK and SM contributed to experimental design, conducted the experiments and participated in analysis of the data. All authors commented on and approved the final draft of the MS.

Acknowledgements

This research was supported by funding to EPZ from the Natural Sciences and Engineering Research Council of Canada and the NIKE Sport Research Laboratory. RAM was supported by BEPE program (proc. no. 2012/05304-5) from FAPESP (Fundação de Amparo à Pesquisa do Estado de São Paulo). The authors thank Kristy Inouye and Kate Scarth for assistance on the figures.

Author details

[1]Rehabilitation Neuroscience Laboratory, University Victoria, PO Box 3010 STN CSC, Victoria, BC V8W 3P1, Canada. [2]Department of Integrative Physiology, Kyorin University School of Medicine, 6-20-2 Shinkawa, Mitaka, Japan. [3]Laboratory of Signal Processing and Motor Control, College of Physical Education, University of Brasília, Brasília, Brazil. [4]Biomedical Engineering Laboratory, EPUSP, PTC, University of São Paulo, São Paulo, Brazil. [5]Nike Sport Research Laboratory, Beaverton, OR, USA. [6]Department of Health and Sports Sciences, Faculty of Education, Chiba University, Chiba, Japan. [7]Human Discovery Science, International Collaboration on Repair Discoveries (ICORD), Vancouver, BC, Canada. [8]Centre for Biomedical Research, University of Victoria, Victoria, BC, Canada. [9]Division of Medical Sciences, University of Victoria, Victoria, BC, Canada.

References

1. Inglis JT, Kennedy PM, Wells C, Chua R: **The role of cutaneous receptors in the foot.** *Adv Exp Med Biol* 2002, **508**:111–117.
2. Kennedy PM, Inglis JT: **Distribution and behaviour of glabrous cutaneous receptors in the human foot sole.** *J Physiol* 2002, **538**(3):995–1002.
3. Zehr EP, Stein RB: **What functions do reflexes serve during human locomotion?** *Prog Neurobiol* 1999, **58**:185–205.
4. Zehr EP, Komiyama T, Stein RB: **Cutaneous reflexes during human gait: electromyographic and kinematic responses to electrical stimulation.** *J Neurophysiol* 1997, **77**(6):3311–3325.
5. Van Wezel BM, Ottenhoff FA, Duysens J: **Dynamic control of location-specific information in tactile cutaneous reflexes from the foot during human walking.** *J Neurosci* 1997, **17**(10):3804–3814.
6. Nurse MA, Nigg BM: **The effect of changes in foot sensation on plantar pressure and muscle activity.** *Clin Biomech (Bristol, Avon)* 2001, **16**(9):719–727.
7. Haridas C, Zehr EP, Misiaszek JE: **Postural uncertainty leads to dynamic control of cutaneous reflexes from the foot during human walking.** *Brain Res* 2005, **1062**(1–2):48–62.
8. Rossignol S, Dubuc R, Gossard JP: **Dynamic sensorimotor interactions in locomotion.** *Physiol Rev* 2006, **86**(1):89–154.

9. Duysens J, Tax AA, Trippel M, Dietz V: **Phase-dependent reversal of reflexly induced movements during human gait.** *Exp Brain Res* 1992, **90**(2):404–414.
10. Yang JF, Stein RB: **Phase-dependent reflex reversal in human leg muscles during walking.** *J Neurophysiol* 1990, **63**(5):1109–1117.
11. Zehr EP, Stein RB, Komiyama T: **Function of sural nerve reflexes during human walking.** *J Physiol* 1998, **507**(Pt 1):305–314.
12. Zehr EP, Fujita K, Stein RB: **Reflexes from the superficial peroneal nerve during walking in stroke subjects.** *J Neurophysiol* 1998, **79**(2):848–858.
13. Nakajima T, Sakamoto M, Tazoe T, Endoh T, Komiyama T: **Location-specific modulations of plantar cutaneous reflexes in human (peroneus longus muscle) are dependent on co-activation of ankle muscles.** *Exp Brain Res* 2009, **195**(3):403–412.
14. Nakajima T, Sakamoto M, Tazoe T, Endoh T, Komiyama T: **Location specificity of plantar cutaneous reflexes involving lower limb muscles in humans.** *Exp Brain Res* 2006, **175**(3):514–525.
15. Haridas C, Zehr EP: **Coordinated interlimb compensatory responses to electrical stimulation of cutaneous nerves in the hand and foot during walking.** *J Neurophysiol* 2003, **90**:2850–2861.
16. Lamont EV, Zehr EP: **Earth-referenced handrail contact facilitates interlimb cutaneous reflexes during locomotion.** *J Neurophysiol* 2007, **98**(1):433–442.
17. Zehr EP, Loadman PM: **Persistence of locomotor-related interlimb reflex networks during walking after stroke.** *Clin Neurophysiol* 2012, **123**(4):796–807.
18. Zehr EP, Komiyama T, Stein RB: **A method for the functional quantification of the reflex effect of human peripheral nerve stimulation.** *Adv Exerc Sports Physiol* 2000, **6**(1):25–32.
19. Klimstra MD, Thomas E, Paul Zehr E: **Biomechanical outcomes and neural correlates of cutaneous reflexes evoked during rhythmic arm cycling.** *J Biomech* 2011, **44**(5):802–809.
20. Lamont EV, Zehr EP: **Task-specific modulation of cutaneous reflexes expressed at functionally relevant gait cycle phases during level and incline walking and stair climbing.** *Exp Brain Res* 2006, **173**(1):185–192.
21. Parsons FG: **On the morphology of the tendo-achillis.** *J Anat Physiol* 1894, **28**:414–418.
22. Andersen OK, Sonnenborg F, Matjacic Z, Arendt-Nielsen L: **Foot-sole reflex receptive fields for human withdrawal reflexes in symmetrical standing position.** *Exp Brain Res* 2003, **152**(4):434–443.
23. Andersen OK, Sonnenborg FA, Arendt-Nielsen L: **Modular organization of human leg withdrawal reflexes elicited by electrical stimulation of the foot sole.** *Muscle Nerve* 1999, **22**(11):1520–1530.
24. Andersen OK, Sonnenborg FA, Arendt-Nielsen L: **Reflex receptive fields for human withdrawal reflexes elicited by non-painful and painful electrical stimulation of the foot sole.** *Clin Neurophysiol* 2001, **112**(4):641–649.
25. Sonnenborg FA, Andersen OK, Arendt-Nielsen L: **Modular organization of excitatory and inhibitory reflex receptive fields elicited by electrical stimulation of the foot sole in man.** *Clin Neurophysiol* 2000, **111**(12):2160–2169.
26. Spaich EG, Arendt-Nielsen L, Andersen OK: **Modulation of lower limb withdrawal reflexes during gait: a topographical study.** *J Neurophysiol* 2004, **91**(1):258–266.
27. Zehr EP, Collins DF, Chua R: **Human interlimb reflexes evoked by electrical stimulation of cutaneous nerves innervating the hand and foot.** *Exp Brain Res* 2001, **140**:495–504.

17

Relationship of post-exercise muscle oxygenation and duration of cycling exercise

Fabian Stöcker[1*], Christoph Von Oldershausen[1], Florian Kurt Paternoster[2], Thorsten Schulz[3] and Renate Oberhoffer[3]

Abstract

Background: Aerobic adaptations following interval training are supposed to be mediated by increased local blood supply. However, knowledge is scarce on the detailed relationship between exercise duration and local post-exercise blood supply and oxygen availability. This study aimed to examine the effect of five different exercise durations, ranging from 30 to 240 s, on post-exercise muscle oxygenation and relative changes in hemoglobin concentration.

Methods: Healthy male subjects ($N = 18$) performed an experimental protocol of five exercise bouts (30, 60, 90, 120, and 240 s) at 80 % of peak oxygen uptake ($\dot{V}O_{2peak}$) in a randomized order, separated by 5-min recovery periods. To examine the influence of aerobic fitness, we compared subjects with gas exchange thresholds (GET) above 60 % $\dot{V}O_{2peak}$ (GET60+) with subjects reaching GET below 60 % $\dot{V}O_{2peak}$ (GET60–). $\dot{V}O_2$ and relative changes in concentrations of oxygenated hemoglobin, deoxygenated hemoglobin, and total hemoglobin were continuously measured with near-infrared spectroscopy of the vastus lateralis muscle.

Results: Post-exercise oxygen availability and local blood supply increased significantly until the 90-s exercise duration and reached a plateau thereafter. Considering aerobic fitness, the GET60+ group reached maximum post-exercise oxygen availability earlier (60 s) than the GET60– group (90 s).

Conclusions: Our results suggest that (1) 90 s has evolved as the minimum interval duration to enhance local oxygen availability and blood supply following cycling exercise at 80 % $\dot{V}O_{2peak}$; whereas (2) 60 s is sufficient to trigger the same effects in subjects with GET60 + .

Keywords: Muscle oxygenation, Hyperemia, Near-infrared spectroscopy, Interval training, Prior exercise

Background

High-intensity training (HIT) and high-intensity interval training or aerobic interval training (HIIT or AIT) are commonly accepted stimuli for improving anaerobic [1, 2] and aerobic [3–7] functions. Although the terms HIT and HIIT are sometimes used interchangeably, HIT usually refers to near-maximal or supramaximal exercise intensities (>90 % peak rate of oxygen uptake, $\dot{V}O_{2peak}$) [6], whereas HIIT or AIT is often used in the context of exercise intensities between 80 % and 90 % $\dot{V}O_{2peak}$ [3, 7, 8].

Acute microvascular responses to exercise (e.g., enhanced blood flow and local blood supply of small vessels in active tissue [9, 10]) have also been reported as long-term adaptations following HIT (e.g., by increased vasodilatory capacity [9] and augmented capillarization [5, 11]). Fu et al. showed these effects to be superior to those of moderate continuous training in patients with heart failure [7]. Furthermore, several studies have suggested that aerobic adaptations are facilitated by the above-mentioned microvascular mechanisms following HIIT/AIT [3, 4, 7].

Although the literature contains substantial knowledge on the acute effects of exercise on local muscle perfusion in general [10, 12–15], the acute post-exercise effects of different exercise durations on local muscle oxygen availability and blood supply have not yet been sufficiently examined. Most studies have focused on the influence of exercise intensity [16–19] or examined the

* Correspondence: fabian.stoecker@tum.de
[1]Center for Teaching and Learning, Technische Universität München, Connollystraße 32, 80809 München, Germany
Full list of author information is available at the end of the article

effect of complete training sessions with only two different work-interval durations [20].

Relative changes in local, total hemoglobin concentration (ΔTHb) is a widely used parameter for blood-volume changes in terms of capillary filling [21–23] and vasodilation [24] and can be noninvasively monitored using near-infrared spectroscopy (NIRS) [22]. With continuous-wave spectrometers, relative changes in the THb and deoxygenated (HHb) and oxygenated Hb (O_2Hb) concentrations can be observed because of the distinct relative transparency of HHb and O_2Hb for specific, near-infrared light wavelengths.

The potential of exercise to prolong augmentation of the local blood supply could be an important determinant for metabolic adaptations. The aim of our study was to identify the association between durations of HIIT/AIT exercise bouts and relative changes in post-exercise concentrations of THb, O_2Hb, and HHb to examine (1) the post-exercise blood supply and (2) local oxygen availability.

Methods

Subjects

A total of 18 healthy, physically active males volunteered to participate in the present study (see Table 1). Participants exercised at least 2 times per week in various sports, whereas aerobic exercise contributed an average of 4 ± 3 h per week. The inclusion criteria included age (18–35 years) and a physically active background. Exclusions included acute or chronic diseases (such as chronic heart disease), diabetes type II, epilepsy, and relevant diseases of the liver and kidney, as well as smoking and excessive alcohol consumption. All subjects were familiar with cycling exercise and exhaustive exercise testing. They received detailed information on the purpose and procedures of the study and their written informed consent was obtained. The local Ethics Committee of the Technische Universität München approved the study protocol (#67/14).

Table 1 Subject data

Parameter	
N	18
Age (years)	28 ± 5
Weight (kg)	77.7 ± 4.9
Height (cm)	181.3 ± 5.2
Skinfold thickness (mm)	7.8 ± 2.9
$\dot{V}O_{2peak}$ ($ml \cdot kg^{-1} \cdot min^{-1}$)	50.4 ± 5.7
GET (% $\dot{V}O_{2peak}$)	58 ± 13
n GET60+	7
n GET60–	11

Values are expressed as mean ± SD

Test design and procedures

Subjects reported to the laboratory for two sessions. We conducted preliminary tests (see section *preliminary maximal testing*) during the first session. During the second session, we aimed to examine the local blood supply in relation to exercise duration. Both sessions had to be completed within one week and had to be separated by at least 48 h to enable full recovery. The subjects were instructed not to perform exhaustive activity 24 h before each session and to avoid caffeinated and high-carbohydrate beverages 2 h before each session. Special bicycle shoes and pedals were not allowed during the ergometer tests to reduce the influence of cycling technique.

Preliminary maximal testing

During the first visit, all subjects performed an incremental test to exhaustion on an electrically braked cycle ergometer (Lode Excalibur; Lode, Groningen, The Netherlands) to determine $\dot{V}O_{2peak}$ and gas-exchange threshold (GET), according to the v-slope method [25]. The 60-W load was increased by 10 W every 30 s and led to volitional exhaustion within 14.8 ± 1.5 min, which has been reported as a suitable time span for reaching maximum aerobic contribution [26]. Subjects were allowed to individually choose the cadence during the cycle ergometer trials but were asked to maintain a minimum cadence of >70 revolutions/min. The test was terminated when pedaling frequency could no longer be maintained. Although all subjects were physically active, healthy, and familiar with exhaustive exercise, $\dot{V}O_2$ did not attain a plateau in two subjects. Thus, we measured $\dot{V}O_{2peak}$ instead of maximum oxygen uptake ($\dot{V}O_{2max}$). However, Day et al. showed that $\dot{V}O_{2peak}$ and $\dot{V}O_{2max}$ do not differ in a healthy, physically active population when maximum effort is put forth [27]. To ensure maximum effort, we verbally motivated subjects at the end of the test and datasets were included only if a maximum respiratory exchange ratio >1.1 had been attained.

Experimental testing

Subjects were asked to complete a randomized protocol consisting of five exercise bouts with different durations (30, 60, 90, 120, and 240 s), separated by 5-min passive, recovery periods. Exercise intensity was determined corresponding to 80 % $\dot{V}O_{2peak}$, based on the data of the preliminary maximal test. Consequently, $\dot{V}O_2$ did not attain 80 % during the 30-s and 60-s exercise bouts because of the finite $\dot{V}O_2$ -kinetics during exercise on transitions [28]. On the other hand, $\dot{V}O_2$ exceeded 80 % slightly during the 240-s bout because of the slow component of $\dot{V}O_2$ [28] (Table 2). The exercise bouts were

Table 2 Recovery parameters for ΔO2Hb, ΔHHb, and ΔTHb

Exercise duration	30 s	60 s	90 s	120 s	240 s
OS_THb ($\Delta\mu mol \cdot l^{-1}$)	3.05 ± 1.26	6.00 ± 2.78	6.97 ± 2.11	6.98 ± 2.30	7.25 ± 3.03
OS_O_2Hb ($\Delta\mu mol \cdot l^{-1}$)	1.09 ± 1.32	4.79 ± 2.37	6.34 ± 1.88	6.54 ± 2.90	5.98 ± 2.75
GET60+: OS_O_2Hb ($\Delta\mu mol \cdot l^{-1}$)	1.14 ± 1.60	6.00 ± 2.70	7.02 ± 2.11	-	6.08 ± 2.15
GET60–: OS_O_2Hb ($\Delta\mu mol \cdot l^{-1}$)	1.06 ± 1.19	4.02 ± 1.88	5.91 ± 1.67	-	5.91 ± 3.18
Recovery of ΔTHb (s)	198 ± 86	206 ± 82	199 ± 65	210 ± 57	234 ± 37
Recovery of ΔO_2Hb (s)	243 ± 56	222 ± 66	239 ± 23	195 ± 71	227 ± 56
Recovery of ΔHHb (s)	212 ± 88	210 ± 76	206 ± 79	185 ± 84	243 ± 31
SD_REC_ ΔTHb ($\Delta\mu mol \cdot l^{-1}$)	0.18 ± 0.21	0.36 ± 0.27	0.24 ± 0.12	0.21 ± 0.14	0.26 ± 1.23
SD_REC_ ΔO_2Hb ($\Delta\mu mol \cdot l^{-1}$)	0.19 ± 0.13	0.34 ± 0.28	0.34 ± 0.12	0.20 ± 0.09	0.28 ± 0.25
SD_REC_ ΔHHb ($\Delta\mu mol \cdot l^{-1}$)	0.11 ± 0.09	0.20 ± 0.09	0.11 ± 0.05	0.15 ± 0.09	0.12 ± 0.04
Time-to-peak ΔTHb (s)	57 ± 29	65 ± 50	79 ± 57	71 ± 37	72 ± 44
Time-to-peak ΔO_2Hb (s)	151 ± 81*	103 ± 59	81 ± 26	91 ± 48	94 ± 39
End-exercise % $\dot{V}O_2$ (%)	43 ± 8*	73 ± 5	81 ± 6	82 ± 6	86 ± 5

$n = 18$ (except GET60+/−); values are expressed as mean ± SD; Significant results for OS_THb/O_2Hb are presented in Fig. 4; SD_REC_ΔTHb/O_2Hb/HHb represent the average standard deviation of the last 30 s of recovery; Time-to-peak values indicate the time from cessation of exercise to the highest value reached during the subsequent recovery period (asterisks indicate significant higher values compared to the other values, ** $P < 0.01$); End-exercise % $\dot{V}O_2$ values are averaged values obtained from the final 10 s of each bout

randomly assigned. It is worth pointing out that Buchheit et al. used 3-min recovery periods for similar measurements [29]. However, we noted that the recovery times of HHb and O_2Hb exceeded 180 s (Table 2), so we decided to use 5-min recovery periods instead. The applied exercise durations, which are commonly used in HIIT/AIT prescriptions, represent interval bouts that range from short to long duration [1]. The exercise intensity of 80 % $\dot{V}O_{2peak}$ is commonly used for HIIT/AIT in combination with long-duration intervals, while short-exercise bouts up to 60 s are associated with supramaximal work rates [3]. In spite of that, a shorter interval (30 s) was included in this setup to obtain a detailed overview on the relationship of exercise duration and post-exercise blood supply.

A 3-min baseline measurement ($BASE_0$) was conducted prior to the first interval with the subject sitting passively on the ergometer. This measurement was followed by a warm-up, consisting of 1 min at 60 % $\dot{V}O_{2peak}$ and 3 min at 80 % $\dot{V}O_{2peak}$. Prior observations revealed that O_2Hb levels would be markedly elevated, following the first exercise bout but would attain similar values between subsequent exercise bouts, which could be due to increased skin blood flow [30]. Furthermore, pre-exercise affects the speed of aerobic metabolism during subsequent exercise on-transitions [31]. Hence, pre-exercise was used to activate muscle blood flow and metabolism to avoid order effects for the first experimental condition. During $BASE_0$, as well as during recovery periods, subjects had to maintain a standardized position, keeping the right foot on a bar between the pedals to minimize movement artifacts by unwanted muscular activity on the NIRS signal.

An exemplary scheme of the experimental protocol is displayed in Fig. 1.

Gas exchange and heart rate measurement

Heart rate was monitored (Polar Team[2,] Polar Electro, Kempele, Finland) throughout all sessions and respiratory parameters were measured continuously with a breath-by-breath metabolic cart (ZAN 600USB; Nspire Health, Oberthulba, Germany), which had been used and validated previously [32, 33]. The oxygen-uptake ($\dot{V}O_2$) curve was smoothed with a 30-s moving average and heart-rate data were smoothed with a 5-s moving average. $\dot{V}O_{2peak}$ was determined as the highest value reached during exercise and was expressed relative to body weight ($ml \cdot kg^{-1} \cdot min^{-1}$). GET was determined using the v-slope method [25] and was confirmed with ventilatory equivalents for O_2 and CO_2. Peak heart rate was recorded for each exercise bout.

NIRS

A wireless continuous-wave NIRS device (PortaMon, Artinis Medical Systems, Zetten, The Netherlands) was used to measure local changes in Hb concentration in the right, vastus lateralis muscle during all sessions. NIRS data were collected using the software Oxysoft (Artinis Medical Systems) and were sampled with a frequency of 10 Hz and expressed as $\Delta\mu mol \cdot L^{-1}$. The PortaMon probe consists of three light sources (wavelengths: 760 nm and 850 nm) separated by 3, 3.5, and 4 cm from the receiving optode, while only data measured with the 3.5 cm optode distance were taken into account, corresponding to a penetration depth of approximately 1.75 cm [17, 34]. The probe,

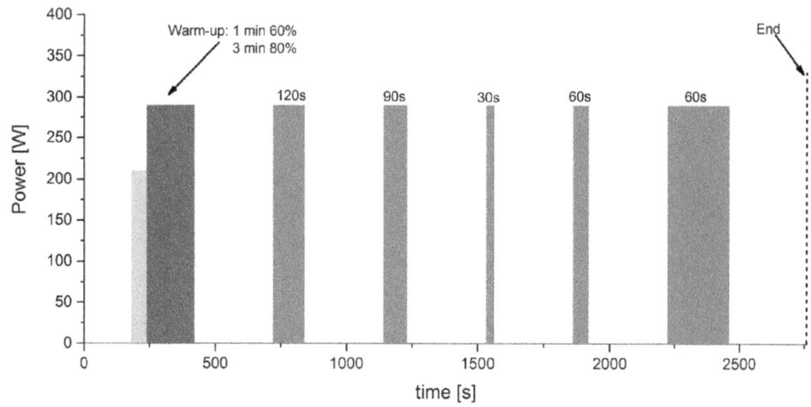

Fig. 1 Scheme of an exemplary experimental protocol. Subjects had to maintain a standardized recovery position, sitting on the ergometer during baseline measurement prior to the warm-up and recovery periods between exercise bouts

which was firmly attached with adhesive tape to the shaved skin above the distal part of the right vastus lateralis muscle, was covered with a lightproof cloth to prevent any influences of ambient light. The position of the probe was marked with a surgical marker to detect possible shifts (of the probe) during the test.

The PortaMon probe simultaneously uses the modified Lambert–Beer law and spatially resolved spectroscopy [22], which enables the observation of relative changes in O_2Hb, HHb, and THb. Because the exact path-length of the photons which penetrate the tissue is unknown when using continuous-wave spectroscopy, a differential path-length factor has to be used [22]. In the present study, we used a differential path-length factor of 4, which has been applied by other studies in measurements of muscle tissue [29, 34]. However, we are aware of the uncertainty of the differential path-length factor for muscle tissue and, hence, have reported all changes relative to individually measured baseline values (ΔTHb/O2Hb/HHb). Due to the equal absorption properties of Hb and myoglobin (Mb), it is not possible to distinguish between their contributions on the NIRS signal. However, the contribution of Mb to the NIRS signal is assumed to be minimal [22]. For simplification, "Hb + Mb" are termed "Hb" in the present study.

After collection, the data were smoothed with a 1-s moving average. The data of the last 30 s of $BASE_0$ were averaged. Baseline values were measured again for each exercise bout in the last 30 s of the previous recovery period ($BASE_{30-240}$). The recovery time of ΔTHb/O2Hb/HHb was determined by assessing the time elapsed from cessation of exercise and the point where the value reached the average of the last 30 s of recovery ±5 standard deviations for the first time (Table 2). We chose five standard deviations because the behavior of the NIRS parameters was not completely stable, even in the end of each recovery period, due to subjects' involuntary movements. End-exercise values (averaged over the last 10 s of exercise) were assessed and expressed in relation to the respective baseline values for each exercise bout (EE_O2Hb/HHb/THb). The early post-exercise overcompensation appears as an overshoot (OS) of ΔO_2Hb and ΔTHb after termination of exercise and was also expressed in relation to baseline values (Fig. 2), as well as the time-to-peak from cessation of exercise (Table 2). To control possible changes of BASE, we calculated the difference between the baseline before and after each exercise bout (ΔBASE40–90).

Statistical analyses

Statistical analyses were performed using the statistical software package, SPSS version 20 (SPSS Inc., Chicago,

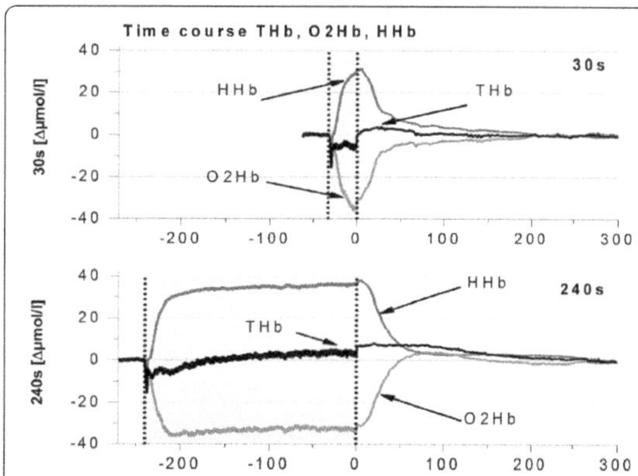

Fig. 2 Typical kinetics of ΔO_2Hb, ΔHHb, and ΔTHb during and after 30-s and 240-s cycling at 80 % $\dot{V}O_{2peak}$ in relation to baseline values (set to zero). Note the marked overshoot in ΔO_2Hb following the 240-s exercise interval compared to the 30-s interval

IL, USA). We used repeated measures analysis of variance (ANOVA) to detect possible differences in the effect of the various exercise durations on OS_O_2Hb/THb, end-exercise concentrations of $\Delta O_2Hb/\Delta HHb/\Delta THb$, peak heart rate, time-to-peak for ΔO_2Hb, and ΔTHb, as well as ΔBASE for $\Delta O_2Hb/\Delta HHb/\Delta THb$. Data were tested for sphericity with Mauchly's test and were corrected using the Greenhouse–Geisser method [35] when necessary. If ANOVA showed a significant main effect, pairwise comparisons were performed with Bonferroni–Holm corrected post-hoc tests. For OS_O_2Hb and OS_THb, the relative aerobic fitness was considered a group factor, whereby subjects with GET below 60 % $\dot{V}O_{2peak}$ and above 60 % $\dot{V}O_{2peak}$ were assigned as "GET60 –" and "GET60+", respectively. The cut-off point was chosen as 60 % $\dot{V}O_{2peak}$ because this approximately corresponds to the mean GET for the entire sample (Table 1). Separate ANOVAs were performed for each level of aerobic fitness when a significant interaction of *time* × *aerobic fitness* could be observed, whereas the differences between 30, 60, 90, and 240 s of exercise were focused on. "Pre-exercise" values of ΔO_2Hb and ΔTHb were individually compared with the corresponding post-exercise peak values (which have been used to calculate OS) using *t*-tests. The purpose of the individual comparisons was to verify whether the post-exercise elevation in both parameters was significant. The same procedure was conducted to compare baseline values before and after particular exercise bouts to test for possible baseline drifts. A *P* value of ≤0.05 was considered statistically significant.

Results

Parameters during exercise

Figure 2 shows a representative time course of one subject showing post-exercise ΔHHb, ΔO_2Hb, and ΔTHb kinetics during and following 30-s to 240-s exercise bouts at 80 % $\dot{V}O_{2peak}$. An ANOVA revealed a significant effect of the factor *time* on end-exercise ΔO_2Hb ($F_{4,68} = 4.1$; $P = 0.005$), ΔHHb ($F_{3,54} = 22.5$; $P < 0.001$), and ΔTHb values ($F_{3,42} = 24.7$; $P < 0.001$, Fig. 3). For ΔO2Hb, post hoc tests showed significantly lower values at the end of the 60-s exercise bouts than in the 120-s and 240-s exercise bouts ($P \leq 0.010$). The end-exercise ΔTHb values increased significantly with increasing exercise duration ($P \leq 0.042$). End-exercise ΔHHb showed a similar time course (i.e., one that increased significantly with increasing exercise duration [$P \leq 0.046$]), except when the value at 90 s was compared with that at 120 s.

Heart-rate values were also affected by exercise duration ($F_{3,41} = 116$; $P < 0.001$) and increased significantly with this factor ($P < 0.001$, Fig. 4a).

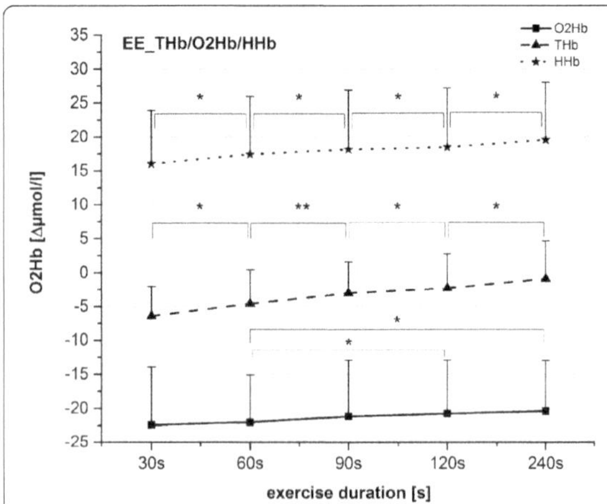

Fig. 3 End-exercise (EE) values (mean ± SD) of ΔO2Hb (*solid line*), ΔHHb (*dotted line*), and ΔTHb (*broken line*). *Asterisks* represent results from post-hoc tests in relation to values marked with double lines; * = $P < 0.05$; ** = $P < 0.01$; *** = $P < 0.001$

Post-exercise parameters

Immediately after cessation of the exercise bouts, ΔO_2Hb, ΔHHb, and (as a consequence) ΔTHb increased abruptly due to the relaxation of the working muscle. Afterward, ΔHHb decreased in an exponential manner and reached a stable level without showing any clear and systematic undershoot. ΔO_2Hb increased inversely following 30 s of exercise. Following 60, 90, 120, and 240 s, of exercising at 80 % $\dot{V}O_{2peak}$, the ΔO_2Hb increased abruptly and reached an overshoot (OS_O_2Hb), relative to the pre-exercise values ($P < 0.001$) within 80 s. This time-to-peak was significantly longer following 30-s of exercise (ANOVA: $F_{4,68} = 6.0$; $P = 0.008$; post-hoc: $P \leq 0.018$, see Table 2). Subsequently, ΔO_2Hb decreased to baseline level. Although there was no overcompensation with a subsequent decrease in ΔO_2Hb after 30-s exercise (Fig. 2), the highest post-exercise value (which actually occurred in the end of the recovery period) was determined as OS_O_2Hb_{30}. Because there were small increases in baseline values throughout the trial, the overshoot following 30 s was also significantly higher ($P = 0.003$) than the pre-exercise baseline values (changes in baseline values were not related to exercise duration). The post-exercise overcompensation also occurred for ΔTHb after all exercise bouts ($P < 0.001$), whereas time-to-peak was not significantly related to exercise duration (Table 2).

ANOVA showed significant effects of the factor *time* on OS_O_2Hb ($F_{3,53} = 26.6$; $P < 0.001$) and OS_THb ($F_{2,40} = 23.2$; $P < 0.001$). Based on post-hoc tests, the OS_O_2Hb increased with increasing length of the exercise bouts up to 90-s exercise duration ($P \leq 0.005$) (Fig. 4b). Also,

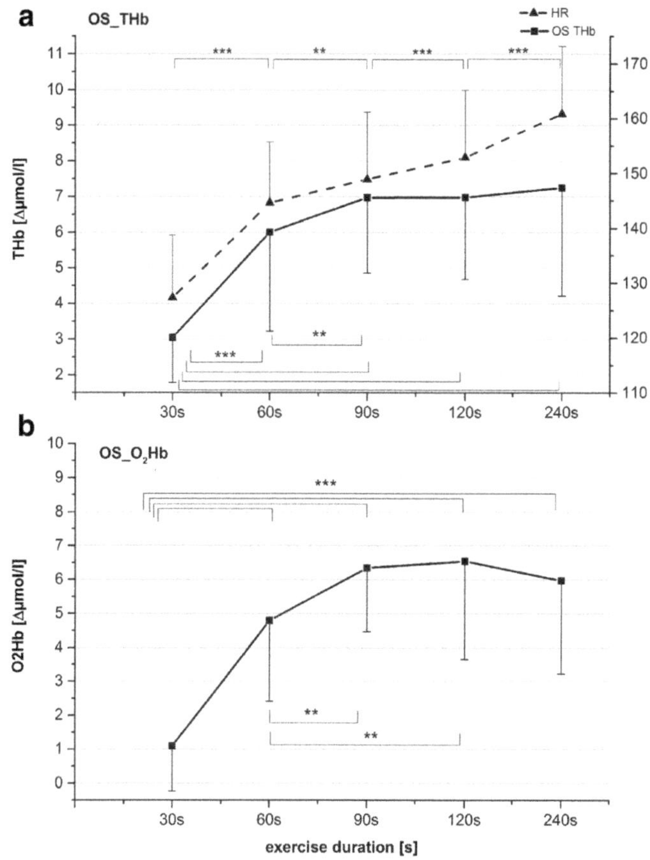

Fig. 4 **a** Overshoot values of ΔTHb (*solid line*) and end-exercise (EE) heart rate values (*broken line*) (mean ± SD) after the five exercise bouts. **b** Overshoot values of ΔO2Hb (mean ± SD) after five exercise bouts. *Asterisks* represent results from post-hoc tests in relation to values marked with double lines; * $P < 0.05$; ** $P < 0.01$; *** $P < 0.001$. Heart-rate values all differed significantly from each other at $P < 0.001$

OS_O_2Hb values following the 120-s and 240-s exercise bouts were not significantly different from those following the 60-s bout.

OS_THb had a similar time course to OS_O_2Hb. OS_THb_{60} was significantly higher ($P \leq 0.005$) than OS_THb_{30} and was significantly lower than OS_THb_{120} ($P \leq 0.008$). However, OS_THb_{90} was not different from OS_THb_{60} and OS_THb_{120} (Fig. 4a). OS_THb_{240} was not different from OS_THb_{120}.

We noted a significant interaction of *time* × *aerobic fitness* in OS_O_2Hb ($F_{3,51} = 4.1$; $P = 0.011$). In the GET60+ group, OS_O_2Hb was significantly influenced by the factor *time* ($F_{3,18} = 17.3$; $P < 0.001$). Post hoc tests showed significantly lower values for OS_O_2Hb following 30 s of exercise than those for the other exercise intensities ($P \leq 0.007$). The factor *time* also affected OS_O_2Hb in the GET60− group ($F_{3,30} = 16.5$; $P < 0.001$), but contrary to the GET60+ group, this parameter increased progressively from 30 s to 90 s in exercise duration ($P \leq 0.015$) and did not change significantly thereafter (Fig. 5).

However, no significant interaction of *time* × *aerobic fitness* could be found for OS_THb ($F_{3,34} = 2.9$; $P = 0.068$).

All parameters (ΔO_2Hb, ΔHHb, and ΔTHb) reached stable values at the end of each recovery period (which was defined as the new baseline for the subsequent exercise bout). These new baseline values did not show any significant exercise "duration-related" differences; neither when sorted by exercise intensity nor by chronological order of the exercise bouts (Table 3).

Discussion

The data of the present study show that cycling exercise at 80 % $\dot{V}O_{2peak}$ triggers post-exercise hyperemia, which is indicated by an overshoot in ΔTHb following exercise bouts in relation to pre-exercise values. ΔTHb has been

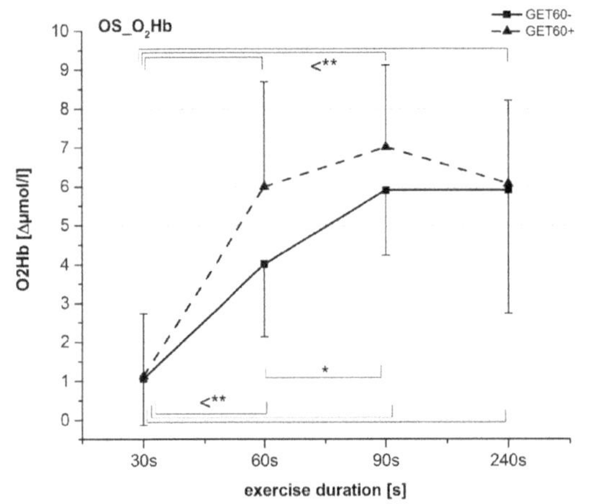

Fig. 5 Overshoot values of ΔO2Hb (mean ± SD) for GET60+ and GET60−. *Asterisks* represent results from post-hoc tests in relation to values marked with double lines; **P* < 0.05; ** *P* < 0.01; *** *P* < 0.001

used as an indirect measure for blood volume previously [21–23]. When we considered the five different exercise durations, the 30-s and 60-s exercise bouts evoked significantly lower overshoot values than the longer exercise bouts.

Because the relationship of post-exercise overshoots of ΔTHb and ΔO_2Hb evolved similarly, we suggested that the arterial blood supply primarily accounts for the increased post-exercise ΔTHb. A reduced outflow would be expected to emerge as a concomitant increase in post-exercise ΔHHb at the point of OS. Like OS_THb, OS_O_2Hb increased stepwise from 30 to 60-s and from 60 to 90-s exercise, indicating an increasing availability of oxygen in the area of interrogation up to exercise durations ≥90 s.

To the best of our knowledge, the present study is the first to investigate post-exercise muscle reoxygenation in relation to single exercise bouts of different durations as they are used in interval-training regimens. In general, a number of studies have reported on post-exercise hyperemia following single exercise bouts of similar durations as they were applied in the present study [16, 17, 19]. Furthermore, Danduran et al. [18] observed hyperemia using NIRS following a graded exercise test design in healthy children. Post-exercise reoxygenation was analyzed in various studies. A significant dependency of post-exercise Hb and muscle oxygenation recovery kinetics on exercise intensity (in terms of a forced reoxygenation following higher exercise intensities) has been reported previously [16, 17, 19]. Despite this dependence, reoxygenation time is apparently not influenced by exercise intensity [19, 29]. When Belfry et al. [36] compared interval-training regimens with constant-load exercise at equal intensity, they found a better matching of O_2 delivery to O_2 utilization during exercise for the interval regimens than that in constant-load exercise. O_2 delivery during interval training was enhanced when recovery was applied in the moderate intensity domain in comparison to "low-intensity" active recovery. Besides the muscle-pump effect, which was presumably increased during interval training with "moderate intensity" recovery, the authors suggested enhanced local vasodilation to be an important determinant for those results.

Zafeiridis et al. [20] were also able to find improved local oxygen delivery during exercise. In contrast to Belfry et al., they found no differences between constant-load exercise and two interval-training regimens with different work-interval durations. The different results in these two studies could likely be attributed to differences in the two study protocols. As we did in the present study, Zafeiridis et al. examined the effect of different work-interval durations. They used work intervals of 30 s with an intensity of 110 % of the power output corresponding to $\dot{V}O_{2\,max}$ and 120-s intervals with an intensity of 95 % $\dot{V}O_{2\,max}$ and did not find significantly different local-oxygen delivery during both interval-training regimens. This finding of Zafeiridis et al. is

Table 3 Baseline drifts

A. Exercise duration	ANOVA	30 s	60 s	90 s	120 s	240 s
ΔBASE_THb (Δµmol·l^{-1})	*P* = 0.182	0.79 ± 1.18	0.76 ± 2.84	1.06 ± 1.26	1.17 ± 0.98	0.83 ± 1.14
ΔBASE_O_2Hb (Δµmol·l^{-1})	*P* = 0.069	−1.54 ± 1.98	−0.62 ± 4.37	0.95 ± 2.31	1.95 ± 1.64	0.65 ± 1.00
ΔBASE_HHb (Δµmol·l^{-1})	*P* = 0.086	0.97 ± 1.24	0.51 ± 2.01	−0.09 ± 1.22	−0.41 ± 0.75	0.72 ± 1.52
B. No. of exercise bout		1	2	3	4	5
ΔBASE_THb (Δµmol·l^{-1})	*P* = 0.564	0.87 ± 3.05	1.16 ± 1.13	0.34 ± 1.24	1.34 ± 1.20	0.17 ± 1.29
ΔBASE_O_2Hb (Δµmol·l^{-1})	*P* = 0.271	0.18 ± 3.30	1.14 ± 1.82	0.77 ± 1.69	1.76 ± 1.75	−0.87 ± 2.43
ΔBASE_HHb (Δµmol·l^{-1})	*P* = 0.218	0.69 ± 1.40	−0.20 ± 1.23	−0.43 ± 0.63	−0.42 ± 1.54	1.04 ± 1.34

n = 18; values are expressed as mean ± SD; ΔBASE values are the differences between the baseline values before and after the exercise bouts; Panel A shows baseline drifts sorted by exercise duration while panel B shows baseline drifts sorted by chronological order of the exercise bouts contrary to our findings, which showed significantly higher post-exercise oxygen availability and blood supply following 120 s of exercise than that following 30 s of exercise with 80 % $\dot{V}O_{2peak}$. We cite two possible explanations for this difference. First, the dependency of post-exercise blood supply and oxygen availability on exercise duration, as it is shown in the present study, appears to be valid only within a certain exercise intensity range. In a previous study, we examined the effect of exercise intensity on post-exercise blood supply and oxygen availability and observed a non-linear relationship [19]. We found no differences between 80 and 90 % $\dot{V}O_{2peak}$, but did not include higher exercise intensities; therefore, it might be possible that our results are not valid for supramaximal exercise. Second, Zafeiridis et al. used different recovery durations between work intervals, which could have contributed to different results. It could be that 30-s work intervals cause hyperemia similar to that associated with 120-s intervals, when recovery periods are adjusted appropriately.

Although the methods used in our study do not provide sufficiently detailed information on the complex regulation of local muscle perfusion, we call attention to a few possible explanations for our results. In general, cardiac output and artery flow increase as a response to dynamic exercise [12]. In exercising muscles, two antagonistic mechanisms happen: There is global sympathetic mediated vasoconstriction on the one hand whereas acute vasodilation occurs in active tissue secondary to a promoted release of vasoactive substances on the other hand. Because vasodilation superimposes sympathetic mediated vasoconstriction in active muscles, capillary perfusion is increased [10, 37, 38]. This process is supported mechanically by rhythmic contractions of the muscle during cycle exercise (muscle pump) [12].

Previous research has shown a biphasic response of muscle blood flow to exercise with an early, rapid response within the first 5–7 s and a prolonged, secondary response starting 15–20 s from the onset of exercise [15], while a steady state is reached within 1–3 min. Hence, blood-flow adjustments to exercise occur rather quickly. After termination of exercise, blood-flow recovery has been reported to be slower following heavy exercise than following moderate exercise [13]. This slowing of blood-flow recovery is most likely due to the prolonged presence of vasoactive substances. In rats, it had been shown that acute, vasodilatory responses to exercise can last up to two days or more [39]. Consequently, prolonged, local vasodilation seems to be dependent on the extent of the release of vasoactive substances during the previous exercise bout.

But which mechanisms are crucial for the increased post-exercise oxygen availability between 30 and 90 s of exercise at 80 % $\dot{V}O_{2peak}$? We did not measure cardiac output in this study, but our data reveals some basis for speculation. The local oxygen availability was equal from 90 to 240 s of exercise duration (Fig. 4b), while end-exercise heart rate increased continuously. We assumed accordingly that end-exercise cardiac output also increased continuously with exercise duration (otherwise, stroke volume would have declined, which is unlikely). Hence, if the prolonged recovery of cardiac output would have greater implications on post-exercise hyperemia, then post-exercise hyperemia would have been expected to increase continuously following exercise durations >90 s. In a previous study, we observed similar characteristics in the relationship of local blood supply and exercise intensity [19]. Among local mechanisms, the muscle pump is neglectable as an explanation of our results as it stops with cessation of exercise, which leads to an abrupt drop in muscle blood flow [13].

Local Vasodilation remains as the most plausible determinant for the hyperemia and increased post-exercise oxygen availability following cycling exercise ≥90 s at 80 % $\dot{V}O_{2peak}$. Factors that trigger vasodilation are various. Among those factors, chemically and flow mediated vasodilation have to be highlighted when discussing exercise induced vasodilation [40]. In particular, adenosine, acetylcholine, and shear stress are presumed to trigger exercise-induced effects on vasodilation [41, 42]. It can be assumed that blood flow during exercise and prolonged vasodilation of small vessels in the post-exercise phase are positively related. It is likely that this effect was more pronounced (in our study) following exercise durations ≥90 s compared to shorter exercise bouts. And again, because we did not measure vasodilating substances or cardiac output and blood flow velocity directly, the implications of the above-mentioned mechanisms for our study results remain speculation-based.

We have shown that oxygen availability following cycling exercise is dependent on exercise duration. Our results demonstrate that this dependency is influenced by the relative aerobic fitness (i.e., GET), expressed as a percentage of $\dot{V}O_{2peak}$. In the GET60+ group, 60 s of exercise were sufficient to evoke a post-exercise overshoot of ΔO_2Hb, which was equal to the overshoots following longer exercise bouts. In the GET60− group, 90 s of exercise were needed to obtain those high values. Hence, adjustments in local vasodilation are possibly faster in subjects showing high relative aerobic power. This means that in subjects with higher aerobic fitness, exercise durations of 60 s are sufficient to evoke an increased post-exercise hyperemia and increased oxygen availability.

Advantages of improved post-exercise O_2 availability

There are several advantages of improved local blood and oxygen supply, as it has been observed following exercise durations >90 s at 80 % $\dot{V}O_{2peak}$. First, gas exchange is facilitated when the functional cross-sectional area of capillaries is increased [9]. Moreover, muscle reoxygenation has been shown to improve with endurance training [43]. A higher local muscle perfusion is associated with enhanced oxidative metabolism, such as fatty acid oxidation [44–46]. Romijn et al. [44] showed reduced fatty acid mobilization during strenuous exercise (85 % $\dot{V}O_{2peak}$), as well as a strongly increased post-exercise plasma fatty-acid availability following strenuous exercise [44, 45]. This increased post-exercise, plasma fatty-acid availability may be one explanation for improvements in fatty-acid oxidation capacity as long-term metabolic adaptations that have been observed following HIT in women [3]. Kimber et al. [47] found a significant dependency of post-exercise fatty-acid oxidation on fatty-acid availability. Exercise that increases fatty-acid availability is, therefore, likely to enhance fatty-acid oxidation after or between exercise bouts. The improved post-exercise blood supply during recovery or, when active recovery is applied, during the relief interval could therefore augment fatty-acid oxidation in particular. However, we reiterate that these suggestions are speculative because we did not measure fatty-acid oxidation.

Study limitations

When using NIRS, the influence of adipose tissue thickness (ATT) has to be considered [34]. If skin and subcutaneous tissue thickness is near to or exceeds the penetration depth of the emitted photons, muscular effects will be blunted. Skin and subcutaneous thickness was approximately 3.75 mm (7.5 ± 3.1 mm skinfold thickness, measured with a caliper). Because penetration depth has been shown to be approximately half of the optode distance [22, 34], it can be concluded that NIRS signal was capable for measuring muscle oxidation in our study as the inter-optode distance was 3.5 cm, enabling a penetration depth of 1.75 cm.

Another point to mention is the 5-min recovery period in-between exercise bouts, which was too short to enable a full recovery of ΔO_2Hb and ΔTHb. It therefore has to be considered, that prior exercise bouts influenced the subsequent exercise bouts [31] First, this baseline drift in ΔO_2Hb and ΔTHb did not show any relationship to exercise duration. Second, we randomized the order of the exercise bouts and placed an intensive warm-up in front of the first experimental exercise bout. Consequently, this issue should not have influenced our results.

We recruited only male subjects to reduce variability in subject characteristics and because of the minor adipose tissue thickness in males relative to that in females, which apparently affects NIRS signals [34]. Hence, the relevance of our results on females is limited.

Work intervals within interval-training regimens are described by interval duration and interval intensity. We investigated the influence of exercise intensity on local muscle O_2 availability and blood supply in an earlier study [19]. The present study aimed to examine the effect of duration, using isolated, "interval-training-associated" exercise bouts. But besides the work interval, several other variables in interval-training prescriptions, such as intensity and duration of the recovery interval and number of repetitions, should be noted. The latter is of particular importance. Because HIT consists of repeated sets of transitions from high to low intensity, work-interval durations <90 s also are potentially effective to increase post-exercise oxygen availability due to a cumulative effect. This "repeated bout" effect could occur when low intervals are too short to provide an adequate recovery. It is therefore conceivable that effects of HIT on local oxygen availability could be similar across different exercise durations, for example when the work-to-rest ratio is kept constant. It has to be highlighted that all intervals in our study had been carried out with the same exercise intensity. Usually, work intervals are prescribed with higher intensity during "short-interval" HIT-regiments [1]. As a consequence, the low interval has to be extended to provide sufficient recovery to enable the completion of the following work interval. Consequently, the relationship between interval intensity, duration and recovery has to be focused in future research.

Finally, the post-exercise O_2 availability and blood supply are two of several determinants causing aerobic adaptations. Investigation of other determinants may require other, optimal "work-interval" durations.

Conclusion

Exercise duration in HIT has a significant impact on post-exercise oxygen availability following cycling exercise with 80 % $\dot{V}O_{2peak}$. The highest post-exercise oxygen availability is induced with exercise durations of 90 s and longer, whereas no further increase is evoked by longer exercise durations up to 240 s. Post-exercise oxygen availability is dependent on aerobic fitness. Subjects, who reached GET below 60 % $\dot{V}O_{2peak}$ needed 90 s to reach the maximum post-exercise oxygen availability, while subjects who reached GET above 60 % $\dot{V}O_{2peak}$ reached the maximum post-exercise oxygen availability following 60 s exercise. To facilitate oxidative adaptations, work intervals within interval-training regimens should be prescribed with a minimum length of 60 s, depending on aerobic fitness, whereas it has to be reiterated that the transferability of our findings to exercise intensities that are different to 80 % $\dot{V}O_{2peak}$ may be limited.

Ethics approval and consent to participate

The study protocol was approved by the local Ethics Committee of the Technische Universität München, Klinikum Rechts der Isar (#67/14). All subjects received detailed information on the purpose and procedures of the study and gave their written informed consent.

Consent for publications

Not applicable.

Abbreviations

AIT: aerobic interval training; ANOVA: analysis of variance; ATT: adipose tissue thickness; BASE: baseline; GET: gas exchange threshold; GET60+: subjects with GET above 60 % $\dot{V}O_{2peak}$; GET60–: subjects with GET below 60 % $\dot{V}O_{2peak}$; HHb: deoxygenated hemoglobin; HIIT: high intensity interval training; HIT: high intensity training; NIRS: near-infrared spectroscopy; $\dot{V}O_2$: oxygen uptake; O_2Hb: oxygenated hemoglobin; $\dot{V}O_{2max}$: maximal oxygen uptake; $\dot{V}O_{2peak}$: peak oxygen uptake; OS: postexercise overshoot; THb: total hemoglobin.

Competing interests

The authors declare that they have no competing interests.

Authors' contribution

FS was responsible for the present study's concept and design, as well as for data acquisition, analysis, and interpretation. Furthermore, he was largely responsible for drafting of the manuscript. CvonO collaborated substantially with data acquisition. FKP was deeply involved in drafting and reviewing the manuscript. TS contributed during the preparation of the study's concept and design and reviewed the manuscript. RO supervised the entire study and manuscript processing, was responsible for the ethical proposal, and gave the final approval for submission of the manuscript.

Authors' information

Stöcker, Fabian: Research associate and lecturer. Main topic: Exercise physiology.
Von Oldershausen, Christoph: Master student.
Paternoster, Florian Kurt: Research associate and lecturer. Main topic: Biomechanics.
Schulz, Thorsten: Phd, Senior Researcher and lecturer. Main topic: Endocrinology.
Oberhoffer, Renate: Professor, MD. Main topic: Cardiology, Pediatrics.

Acknowledgements

The authors thank all subjects for their cooperation in this study.

Funding

No external funding was received for this study.

Author details

[1]Center for Teaching and Learning, Technische Universität München, Connollystraße 32, 80809 München, Germany. [2]Department for Biomechanics in Sports, Technische Universität München, München, Germany. [3]Department for Preventive Pediatrics, Technische Universität München, München, Germany.

References

1. Buchheit M, Laursen PB. High-intensity interval training, solutions to the programming puzzle. Sports Med. 2013;43:927–54.
2. Weston AR, Myburgh KH, Lindsay FH, Dennis SC, Noakes TD, Hawley JA. Skeletal muscle buffering capacity and endurance performance after high-intensity interval training by well-trained cyclists. Eur J Appl Physiol Occup Physiol. 1996;75:7–13.
3. Talanian JL, Galloway SDR, Heigenhauser GJF, Bonen A, Spriet LL. Two weeks of high-intensity aerobic interval training increases the capacity for fat oxidation during exercise in women. J Appl Physiol. 2006;102: 1439–47.
4. Laursen PB, Jenkins DG. The scientific basis for high-intensity interval training. Sports Med. 2002;32:53–73.
5. Esfarjani F, Laursen PB. Manipulating high-intensity interval training: effects on VO2 max, the lactate threshold and 3000 m running performance in moderately trained males. J Sci Med Sport. 2007;10:27–35.
6. Buchheit M, Laursen PB. High-intensity interval training, solutions to the programming puzzle. Sports Med. 2013;43:313–38.
7. Fu T-C, Wang C-H, Lin P-S, Hsu C-C, Cherng W-J, Huang S-C, Liu M-H, Chiang C-L, Wang J-S. Aerobic interval training improves oxygen uptake efficiency by enhancing cerebral and muscular hemodynamics in patients with heart failure. Int J Cardiol. 2011;167:41–50.
8. Peake JM, Tan SJ, Markworth JF, Broadbent JA, Skinner TL, Cameron-Smith D. Metabolic and hormonal responses to isoenergetic high-intensity interval exercise and continuous moderate-intensity exercise. AJP: Endocrinology and Metabolism. 2014;307:E539–52.
9. Calbet JAL, Lundby C. Skeletal muscle vasodilatation during maximal exercise in health and disease. J Physiol Lond. 2012;590:6285–96.
10. Huonker M, Halle M, Keul J. Structural and functional adaptations of the cardiovascular system by training. Int J Sports Med. 1996;17:S164–72.
11. Messonnier L, Freund H, Denis C, Dormois D, Dufour A-B, Lacour J-R. Time to exhaustion at VO(2)max is related to the lactate exchange and removal abilities. Int J Sports Med. 2002;23:433–8.
12. Saltin B, Rådegran G, Koskolou MD, Roach RC. Skeletal muscle blood flow in humans and its regulation during exercise. Acta Physiol Scand. 1998;162:421–36.
13. Ferreira LF, Harper AJ, Townsend DK, Lutjemeier BJ, Barstow TJ. Kinetics of estimated human muscle capillary blood flow during recovery from exercise. Exp Physiol. 2005;90:715–26.
14. Belardinelli R, Barstow TJ, Porszasz J, Wasserman K. Changes in skeletal muscle oxygenation during incremental exercise measured with near infrared spectroscopy. Eur J Appl Physiol. 1995;70:487–92.
15. Tschakovsky ME. Immediate exercise hyperemia: contributions of the muscle pump vs. rapid vasodilation. J Appl Physiol. 2004;97:739–47.
16. Bhambhani YN, Buckley S, Susaki T. Muscle oxygenation trends during constant work rate cycle exercise in men and women. Med Sci Sports Exerc. 1999;31:90–8.
17. Chance BB, Dait MTM, Zhang CC, Hamaoka TT, Hagerman FF. Recovery from exercise-induced desaturation in the quadriceps muscles of elite competitive rowers. Am J Physiol. 1992;262:C766–75.
18. Danduran MJ, Dixon JE, Rao RP. Near infrared spectroscopy describes physiologic payback associated with excess postexercise oxygen consumption in healthy controls and children with complex congenital heart disease. Pediatr Cardiol. 2012;33:95–102.
19. Stöcker F, Von Oldershausen C, Paternoster FK, Schulz T, Oberhoffer R. End-exercise ΔHHb/ΔVO 2and post-exercise local oxygen availability in relation to exercise intensity. Clin Physiol Funct Imaging. 2015 [Epub ahead of print].
20. Zafeiridis A, Kounoupis A, Dipla K, Kyparos A, Nikolaidis M, Smilios I, Vrabas I. Oxygen delivery and muscle deoxygenation during continuous, long- and short-interval exercise. Int J Sports Med. 2015;36:872–80.
21. Costes F, Prieur F, Féasson L, Geyssant A, Barthélémy J-C, Denis C. Influence of training on NIRS muscle oxygen saturation during submaximal exercise. Med Sci Sports Exerc. 2001;33:1484.
22. Ferrari M, Mottola L, Quaresima V. Principles, techniques, and limitations of near infrared spectroscopy. Can J Appl Physiol. 2004;29:463–87.
23. Ihsan M, Abbiss CR, Lipski M, Buchheit M, Watson G. Muscle oxygenation and blood volume reliability during continuous and intermittent running. Int J Sports Med. 2013;34:637–45.
24. Watanabe S, Ishii C, Takeyasu N, Ajisaka R, Nishina H, Morimoto T, Sakamoto K, Eda K, Ishiyama M, Saito T, Aihara H, Arai E, Toyama M, Shintomi Y, Yamaguchi I. Assessing muscle vasodilation using near-infrared spectroscopy in cardiac patients. Circ J. 2005;69:802–14.
25. Beaver W, Wasserman K, Whipp BJ. A new method for detecting anaerobic threshold by gas exchange. J Appl Physiol. 1986;60:2020–7.
26. Midgley AW, Bentley DJ, Luttikholt H, McNaughton LR, Millet GP. Challenging a dogma of exercise physiology: does an incremental exercise

test for valid VO 2 max determination really need to last between 8 and 12 minutes? Sports Med. 2008;38:441–7.
27. Day JR, Rossiter HB, Coats EM, Skasick A, Whipp BJ. The maximally attainable V̇o 2during exercise in humans: the peak vs. maximum issue. J Appl Physiol. 2003;95:1901–7.
28. Burnley M, Jones AM. Oxygen uptake kinetics as a determinant of sports performance. European J Sport Sc. 2007;7:63–79.
29. Buchheit M, Ufland P, Haydar B, Laursen PB, Ahmaidi S. Reproducibility and sensitivity of muscle reoxygenation and oxygen uptake recovery kinetics following running exercise in the field. Clin Physiol Funct Imaging. 2011;31: 337–46.
30. Davis SL, Fadel PJ, Cui J, Thomas GD, Crandall CG. Skin blood flow influences near-infrared spectroscopy-derived measurements of tissue oxygenation during heat stress. J Appl Physiol. 2006;100:221–4.
31. Jones AM, Koppo K, Burnley M. Effects of prior exercise on metabolic and gas exchange responses to exercise. Sports Med. 2003;33:949–71.
32. Bringard A, Layec G, Micallef J-P, Bendahan D, Perrey S. Gas exchange measurements within a magnetic environment: validation of a new system. Respir Physiol Neurobiol. 2012;182:37–46.
33. Kusch M, Vogt A, Hoffmann U. Quality control of various ergospirometric measuring parameters by means of a gas exchange simulating system. J Kardiol. 2003;10:405.
34. van Beekvelt MC, Borghuis MS, van Engelen BG, Wevers RA, Colier WN. Adipose tissue thickness affects in vivo quantitative near-IR spectroscopy in human skeletal muscle. Clin Sci. 2001;101:21–8.
35. Greenhouse SW, Geisser S. On methods in the analysis of profile data. Psychometrika. 1959;24:95–112.
36. Belfry GR, Paterson DH, Murias JM. The effects of short recovery duration on VO2 and muscle deoxygenation during intermittent exercise-Springer. Eur J Appl Physiol. 2012;112:1907–15.
37. Laughlin MH, Korzick DH. Vascular smooth muscle: integrator of vasoactive signals during exercise hyperemia. Med Sci Sports Exerc. 2001;33:81–91.
38. Murias JM, Kowalchuk JM, Paterson DH. Speeding of VO2 kinetics with endurance training in old and young men is associated with improved matching of local O2 delivery to muscle O2 utilization. J Appl Physiol. 2010; 108:913–22.
39. Haram PM, Adams V, Kemi OJ, Brubakk AO, Hambrecht R, Ellingsen O, Wisløff U. Time-course of endothelial adaptation following acute and regular exercise. Eur J Cardiovasc Prev Rehabil. 2006;13:585–91.
40. Joyner MJ, Casey DP. Regulation of increased blood flow (hyperemia) to muscles during exercise: a hierarchy of competing physiological needs. Physiol Rev. 2015;95:549–601.
41. Hellsten Y, Nyberg M, Jensen LG, Mortensen SP. Vasodilator interactions in skeletal muscle blood flow regulation. J Physiol Lond. 2012;590:6297–305.
42. Gielen S, Schuler G, Adams V. Cardiovascular effects of exercise training: molecular mechanisms. Circulation. 2010;122:1221–38.
43. Buchheit M, Ufland P. Effect of endurance training on performance and muscle reoxygenation rate during repeated-sprint running. Eur J Appl Physiol. 2010;111:293–301.
44. Romijn JA, Coyle EF, Sidossis LS, Gastaldelli A, Horowitz JF, Endert E, Wolfe RR. Regulation of endogenous fat and carbohydrate metabolism in relation to exercise intensity and duration. Am J Physiol. 1993;265:E380–91.
45. Horowitz JF. Fatty acid mobilization from adipose tissue during exercise. Trends Endocrinol Metab. 2003;14:386–92.
46. Laaksonen MS, Kemppainen J, Kyröläinen H, Knuuti J, Nuutila P, Kalliokoski KK. Regional differences in blood flow, glucose uptake and fatty acid uptake within quadriceps femoris muscle during dynamic knee-extension exercise. Eur J Appl Physiol. 2013;113:1775–82.
47. Kimber NE, Cameron-Smith D, McGee SL, Hargreaves M. Skeletal muscle fat metabolism after exercise in humans: influence of fat availability. J Appl Physiol. 2013;114:1577–85.

18

The association between generalized joint hypermobility and active horizontal shoulder abduction in 10–15 year old competitive swimmers

Tina Junge[1,2,3*], Peter Henriksen[2,3], Heidi Lund Andersen[1], Linette Dyg Byskov[1], Hans Kromann Knudsen[1] and Birgit Juul-Kristensen[3,4]

Abstract

Background: Increased shoulder mobility and Generalised Joint Hypermobility (GJH) are assumed to be predisposing risk factors for shoulder injuries. The association between GJH and shoulder mobility among competitive swimmers is unknown. The aim was to study the association between GJH and active horizontal shoulder abduction (AHSA) in young, competitive swimmers and to describe normative values of AHSA in this group.

Methods: In total, 92 swimmers (10–15 years) without shoulder pain participated. GJH was evaluated with the Beighton Tests (BT) for joint hypermobility. Shoulder mobility was measured as maximum AHSA. A multiple regression model was used to assess associations between GJH and AHSA.

Results: Overall, positive associations were found between GJH and AHSA. An increase of BT score was associated with an increase of AHSA, seen as an increased AHSA of 3.9°, 5.7° and 7.9° by BT cut off points ≥5/9, ≥6/9 and ≥7/9, respectively. Normative values for AHSA ranged from 40° to 52°, depending on age.

Conclusions: Positive associations were found between GJH and AHSA, as maximum AHSA range increased with increasing BT scores. Due to lack of shoulder mobility tests in the BT scoring system, the AHSA test seems to be a promising supplemental test.

Keywords: Competitive swimmers, Generalized joint hypermobility, Active horizontal shoulder abduction, Shoulder injuries

Background

A competitive swimmer swims 9–110 km a week, depending on age, fitness level and training requirements [1]. This amount leads to a large amount of repetitive movements, which may result in overuse injuries of the shoulder [2]. Although competitive swimming attracts a large number of children and adolescents, there are almost no epidemiological studies on adolescent shoulder injuries for children or adolescents within this sport [3]. The prevalence of shoulder injuries in adult competitive swimmers varies from 40 to 91 %, partly due to inconsistency in definition of injury, study design and data collection methods [2].

Freestyle stroke is a whole body movement, but with the upper extremities producing 90 % of the propulsive power [4], requiring shoulder strength, endurance and stability. Biomechanical challenges of the shoulder for the freestyle stroke may occur during the recovery phase, which demands a large Range Of Motion (ROM). A large ROM is anticipated to be advantageous by allowing the swimmer to achieve a body position that permits a larger stroke length, positively associated with swimming speed [2]. Consequently, the shoulder is repetitively forced into extension, horizontal abduction and internal rotation. Thus, swimming induces a large amount of stress on the

* Correspondence: tjunge@health.sdu.dk
[1]Department of Physiotherapy, University College Lillebaelt, Odense, Denmark
[2]Health Sciences Research Centre, University College Lillebaelt, Odense, Denmark
Full list of author information is available at the end of the article

anterior capsule and ligaments of the glenohumeral joint, which may lead to local shoulder laxity and/or an increased shoulder ROM [2, 5].

Increased shoulder ROM may be a genetic predisposition or an adaptation to the repetitive and excessive overhead movements in swimming. A condition in individuals with hereditary increased ROM is Generalised Joint Hypermobility (GJH), in which the ligaments and capsules are more lax compared with the normal population [6]. GJH is frequently present in swimmers, since as many as 20 % of male and female adult swimmers are classified with GJH [7]. Also, a higher prevalence of GJH is found in young, competitive swimmers compared with non-competitive swimmers [5, 8]. Increased shoulder ROM alone and GJH including shoulder hypermobility may play an important role in development of shoulder pain and injuries, and the extent of both conditions must be described as part of an injury sequence prevention strategy, focusing on underlying mechanisms [9].

GJH is most often assessed by the Beighton Tests (BT), involving a score from 0 to 9, with a suggested cut off point for classification of GJH of ≥4/9 in adults [10]. A cut off point for classifying children or adolescents with GJH has not been established, which is why the cut off point for GJH varies between studies [8, 11, 12]. The BT for hypermobility includes the 1st and 5th fingers, the elbows, the knees and forward bending, but there is no test for shoulder hypermobility [6]. The Active Horizontal Shoulder Abduction test (AHSA) (Illustration 1) could be a relevant shoulder mobility test for swimmers, simulating a swim-related stressful situation like the recovery phase of the freestyle stroke. Since the BT score is closely related to the general mobility of all joints [6] [13], the AHSA as supplemental test may provide a more comprehensive profile of the single swimmer's shoulder joint mobility.

In order to compare AHSA between different populations, normative data is required for young, competitive swimmers, taking into account age and sex. Such data exists for 15–21 year olds [14], however, no reference material covering younger swimmers between the ages of 10 to 15 years.

Thus, the aims of this study were to examine the association between shoulder ROM, defined by the Horizontal Shoulder Abduction test (AHSA) and the BT score, and to present normative values for AHSA in young, competitive swimmers between the ages of 10–15 years.

Methods

Participants

In total, 116 young, competitive swimmers aged 10–15 years were invited to take part in the current study, a substudy of the longitudinal cohort study, the *"Physical Performance in Young Competitive Swimmers"* (PPYCS). PPYCS involves young, competitive swimmers from 5 different swim teams at Funen, Denmark. The overall purpose of PPYCS is to assess development of mobility, physical fitness, motor performance and sports-related injuries longitudinally, within this specific cohort.

The inclusion criteria were healthy swimmers aged 10–15 years, participating in competitive swim teams, defined as a swimmer taking part in competitions at a level corresponding to a local district, a larger region or at national level. Exclusion criteria were musculoskeletal pain, injury or illness preventing the swimmer from participating on the day of testing.

Testers

Testers were last semester physiotherapy students, who carried out this study as part of their final thesis. Prior to testing, the testers undertook a supervised training phase by two experienced physiotherapists (HKK & TJ) in order to standardise test instructions and procedures and to approve a satisfactory inter- and intra tester reproducibility. The training phase included testing of approximately 100 adolescents aged 10–18 years. For both the BT and the AHSA test, the testers gave instructions to the swimmers according to the standardized protocol, along with visual demonstrations. The testers performing the AHSA test were blinded to the status of the swimmers being GJH or controls. All swimmers were tested with the BT and afterwards with the AHSA test.

Beighton tests (BT)

GJH was evaluated according to the BT score [6, 15]. The BT consists of five manoeuvres: 1) passive dorsiflexion of the little fingers beyond 90°, 2) passive apposition of the thumbs to the flexor aspects of the forearm, 3) hyperextension of the elbows beyond 10°, 4) hyperextension of the knees beyond 10° and 5) forward flexion of the trunk with the knees straight, resting the palms easily on the floor. One point was allocated for each of the tests being positive as described, bilaterally for manoeuvres 1–4, with a total score ranging from 0 to 9 [6]. The reliability of the Beighton score has been examined for the current test procedures in a corresponding age population with good to excellent inter and intra tester reproducibility [15]. Children were classified with GJH at different BT cut off points of ≥5/9, ≥6/9 and ≥7/9. The control group included children with a BT score ≤4/9.

Test for active horizontal shoulder abduction (AHSA)

AHSA was measured in prone using a Saunder Digital Inclinometer (Illustration 1). Each swimmer was lying in a prone starting position with the upper arm placed horizontally, 90° elbow flexion, fingertips pointing towards the floor and the head turned in the opposite

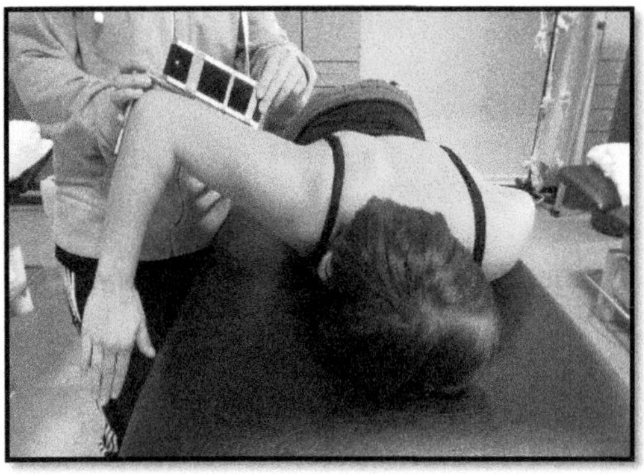

Illustration 1 Test of the horizontal shoulder abduction

direction of the shoulder being tested to avoid rotation of the spine. The Digital Inclinometer was mounted at the proximal end of an angle hinge, perpendicular to the distal end. The distal end was aligned to the forearm and the proximal to the upper arm, so that the elbow joint was kept in 90° angle, to secure stabilization during measurements and to optimize standardization during measurements (Illustration 2). The swimmer was asked to lift the elbow as far as possible towards the ceiling. The test was performed three times actively for both shoulders, and the maximum angle of the upper arm in horizontal shoulder abduction was recorded in degrees.

Data analysis

Data was tested for Normality with Shapiro-Wilks tests. Since no significant difference was found between left and right shoulder in the AHSA test ($p = 0.09$), a mean of AHSA for both shoulders was used for further analyses. A multiple linear regression model was used to test the association between AHSA and the BT score, using the three different BT cut off points at ≥5/9, ≥6/9 and ≥7/9, adjusted for sex and age.

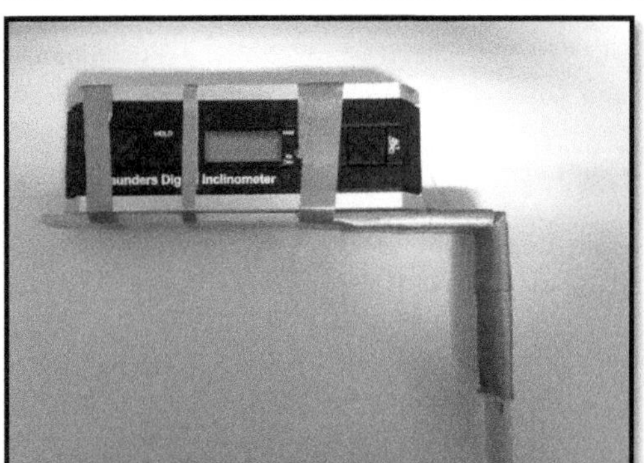

Illustration 2 Device with inclinometer

When calculating normative data of AHSA, age was found to be significantly or close to significant associated with the maximum AHSA for cut off point ≥6/9 ($p = 0.04$) and ≥7/9 ($p = 0.052$), for which reason data were stratified by age. There was no statistically significant effect of sex on maximum AHSA, hence data for boys and girls were merged and presented for the entire sample.

A p-value of 0.05 or less was considered statistically significant. All statistical analyses were conducted in SPSS version 20 (IBM SPSS Inc, Chicago, IL, USA, 2012).

Results

In total, 92 young, competitive swimmers (mean age 13 years; 49 girls), with no shoulder pain participated.

In demographic variables, the only significant difference were height, with the GJH group being shorter (Table 1). A larger prevalence of girls was found in the GJH group, no matter the cut-off point (Tables 1 and 2).

Significant positive associations were found between the BT score and AHSA, adjusted for sex and age (Table 3). An increasing degree of AHSA was found with an increasing BT score for all cut-off points. Swimmers with BT at cut-off point ≥5/9 had an AHSA which was 3.98° higher than controls. For the BT score of ≥7/9, the difference in AHSA increased to 7.90° between groups. There was no effect of gender. A significant negative effect on maximum AHSA with age was only found at cut-off point ≥6/9.

Normative data for the AHSA test were from 40.02° to 51.83° (mean 43.95°) across all age groups, for both controls and at all cut-off points for the GJH group, with the highest value and range of shoulder mobility for the youngest age groups, decreasing by age (Table 4).

Discussion

In the current study, a significant positive association was found between GJH and AHSA, with AHSA ranging from 5° to 8° higher than controls, with an increased BT

Table 1 Characteristics of participants with Generalised Joint Hypermobility (GJH), and without GJH (controls)

	GJH ($n = 29$) (mean, SD)	Controls ($n = 63$) (mean, SD)	*p-value*
Sex (no. girls)	20	29	0.04[a]
Age (years)	12.62 ± 1.6	12.88 ± 1.2	0.37
Height (m)	1.61 ± 11.7	1.66 ± 10.6	0.05[b]
Mass (kg)	50.01 ± 11.7	53.51 ± 10.2	0.14
Right AHSA (degree)	45.55 ± 9.55	43.23 ± 13.6	0.41
Left AHSA (degree)	44.06 ± 9.68	41.03 ± 9.0	0.14

AHSA Active Horizontal Shoulder Abduction
[a]Significant difference between sexes
[b]Significant difference between groups

Table 2 Prevalence stratified by sex for participants with Generalised Joint Hypermobility (GJH) at cut-off points 5/9, 6/9 and 7/9, and for controls

	Participants (*n*)	GJH (%)	Controls (%)
Cut off point ≥5/9			
Boys	43	9 (21)	34 (37)
Girls	49	20 (41)	29 (31)
Total	92	29 (32)	63 (68)
Cut off point ≥6/9			
Boys	43	5 (12)	38 (41)
Girls	49	14 (29)	35 (38)
Total	92	19 (21)	73 (79)
Cut off point ≥7/9			
Boys	43	3 (7)	40 (43.5)
Girls	49	9 (18)	40 (43.5)
Total	92	12 (13)	80 (87)

score. Normative data for AHSA ranged from 40° to 52°, depending on age.

Swimmers with GJH ≥7/9 presented with 15 and 20 % higher maximum AHSA mobility than controls at the age of 10 and 14, respectively. These findings are in contrast to a previous study, where no association was found between GJH and shoulder rotation and extension in young swimmers, with only 4 swimmers classified as GJH at cut off point ≥5/9 [16]. Likewise, in non sport-specific adults, there was no association between number of positive BT and passive glenohumeral ROM values [17, 18]. The current data, however, indicates that maximum AHSA is associated with GJH in adolescent swimmers, and that this test may reveal increased shoulder mobility in this group.

Increased ROM of the shoulder is often seen in swimmers, and is generally considered a potential risk factor for shoulder pain and/or injuries. However, such relationship has not yet been confirmed [3, 19–21]. In a

Table 3 Association of Active Horizontal Shoulder Abduction in degrees and the Beighton tests score by cut off point ≥5/9, ≥6/9 and ≥7/9

Beighton tests score	Estimate (degrees)	95 % CI	*p*-value
Cut off point ≥5/9	3.98	[−0.12–8.07]	0.057
Age	−1.28	[−2.66–0.10]	0.069
Girls	−2.22	[−6.02–1.59]	0.251
Cut off point ≥6/9	5.71	[1.02–10.42]	0.018[a]
Age	−1.43	[−2.80–0.07]	0.040[a]
Girls	−2.49	[−6.27–1.29]	0.194
Cut off point ≥7/9	7.90	[2.27–13.52]	0.007[a]
Age	−1.34	[−2.69–0.01]	0.052
Girls	−2.44	[−6.15–1.26]	0.194

[a]Significant results, with $p \leq 0.05$

Table 4 Normative data for the Active Horizontal Shoulder Abduction (AHSA) test in degrees for both the GJH group at all cut off points and controls

Age	Mean ± SD (degree)	95 % CI (degree)
10	51.83 ± 10.05	26.86–76.81
11	45.60 ± 7.19	41.62–49.58
12	40.71 ± 10.22	36.06–45.37
13	43.31 ± 7.73	39.79–46.83
14	40.02 ± 8.11	36.43–43.62
15	42.25 ± 11.32	34.15–50.35

cross-sectional study of 32 competitive swimmers aged 15 to 21 years, no association was seen between horizontal abduction and actual shoulder pain, however, classification of GJH was not included in the test battery [14]. Similarly, no association was found between shoulder internal and external ROM and the occurrence of pain in a cross-sectional study including15 participants, with six of these categorised as having shoulder laxity, but none with GJH [22]. The decreased passive stability in GJH along with a higher degree of AHSA requires a large contribution of active stability provided by the rotator cuff muscles to control for glenohumeral translation. Increased demands for active stability may hypothetically result in muscle fatigue, leading to repetitive micro trauma seen as overuse injuries.

At cut off point ≥7/9, maximum AHSA was increased by 8° compared to controls, and a question to be considered is whether GJH and increased shoulder ROM is predictive of shoulder injury and/or pain. The ability to establish a relationship between the BT score including maximum AHSA and shoulder injury in young competitive swimmers is limited by the cross-sectional design of the current study.

The current normative values are in line with a previous study of AHSA in 15–21 year old competitive swimmers [14], however, not tested with BT, but with AHSA presented for the whole group (left shoulder 44° ±14° and right shoulder 44° ±16° versus the current range of 40–51°). The current study included both swimmers with and without GJH in the normative values, representing a typical population of swimmers.

The prevalence of girls at 12 years (mean age) with GJH in the current population of swimmers was about twice as high as found in a normal population (different sports) at similar age; 41 % vs. 20 %, 29 % vs. 15 % and 18 % vs. 5 % for cut off points ≥5/9, ≥6/9 and ≥7/9, respectively [8]. The same pattern was seen for the current 12 year old boys, with a prevalence of GJH also being about twice as high than the normal population of age-matched boys being 19 % vs. 9 %, 10 % vs. 6 % and 5 % vs. 1 % for the three different cut off points, respectively [8]. However, the current high prevalence of GJH is in line with a previous study of adult, competitive swimmers, with prevalence of 20 % for GJH 4≥/9 [7]. Contrary, a previous study of children participating in swimming, found girls aged 9 to have lower BT score than controls (median 2 vs. 3), with no group differences for girls aged 12, but with boys (aged 9 and 12) displaying higher BT score than controls (median 4 vs. 2, and median 2 vs. 1, respectively) [19]. The high prevalence of GJH in the current study of competitive swimmers may be due to the fact that large shoulder mobility with respect to stroke length is recognised as an advantage for competitive swimmer, thereby being seen more prevalent in this sport for those with GJH, as also previously reported [7].

The current study is in line with previous studies showing the prevalence of GJH increasing by age for girls and decreasing by age for boys [8, 23, 24]. Thus, the choice of cut off points for classification of GJH may vary from ≥4/9 to ≥6/9 within this age group [8, 11, 12, 25]. With cut off point ≥6/9 for GJH, almost 33 % of the current girls are considered to have GJH. This is recognised as a relatively high prevalence compared with a normal child population (mean age 13.8 years), where only 7 % of the girls were classified GJH at this cut off point [25]. It seems difficult to determine a single cut off point for children and adolescents, since joint mobility represents a variable fluctuating condition during maturation [24]. It is therefore recommended that future studies present data of GJH prevalence with different cut off points, in addition to age and gender, as presented in the current study.

The limitations of the current study are mainly the unknown reliability and validity for the AHSA test. Previous studies found excellent reliability for inclinometer measurements of shoulder abduction ROM, when tested in a seated position [26]. The purpose of the current test was to measure shoulder mobility, expressed as AHSA, but as AHSA is a coupled motion performed actively, the outcome may rather indicate the swimmers ability to move the arm against gravity, than the actual and specific shoulder ROM. The concurrent validity of the current clinical AHSA test, therefore, remains unknown. However, AHSA was selected due to its similarity with the swimmers freestyle stroke movements, and as such AHSA represents the most swim-related shoulder mobility test.

Another limitation is, that the GJH group accounted for 2/3 girls, which may hamper generalizability. However, since the prevalence of GJH among girls and women is higher in general, the current group may be well representative of the GJH group [27]. The normative values of the current study are distributed by age, but with the small sample sizes in the 10-year-old group (three subjects), the validity of this age group is hampered. A larger sample of this age group is therefore required in future studies for comparison to establish validity.

The strengths of this study are the standardized protocol of the BT and AHSA test, the supervised training phase of the testers and the large sample size. This study was carried out in young, competitive swimmers, making the results largely relevant for this group.

Conclusions

A positive association between AHSA and GJH was found in young, competitive swimmers, regardless of sex, age and cut off point. Normative values for AHSA ranged from 40° to 52°, depending on age. Due to lack of shoulder mobility tests in the BT scoring system, the AHSA test seems to be a promising supplemental test, displaying shoulder mobility conditions more precisely.

Future longitudinal studies should test GJH including AHSA as predicting factors for shoulder injuries.

Abbreviations

AHSA, active horizontal shoulder abduction; BT, beighton tests; GJH, generalised joint hypermobility; PPYCS, physical performance in young competitive swimmers; ROM, range of motion

Acknowledgements

The authors would like to thank physiotherapy students in PPYCS for their thorough assistance in testing the children.

Funding

There was no funding for this study.

Authors' contribution

TJ and HKK contributed to the design of the study. TJ, HLA, LDB and HKK collected the data. TJ, HLA and LDB performed the data management. TJ, HLA and LDB performed the data analysis and TJ, HLA, LDB, PH, HKK and BJK were in charge of data interpretation. TJ, PH and BJK wrote the manuscript. All authors participated in data interpretation and contributed to manuscript revision. All authors read and approved the final version.

Competing interests

The authors declare that they have no competing interests.

Consent for publication

Not applicable.

Ethics approval and consent to participate

For the PPYCS study, The Regional Scientific Ethical Committee for Southern Denmark considered the protocol as non-invasive, since no intervention was performed in this study. Parents of each participating child received written information according to the Declaration of Helsinki, and before examination, each swimmer gave oral consent to participate in the study.

Author details

[1]Department of Physiotherapy, University College Lillebaelt, Odense, Denmark. [2]Health Sciences Research Centre, University College Lillebaelt, Odense, Denmark. [3]Department of Sports Science and Clinical Biomechanics, University of Southern Denmark, Odense, Denmark. [4]Institute of Occupational Therapy, Physiotherapy and Radiography, Bergen University College, Bergen, Norway.

References

1. Gaunt T, Maffulli N. Soothing suffering swimmers: a systematic review of the epidemiology, diagnosis, treatment and rehabilitation of musculoskeletal injuries in competitive swimmers. Br Med Bull. 2012;103(1):45–88.
2. Wanivenhaus F, Fox AJ, Chaudhury S, Rodeo SA. Epidemiology of injuries and prevention strategies in competitive swimmers. Sports health. 2012;4(3):246–51.
3. Kocher MS, Waters PM, Micheli LJ. Upper extremity injuries in the paediatric athlete. Sports Med. 2000;30(2):117–35.
4. Heinlein SA, Cosgarea AJ. Biomechanical considerations in the competitive Swimmer's shoulder. Sports health. 2010;2(6):519–25.
5. Zemek MJ, Magee DJ. Comparison of glenohumeral joint laxity in elite and recreational swimmers. Clin J Sport Med. 1996;6(1):40–7.
6. Beighton P, Solomon L, Soskolne CL. Articular mobility in an African population. Ann Rheum Dis. 1973;32(5):413–8.
7. Pink MM, Tibone JE. The painful shoulder in the swimming athlete. Orthop Clin North Am. 2000;31(2):247–61.
8. Jansson A, Saartok T, Werner S, Renstrom P. General joint laxity in 1845 Swedish school children of different ages: age- and gender-specific distributions. Acta Paediatr. 2004;93(9):1202–6.
9. van Mechelen W, Hlobil H, Kemper HC. Incidence, severity, aetiology and prevention of sports injuries. A review of concepts. Sports Med. 1992; 14(2):82–99.
10. Grahame R, Bird HA, Child A. The revised (Brighton 1998) criteria for the diagnosis of benign joint hypermobility syndrome (BJHS). J Rheumatol. 2000;27(7):1777–9.
11. Juul-Kristensen B, Kristensen JH, Frausing B, Jensen DV, Rogind H, Remvig L. Motor competence and physical activity in 8-year-old school children with generalized joint hypermobility. Pediatrics. 2009;124(5):1380–7.
12. Clinch J, Deere K, Sayers A, Palmer S, Riddoch C, Tobias JH, Clark EM. Epidemiology of generalized joint laxity (hypermobility) in fourteen-year-old children from the UK: a population-based evaluation. Arthritis Rheum. 2011; 63(9):2819–27.
13. Bulbena A, Duro JC, Porta M, Faus S, Vallescar R, Martin-Santos R. Clinical assessment of hypermobility of joints: assembling criteria. J Rheumatol. 1992;19(1):115–22.
14. Beach ML, Whitney SL, Dickoff-Hoffman S. Relationship of shoulder flexibility, strength, and endurance to shoulder pain in competitive swimmers. J Orthop Sports Phys Ther. 1992;16(6):262–8.
15. Junge T, Jespersen E, Wedderkopp N, Juul-Kristensen B. Inter-tester reproducibility and inter-method agreement of two variations of the beighton test for determining generalised joint hypermobility in primary school children. BMC Pediatr. 2013;13:214.
16. Baril B, Bivens B, Brown L, Travis J. The Effects of Generalized Joint Laxity and Shoulder Joint Laxity on Shoulder Joint ROM in Swimmers. In Proceedings of the Fourth Annual GRASP Symposium. Wichita, KS: Wichita State University; 2008. http://soar.wichita.edu/dspace/bitstream/10057/1333/1/grasp-2008-01.pdf. Accessed 15 Jan 2015.
17. Lintner SA, Levy A, Kenter K, Speer KP. Glenohumeral translation in the asymptomatic athlete's shoulder and its relationship to other clinically measurable anthropometric variables. Am J Sports Med. 1996;24(6):716–20.
18. Sauers EL, Borsa PA, Herling DE, Stanley RD. Instrumented measurement of glenohumeral joint laxity and its relationship to passive range of motion and generalized joint laxity. Am J Sports Med. 2001;29(2):143–50.
19. Jansson A, Saartok T, Werner S, Renstrom P. Evaluation of general joint laxity, shoulder laxity and mobility in competitive swimmers during growth and in normal controls. Scand J Med Sci Sports. 2005;15(3):169–76.
20. Warner JJ, Micheli LJ, Arslanian LE, Kennedy J, Kennedy R. Patterns of flexibility, laxity, and strength in normal shoulders and shoulders with instability and impingement. Am J Sports Med. 1990;18(4):366–75.
21. Hovis WD, Dean MT, Mallon WJ, Hawkins RJ. Posterior instability of the shoulder with secondary impingement in elite golfers. Am J Sports Med. 2002;30(6):886–90.
22. Bak K, Magnusson SP. Shoulder strength and range of motion in symptomatic and pain-free elite swimmers. Am J Sports Med. 1997;25(4):454–9.
23. Quatman CE, Ford KR, Myer GD, Paterno MV, Hewett TE. The effects of gender and pubertal status on generalized joint laxity in young athletes. Aust J Sci Med Sport. 2008;11(3):257–63.
24. Junge T, Larsen LR, Juul-Kristensen B, Wedderkopp N. The extent and risk of knee injuries in children aged 9–14 with Generalised Joint Hypermobility and knee joint hypermobility - the CHAMPS-study Denmark. BMC Musculoskelet Disord. 2015;16:143.
25. Tobias JH, Deere K, Palmer S, Clark EM, Clinch J. Joint hypermobility is a risk factor for musculoskeletal pain during adolescence: findings of a prospective cohort study. Arthritis Rheum. 2013;65(4):1107–15.
26. Kolber MJHW. The reliability and concurrent validity of shoulder mobility measurements using a digital inclinometer and goniometer: a technical report. Int J Sports Phys Ther. 2012;7(3):306–13.
27. Remvig L, Jensen DV, Ward RC. Epidemiology of general joint hypermobility and basis for the proposed criteria for benign joint hypermobility syndrome: review of the literature. J Rheumatol. 2007;34(4):804–9.

19

The effectiveness of physiotherapy treatment on balance dysfunction and postural instability in persons with Parkinson's disease

Asmare Yitayeh[1*] and Amare Teshome[2]

Abstract

Background: Balance dysfunction and postural instability in Parkinson's disease are among the most relevant determinants of an impaired quality of life. Physiotherapy interventions are essential to reduce the level of disability by treating balance dysfunction and postural instability. The aim of this systematic review with meta-analysis was to test the effectiveness of conventional physiotherapy interventions in the management of balance dysfunction and postural instability in Persons with idiopathic Parkinson's disease.

Method: A systematic literature search of the Cochrane Library, PubMed/Medline, PEDro, Rehadat, and Rehab Trials were performed by 2 reviewers (AY and AT) independently. Eligible randomised controlled trials published from September 2005 to June 2015 were included. The selected RCTs, which investigated the effects of conventional physiotherapy treatments in the management of postural instability and balance dysfunction in Persons with Parkinson's disease, were assessed on a methodological quality rating scale. Included studies differed clearly from each other with regard to patient characteristics, intervention protocol, and outcome measures. Important characteristics and outcomes were extracted, summarized and analyzed.

Results: Eight trials with a total of 483 participants were eligible for inclusion of which 5 trials provide data for meta-analysis. Benefits from conventional physiotherapy treatment were reported for all of the outcomes assessed. The pooled estimates of effects showed significantly improved berg balance scale (SMD, 0.23; 95 % CI, 0.10–0.36; $P < 0.001$) after exercise therapy, in comparison with no exercise or sham treatment. Exercise interventions specifically addressing components of balance dysfunction demonstrated the largest efficacy with moderate effect size (SMD, 5.98; 95 % CI, 2.29–9.66; $P < 0.001$). Little effects were observed for interventions that specifically targeted Falls efficacy scale. The pooled data indicated that physiotherapy exercises decreased the incidence of falling by 6.73 (95 % CI: −14.00, 0.54, $p = 0.07$) with the overall effect of $Z = 1.81$.

(Continued on next page)

* Correspondence: asmphysio@gmail.com
[1]Department of Physiotherapy, School of Medicine, College of Medicine and Health Sciences, University of Gondar, Gondar, Ethiopia
Full list of author information is available at the end of the article

(Continued from previous page)

Conclusion: Physiotherapy interventions like balance training combined with muscle strengthening, the range of movement and walking training exercise is effective in improving balance in patients with Parkinson's disease and more effective than balance exercises alone. Highly challenging balance training and incremental speed-dependent treadmill training can also be part of a rehabilitation program for management of balance dysfunction and Postural instability in patients with idiopathic Parkinson's disease.

Keywords: Randomized controlled trials, Parkinson's disease, Physiotherapy, Postural instability, Balance dysfunction, Exercise, Equilibrium, Postural control, Rehabilitation

Background

Parkinson's disease (PD) is a debilitating chronic neurodegenerative illness resulting in motor dysfunction, which leads to weakness, pain, and tightness, difficulty in walking, rising from chairs, clumsy movements and a decline in physical activity. It is the second most common neurological disease in the world that affects neurophysiologic function, movement abilities, and quality of life (QOL) [1–5].

Balance dysfunction (BD) and Postural instability (PI) are the common incapacitating symptoms of PD. Untreated BD and PI can lead to increased frequency of falls and injuries which in turn increases the chance of developing Comorbidity and disability by causing alterations in postural control strategies during standing tasks and when performing voluntary movements [5–7]. Balance dysfunction and PI are also associated with a loss of equilibrium, sudden falls, progressive loss of independence and immobility [8–10].

Balance dysfunction and PI usually occur in the middle-later stages of the disease and became a clinical concern since they are not easily amenable to treatment with medication [11, 12]. Although Patients with PD get the best available medications, they still experience a declining of body function, daily activities, participation and weakening in mobility [13].

Recently, a number of systematic reviews assessed the effect of physiotherapy treatments or exercises in the management of balance dysfunction and postural instability among patients with idiopathic PD [14–18]. Although the results seem promising,most studies included in the systematic review have a small number of patients enrolled in their included studies and methodological limitations such as limited quality and a limited set of relevant outcome measures. This makes their result inconclusive about the use of physiotherapy treatments in the management of BD and PI bias [12, 19, 20].

Therefore, this systematic review aimed to evaluate the effectiveness of conventional physiotherapy treatments in improving balance and postural stability among persons with idiopathic PD.

Method

Protocol and registration

The systematic review was done using the preferred reporting items for systematic reviews and Meta-analysis (PRISMA) checklist.

There was no registration done either for the protocol or the systematic review.

Eligibility criteria

A study was included if it met the following criteria:

a) Randomized controlled trial methodology (level 1b evidence according to Oxfords level of evidence criteria [21] (see Table 1).
b) Quality rating of greater than or equal to 5 by PEDro score;
c) The target population was individuals with idiopathic PD of any time duration;
d) The effects of different conventional physiotherapy treatment techniques or exercise interventions were compared with control or comparison groups,
e) The primary outcomes included at least one of the following: postural instability, deficits in balance demanding activities, or risk of falling
f) The article was available in English.

A study was excluded: –If the effects of non-exercise interventions were evaluated (like behavioral interventions), If other study designs than RCT were used and If quality rating was 4 or less as determined by PEDro score.

Data sources and search strategy

Five databases (Cochrane Library, PubMed/Medline, PEDro, Rehadat, and Rehab Trials) were used during article selection process from February 2015 to September 2015. An electronic database search for relevant Randomized controlled trials (RCTs) which examined physiotherapy techniques used to treat, BD and PI among people with PD of any duration and published in international medical journals in the English language from 2005 to June 2015was conducted. We(AY,

Table 1 Hierarchies of evidence for questions of therapy, prevention, aetiology or harm [CEBM]

Level 1a:	Systematic reviews (with homogeneity) of randomized controlled trials (RCTs)
Level 1b:	Individual RCTs (with narrow confidence interval)
Level 1c:	All or none studies
Level 2a:	Systematic reviews (with homogeneity) of cohort studies
Level 2b:	Individual cohort study or low quality RCTs (e.g. <80 % follow-up)
Level 2c:	"Outcomes" Research; ecological studies
Level 3a:	Systematic review (with homogeneity) of case-control studies
Level 3b:	Individual case-control study
Level 4:	Case-series (and poor quality cohort and case-control studies)
Level 5:	Expert opinion without explicit critical appraisal, or based on physiology, bench research or 'first principles'

AT) searched articles using keywords of *RCTs, Parkinson's disease, physiotherapy, postural instability, balance dysfunction, Exercise, equilibrium, postural control, and rehabilitation.*

The relevance of the reviewed studies was checked based on their topic, objectives, and methodology. Preliminary assessments have been made and some articles were excluded at the first step just by looking at the topic. On the second step, abstracts have been seen and were excluded if they did not match to the current study objectives. For the rest, the whole content of the articles was accessed and selected based on the independent and dependent variables under review.

Type of intervention

The intervention was chosen if the RCTs used one of the following conventional physiotherapy treatment techniques: stretching, aerobic training, relaxation and muscle activation, strengthening exercises and treadmill walking.

Type of outcomes

The primary outcomes of this study were changes in berg balance scale and falls efficacy scale among the intervention and control group at the end of the follow-up. However, there are some other secondary outcome measures used in this systematic review with Meta-analysis (Table 2).

Data extraction and analysis

Two reviewers (AY, AT)extracted data from the selected RCT studies using pre-designed forms independently. Any conflict between these two reviewers was resolved by consensus. From the selected studies, the following parameters were extracted; demographic variables (mean age, sample size), Initial and Final results of used outcome measures, and the type of intervention given along with the duration of follow-up (Table 2).

Data which are suitable to meta-analysis were entered and analyzed using RevMan 5.3 software. The difference in percentage in each treatment was recorded. When there is no documented difference, it was calculated by extracting the mean change in the experimental and control group.

Quality assessment

The selected RCTs were critically appraised with 11 items of PEDro scale scores extracted from the Physiotherapy Evidence Database (www.pedro.org.au), 10 of which were scored using explicit decision rules. The PEDro scale assesses the methodological quality of a study based on important criteria, such as concealed allocation, intention-to-treat analysis, and adequacy of follow-up.

These characteristics make the PEDro scale a useful tool to assess the methodological quality of physical therapy and rehabilitation trials. The PEDro scale is based on a Delphi list [22] and consists of 11 items. Items 2–9 refer to the internal validity of a paper, and items 10 and 11 refer to the statistical analysis, ensuring sufficient data to enable appropriate interpretation of the results [23].

Item 1 is related to the external validity and therefore not included in the total PEDro score Item 4 (baseline similarity) was considered to be fulfilled if there were no significance ($p > 0.05$) difference between groups at baseline for one key outcome measure. Only one outcome had to achieve baseline similarity, in the case of more than one outcome is measured by the trials to fulfill item 4 criteria. The trials were rated independently by two investigators. Studies were excluded in the subsequent analysis if the cut-off of 5 points was not reached on PEDro scale score.

The following data were extracted from the included trials: study design, subject information, and description of interventions between the control and experimental group, outcome measures, outcome data, follow-up period. These data were then compiled into a prepared table. The two reviewers who selected the appropriate studies also extracted the data and evaluated the risk of bias. Data at baseline, post-treatment and follow-ups were extracted for interested outcomes.

Data analysis

Qualitative analysis

The necessary information was extracted from each original study by using a format prepared in Microsoft Excel Spreadsheet.

Table 2 Characteristics of included randomized controlled trials

Authors	Participant characteristics	Intervention types and intensity for experiment and control groups	Outcomes
(Ashburn et al. 2007) [7]	• n = 142 (Exp = 70, Control = 72).	Exp group: muscle strengthening, range of movement, balance training, walking training and Strategies for falls prevention, movement initiation and compensation.	• Rates of Falling
	• Sex :male = ___female = ___	Con group: visited by nurse For 6 months	• Functional reach
	• Mean Age of expt. =72.7(9.6)		• BBS timed up and go test
	• Mean Age of control. =71.6(8.8)		
	• Baseline UPDRS: Exp = 19.8(8.3) and Control = 22.2(11.9)		
(Smania et al. 2010) [8]	• n = 64 (Exp = 33, control = 31)	Exp group: Exercises of self-destabilization of the COBM, Inducing destabilization of COBM externally and coordination between leg and arm movements during walking &locomotor dexterity over an obstacle course	• BBS
	• Mean Age of expt. =67.64 (7.41)	Cont.group:- active joint mobilization, muscle stretching, and motor coordination exercises.	• ABC
	• Mean Age of control = 67.26(7.18)	21 treatment sessions of 50 min each for one month.	• UPDRS
	• idiopathic PD and PI (Hoehn and Yahr [H&Y] stage 3–4)		• modified Hoehn and Yahr scale
(Protas et al., 2005) [24]	n = 18(Expt. = 9, Control = 9)	Exp group I: Gait training(walking on a treadmill at a speed greater than over ground walking speed)	Gait parameters
	Mean age of exp. = 71.3(7.4) Mean age of contrl. = 73.7 (8.5)	Exp group II [PNF]: Basic and Gait PNF, movement guidance, support & resistance for 1 h/day, three times per week for 8 weeks	5-step test report of falls
(Schlenstedt et al. 2015) [27]	n = 32(Res. Training : n =17, balance training: n = 15;	2x/week for 7 weeks, Each session lasted 60 min.	Fullerton Advanced Balance (FAB) scale
	Mean age of exp. = 75.7 ± 5.5	Resistance training group: strengthening exercise was given to lower limb muscles	Timed-up-and-go-test (TUG)
	Mean age of contl. = 75.7 ± 7.2	Balance training group : stance- and gait tasks which require feed forward and feedback postural control	UPDRS
(Conradsson et al. 2015) [25]	(n = 100), experimental group = 51	Expt: reactive postural adjustments to control their balance during single-tasking(a 10-week Hi Balance program)	• Mini BESTest,
	Control group =49. Mean Age of expt. =72.9 (6.0)	Control: normal physical activities and participation in ongoing rehabilitation program.	• gait velocity • Falls Efficacy Scale
	Mean Age of control. =73.6 (5.3)		
(Shen and Mak 2014) [29]	n = 51, (Expt., = 26) and (Contrl, = 25).	Expt : technology assisted balance + gait training	• falls rate
	Mean Age of expt. =63.3 (8.0) Mean Age of control. =65.3 (8.5)	Control :- strengthening exercises (3 sessions/week, separated by 4 weeks of selfsupervised home-based training at a frequency of 5 sessions/week	• single-leg-stance time, • stride length
(Allen et al. 2010) [26]	n = 45 (Expt. =21 and Contrl. = 24)	Exp't: Multi component exercise program (home-based)	• falls risk score
	Mean Age of expt. =66 (10)	3 sessions/week/40-60 min/session/week for 30 days for 72 sessions	• timed sit-to-stand
	Mean Age of control. =68 (7)	Control: Usual care (no exercise)	• falls rate
(Cakit et al. 2007) [28]	n = 31 (expt. = 21, control = 10), mean age =71.8 ± 6.4	Experimental group: Incremental speed-dependent treadmill training for 8 weeks.	• UPDRS
	baseline UPDRS 18.14 _ 9.32	control group: not really mentioned	• BBS
			• Dynamic Gait Index
			• FES

Quantitative analysis (Meta-Analysis)

Meta-analysis was performed using the Review manager (RevMan5.3) software. The post-intervention data were used to obtain the pooled estimate of the immediate effect of physiotherapy interventions and effects beyond intervention period. Heterogeneity between trials was assessed using the I^2 statistic. Heterogeneity was considered substantial if I^2 was greater than 50 % and a random effects model applied; otherwise, a fixed effects model was used for the analysis. The pooled data for each outcome were reported as weighted mean differences (MD) with a 95%CI.

Results

Search yield

A total of 346 records were identified from electronic search and additional records but 131 were duplicates. After screening title, abstracts, and references 119 papers were removed. The full-text article was obtained for 33 papers of which 25 papers were eliminated as they did not meet inclusion criteria and therefore, 8Studies included in the qualitative synthesis and 5 of them included in quantitative synthesis (see Fig. 1).

Characteristics of included trials

All 8 trials involved a total of 483 participants and investigated the effectiveness of physiotherapy treatment and Exercise on improving postural stability and balance in Persons with Parkinson's disease. All trials were conducted in between September 2005 and June 2015 (see Table 2).

Quality

The mean PEDro scores of the included trials were 7. Three studies [8, 24, 25] blinded participants, two studies [8, 24] blinded therapists and the other five trials did not, due to innate difficulties. Concealed allocations of participants were stated clearly in only two studies [25, 26] and the intention to treat analysis was considered by only three studies [25–27]. The quality assessment scores and

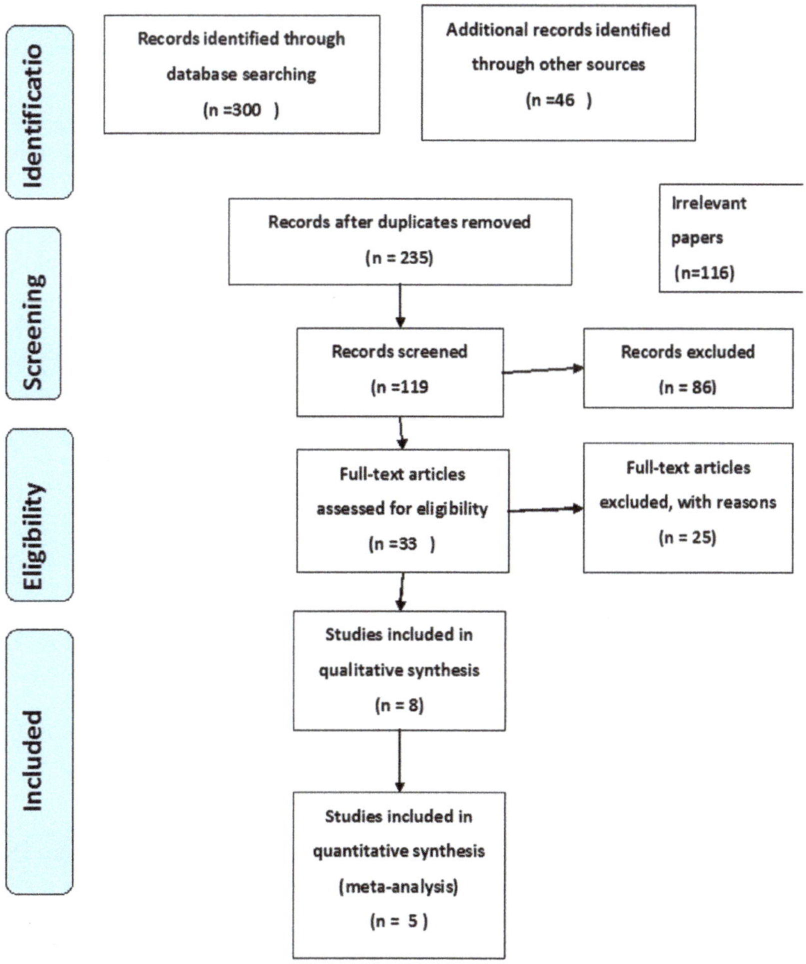

Fig. 1 PRISMA Flow diagram showing the flow of information in the procedure of including studies in systematic review, 2015, Ethopia

the decisions of each item for the included trials are shown in Table 3.

Participants

There were 248 patients (ranged from 9 to 70 patients per study) in the experimental group and 235 patients (ranged from 9 to 72 patients per study) in the control group. Three of the trails [7, 25, 26] recruited community-dwelling participants, two trials recruited their outpatient study participants from medical educational and research centers [24, 28] and the other three trials [8, 27, 29] recruited their study participants from hospitals. The mean age range of the participants was 63.3 ± 8.0 to 75.7 ± 5.5 in the experimental group and 65.3 ± 8.5 to 75.7 ± 7.2 in the control group. In seven of the included articles, the disease severity of their study participants was recorded using the Hoehn and Yahr[H&Y] Scale and Patients with idiopathic PD with a baseline stage between 2 and 4 were recruited as a study participant [7, 8, 24, 25, 27–29].

Interventions

The experimental groups were treated with different treatment approaches. Five studies used postural adjustment and falls prevention strategies and balance training [7, 8, 25–27, 29],three studies used strengthening exercises [7, 26, 27], three studies applied gait training through overground walking and treadmill training [26, 28, 29] only one study [24] used PNF exercise and coordination training has been given for another one study [8].

Balance training was performed in the form of static, dynamic and functional balance training [7], in the form of exercises aimed at improving both feed forward and feedback postural reactions [8], in the form of highly challenging balance training (HiBT) that incorporates both dual-tasking and PD-specific balance components [25],in the form of stance- and gait tasks which require feedforward and feedback postural control [27] and in the form of technology-assisted balance training [29].

Strengthening exercises were performed with the aim to improve hip flexors, hip extensors and abductors, knee flexors and extensors, ankle dorsiflexors and plantar flexors [27], in the form of progressive lower limb strengthening [26], knee and hip extensors and hip abductors muscle strengthening [7].

Participants undertook training for 30 to 60 min per session for 7 to 24 weeks. Participants of the control group received no intervention in two studies [24, 28], visited by nurses [7], given joint mobilization and stretching exercises [8], asked to do physical activities [25], took medication and usual care [26] and provided strengthening exercise in two studies [27, 29].

Outcome measures

Three trails used berg's balance scale of 0–56 scale range to measure the effect of training on balance outcome [7, 8, 28]. Three trials [25, 26, 28] used falls efficacy scale to assess balance and risk of falling. Falls risk in one study [26], UPDRS [27, 28], Fullerton Advanced balance scale [8, 27] and falls rate [8, 29] were also used as outcome measures to assess the level of balance dysfunction, postural instability, and risk of falling among patients with Parkinson's disease (See Table 4).

Table 3 PEDro criteria and summary of quality assessment scores of Included studies ($n = 8$)

Criteria	(Ashburn et al., 2007) [7]	(Smania et al., 2010) [8]	(Protas et al., 2005) [24]	(Schlenstedt et al., 2015) [27]	(Conradsson et al., 2015) [25]	(Shen and Mak, 2014) [29]	(Allen et al., 2010) [26]	(Cakit et al., 2007) [28]
Eligibility criteria	✓	✓	✓	✓	✓	✓	✓	✓
Random allocation	1 Block	1 block	1	1	1	1	1	1
Allocation concealed	1	0	0	0	1	0	1	0
Baseline similarity	1	1	1	1	1	1	1	1
Patient blinding	0	1	1	0	1	0	0	0
Therapist blinding	0	1	1	0	0	0	0	0
Assessor blinding	1	1	1	1	0	1	1	1
<15 % drop outs	1	1	1	0	1	0	1	0
ITT analysis	1	0	0	1	1	0	1	0
Between group comparison reported	1	1	1	1	1	1	1	1
Post intervention point & variability measures	1	1	1	1	1	1	1	1
Total	8/10	8/10	8/10	6/10	8/10	5/10	8/10	5/10

Table 4 Summary of results of included randomized controlled trials ($n = 8$)

Reference	Results
(Ashburn et al. 2007) [7]	1. Functional reach test(cm): – Experimental group at (start/8 weeks/6 months) = 23.2/23.6/23.8
	Control group at (start/8 weeks/6months) = 25.0/24.0/22.5
	2. Berg balance scale(BBS) (o-56) : the higher the score, the risk of falling decreases
	Experimental group at (start/8 weeks/6 months) = 44.3/45.8/45.3
	Control group at (start/8weeks/6months) = 43.6./45.2/44.6
(Smania et al. 2010) [8]	1. BBS(0–56):- Experimental group (before/after/1 month) =44.5/49.8/49.9
	Control group (before/after/1 month) = 41.8/41.0/40.85
	2. Activities-Specific Balance Confidence Scale ABC(0–100):- Experimental group (before/after/1 month) = 54.3/61.3./62.3
	Control group (before/after/1 month) = 49.5/48.2/47.0
	3. Number of falls : Experimental group (before/after/1 month) = 4.3/1.3/1.3
	Control group (before/after/1 month) = 4.6/4.1/4.1
(Protas et al. 2005) [24]	Gait and step perturbation training resulted in a reduction in falls and improvements in gait and dynamic balance.
(Schlenstedt et al. 2015) [27]	1. FAB scale :- resistance group 22.2 ± 4.8
	Balance group 24.5 ± 4.6,(*P* value = 0.123)
(Conradsson et al. 2015) [25]	1. Falls Efficacy scale score:- Experimental group (baseline/post test = 30.1(/27.3
	Control group (baseline/post test = 28.8/26.5
(Shen and Mak 2014) [29]	There were fewer fallers in the expt. than in the Cont. group at Post 3 m, Post 6 m, and Post 12 m (P < .05). In addition, the expt. group had lower fall rate than the Cont. group at Post 3 m, 6 m and 15 m
(Allen et al. 2010) [26]	1. PD falls risk score: Experimental group (baseline(SD)/post test(SD) =34(25)/23(22)
	Control group (baseline(SD)/post test(SD) = 39(34)/38(31)
	2. Falls Efficacy scale score :- Experimental groups(baseline/post test = 28.1(12.1)/25.8(7.9)
	Control groups baseline/post test =29.1(10.3)/30.4(10.8)
(Cakit et al. 2007) [28]	1. BBS : Experimental group (baseline/8 weeks = 37.0 ± 9.41/44.09 ± 7.11
	Control Group (baseline/8 weeks = 42.6 ± 9.37/41.4 ± 10.65
	2. Falls Efficacy Scale : expt. group(baseline/8 weeks. = 37.72 ± 9.29/25.45 ± 7.46
	Control group(baseline/8 weeks. = 26.8 ± 8.06/29.2 ± 9.87

Qualitative analysis of the effect of physiotherapy interventions on different outcomes

The effects of postural adjustment, fall prevention strategies, and balance training exercises on near falls and quality of life have been done by a study done in Southampton. The results showed that there was a tendency towards a reduction in fall events and injurious falls [7].

An RCT conducted in Italy brought that balance training showed significant improvements in declining PI and improving balance in patients with PD [8].

Another study conducted in the USA showed that Gait and step perturbation training can result in a reduction in falls and improvements in gait and dynamic balance for patients with PD [24].

According to a RCT conducted in Sweden, a HiBT regimen that incorporated both dual-tasking and PD-specific balance components (walking tasks on varying surfaces with or without visual constraints and voluntary arm/leg/trunk movements) significantly benefited balance and gait abilities when compared with usual care and showed promising transfer effects to everyday living [25].

Another comparative RCT done in Germany found that it is effective to use both coordinated resistance and balance training to improve balance and postural control for patients with PD [27].

A study done in china on the effectiveness of technology-Assisted Balance and Gait training found that the balance and gait training program assisted by technological devices reduced the number of fallers and the fall rate compared with the strength training program. It supported the clinical use of balance and gait training for reducing fall events in people with PD [29].

The effects of an exercise program on reduction of fall risk factors in People with PD were determined by a study done in Australia. It found that there were trends towards improvement in the exercise group for measures of muscle strength, walking, and fear of falling, but there was a lack of improvement in balance outcomes [26].

A study done in turkey on the effects of incremental speed-dependent treadmill training on postural instability and fear of falling found that specific exercise programs using incremental speed-dependent treadmill training may improve mobility, reduce postural instability and fear of falling in patients with Parkinson's disease [28].

The effects of physiotherapy interventions on different outcome measures are summarized in Table 4.

Meta- analysis on effects of physiotherapy interventions on berg balance scale

The effects of muscle strengthening, range of movement, balance training, walking training, Exercises of self-destabilization of the center of body mass and incremental speed-dependent treadmill training on berg balance scale(BBS)immediately after intervention period was examined by pooling data from three trials involving 239 participants. The pooled data indicated that physiotherapy exercises increased BBS by 5.98 (95 % CI-2.29 to 9.66,$p = 0.001$) than the control group (Fig. 2).

Meta- analysis on effects of physiotherapy interventions on falls efficacy scale

The effects of muscle strength, balance training, freezing and reactive postural adjustments in controlling balance during single-tasking compared with normal physical activities and participation in ongoing rehabilitation program was examined by pooling data from three studies involving 167participants. The pooled data indicated that these physiotherapy exercises decreased the incidence of falling by 6.73: (95 % CI: −14.00, 0.54, $p = 0.07$) with the overall effect of $Z = 1.81$. However, it was not significant. There was heterogeneity between the studies ($I^2 = 99$ %) (See Fig. 3).

Discussion

The objective of this systematic review was to evaluate the current evidence for benefits of physiotherapy treatments for treating balance impairment, postural instability and reducing the tendency and frequency of falling for patients with idiopathic Parkinson's disease.

The overall result of this systematic review of RCTs indicates that multifactorial physiotherapy interventions like muscle strengthening, range of movement, balance training and walking training exercises were found to have a positive effect on treating BD and PI among idiopathic patients with PD. But the effect of training intensity, duration, and modality is variable and inconsistent.

In this systematic review, different balance training techniques were found to be effective in improving balance and they were administered in the form of static, dynamic and functional training [7]. Exercises aimed at improving both feed forward and feedback postural reactions [8], HiBT that incorporates both dual-tasking and PD-specific balance components [25], stance- and gait tasks which require feed forward and feedback postural control [27] and technology assisted balance training exercises [29] also demonstrated a very promising outcome of balance improvement. This finding is supported by a meta-analysis which found that exercises and motor training can improve the performance of balance-related activities in people with PD [12].

Physiotherapy interventions targeted at preventing falls and Exercises of self-destabilization of the Center of body mass during walking and locomotor dexterity have an impact on reinforcing the need to focus attention on maintaining balance when performing mobility tasks in a standing position [7, 8]. This result was found by two studies which have the following limitations: Increasing numbers of control subjects who accessed rehabilitation outside of the trial by 6 months [7], lack of a follow-up assessment at 3 or more months after training and lack of assessment of some important parameters related to balance and PI [8].

This systematic review showed that repetitive exercises, HiBT, and incremental speed-dependent treadmill training will help to improve range of motion, endurance, gait parameters, functional reaching activities and postural stability in particular and balance at large. It also showed that those exercises help to decrease fall rate and fear of falling which could have the direct or indirect contribution in improving balance [7, 24–26, 28]. However, the results of a study done on the effects of HiBT [25] can only be generalized to elderly, specifically community-dwelling individuals with mild- to moderate-stage PD without known cognitive impairments.

Other limitations of these studies include a majority of the participants were recruited by advertisement, a method that can lead to a convenience sample of individuals

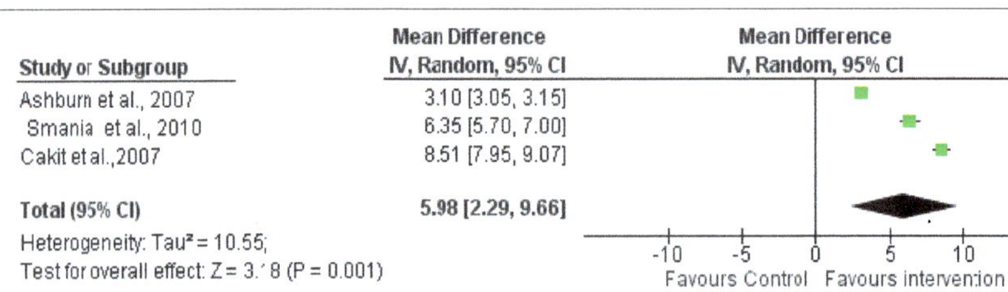

Fig. 2 Comparison of physiotherapy interventions with controls in relation to the Berg balance scale

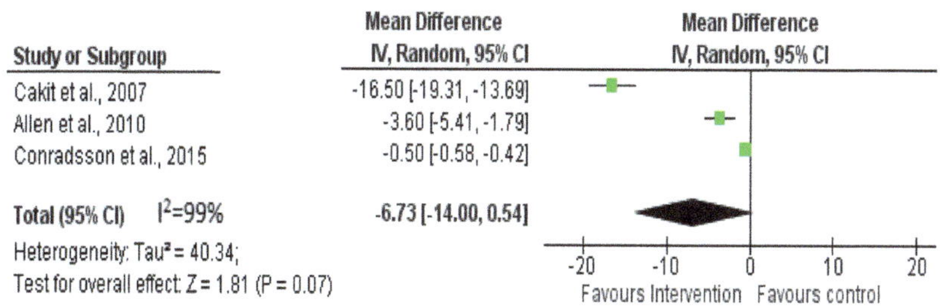

Fig. 3 Comparison of physiotherapy interventions with controls in relation to falls efficacy scale

interested in training and improving balance abilities [25], did not attempt to prevent participants from changing their medications during the study period for ethical reasons [26], relatively small sample size and unable to address the intensity, frequency, and duration of the training intervention [24] and having small sample size [28].

The difference between resistance and balance training to improve postural control and balance in people with PD have also been analyzed in this systematic review and weak evidence was found that freely coordinated resistance training might be more effective than balance training [27]. Nevertheless, the major limitation of this RCT is that training frequency was low and probably under-dosed to detect significant differences between these two competing training types. Second, it had a 20 % drop-out rate which might have been underpowered to detect significant differences. Furthermore, they did not assess fall rates which would be of interest as strength and balance performance are independent risk factors for falls. Finally, they did not include any control group without any intervention which would allow to further interpret the effects of both training types [27].

Technology assisted balance and gait training have been found significant in reducing the number of fallers at Post 3 month, 6 months, and 12 months. In addition, it also showed that a lower fall rate than the Control group was registered [29]. However, the included study has several limitations. First, the sample size and statistical power were not adequate to detect group differences. Second, there was a possible placebo effect since subjects were not blinded to group assignment. Third, all of the subjects were community-dwelling people with a mild to moderate disease level. Fourth, they used monthly phone follow-up registration of fall incidence instead of using a fall diary because most of the subjects did not have education beyond the elementary level and some were even illiterate. Fifth, the dropout rate of 31 % was relatively high. Therefore, the results cannot be generalized to patients with advanced-stage PD or those who have been institutionalized and educated [29].

This meta-analysis indicated that a significant difference was obtained on physiotherapy intervention for improving balance. However, there was not a significant difference was obtained on physiotherapy intervention for improving postural stability.

A meta-analysis of the effects of exercise and motor training on balance and falls in PD supported our finding. It concluded that there was a significant but small benefit of physiotherapy interventions on balance-related performance measures. However, there was no beneficial effect on falls in PD [30].

Limitation of this systematic review

Addressing all important outcome measures was not possible. No attempts were made to source unpublished studies, nor studies published in languages other than English. The authors suggestively agreed that unpublished trials may have poor methodology over the published ones. The review had feasibility constraint over translation for other language trails.

Conclusion

The results of this systematic review with meta-analysis concluded that physiotherapy interventions like balance training combined with muscle strengthening, the range of movement, walking training exercise is effective in improving balance in patients with PD and more effective than balance exercises alone.

HiBT and incremental speed-dependent treadmill training can also be part of a rehabilitation program for management of balance and Postural instability in patients with idiopathic PD.

Clinical application

This review suggests that physiotherapy techniques, exercises, and balance training appear to result in comparable outcomes for balance, postural stability, and reduction in falls. Consequently, prescription of balance and walking training exercise, repetitive exercises, HiBT and incremental speed-dependent treadmill training for idiopathic PD may pledge substantial improvement. Therefore, balance training exercises should be incorporated into a plan of care in conjunction with other necessary interventions to make the patient independent as much as possible.

Abbreviations

ABC, activities-specific balance confidence scale; BBS, berg balance scale; BD, balance dysfunction; BEST, balance evaluation systems test; COBM, center of body mass; FAB, Fullerton advanced balance scale; FES, falls efficacy scale; H&Y, Hoehn and Yahr; HiBT, highly challenging balance training; *P* value (Z), *P* value and corresponding *Z* value; PD, Parkinson's disease; PI, postural instability; QOL, quality of life in persons; RCT, randomized controlled trial; UPDRS, unified Parkinson's disease rating scale

Acknowledgments

We would like to thank the University of Gondar, especially the college of medicine and health sciences for allowing us to use the free internet service during search articles online.

Authors' contributions

Both AY and AT contributed to design the study method, searching strategies, selection of articles, study design, and the data analysis. AY was the main investigator and wrote the first draft of the manuscript AT contributed to the data analysis and wrote the final manuscript. Both authors read and approved the paper.

Competing interests

The authors declare that they have no competing interests.

Ethics approval and consent to participate

Not applicable.

Author details

[1]Department of Physiotherapy, School of Medicine, College of Medicine and Health Sciences, University of Gondar, Gondar, Ethiopia. [2]Department of Dentistry, School of Medicine, College of Medicine and Health Sciences, University of Gondar, Gondar, Ethiopia.

References

1. Morris ME. Movement disorders in people with Parkinson disease: a model for physical therapy. Phys Ther. 2000;80(6):578–97.
2. Jankovic J. Parkinson's disease: clinical features and diagnosis. J Neurol Neurosurg Psychiatry. 2008;79(4):368–76.
3. Rao SS, Hofmann LA, Shakil A. Parkinson's disease: diagnosis and treatment. Am Fam Physician. 2006;74(12):2046–54.
4. Paul SS, Sherrington C, Fung VS, Canning CG. Motor and cognitive impairments in parkinson disease relationships with specific balance and mobility tasks. Neurorehabil Neural Repair. 2013;27(1):63–71.
5. Brod M, Mendelsohn GA, Roberts B. Patients' experiences of Parkinson's disease. J Gerontol B Psychol Sci Soc Sci. 1998;53(4):213–22.
6. Ashburn A, Stack E, Pickering RM, Ward CD. Predicting fallers in a community-based sample of people with Parkinson's disease. Gerontology. 2001;47(5):277–81.
7. Ashburn A, Fazakarley L, Ballinger C, Pickering R, McLellan LD, Fitton C. A randomised controlled trial of a home based exercise programme to reduce the risk of falling among people with Parkinson's disease. J Neurol Neurosurg Psychiatry. 2007;78(7):678–84.
8. Smania N, Corato E, Tinazzi M, Stanzani C, Fiaschi A, Girardi P, et al. Effect of balance training on postural instability in patients with idiopathic Parkinson's disease. Neurorehabil Neural Repair. 2010;24(9):826–34.
9. Mak MK, Pang MY. Balance confidence and functional mobility are independently associated with falls in people with Parkinson's disease. J Neurol. 2009;256(5):742–9.
10. Mak MK, Pang MY. Fear of falling is independently associated with recurrent falls in patients with Parkinson's disease: a 1-year prospective study. J Neurol. 2009;256(10):1689–95.
11. Adkin AL, Frank JS, Jog MS. Fear of falling and postural control in Parkinson's disease. Mov Disord. 2003;18(5):496–502.
12. Allen NE, Sherrington C, Paul SS, Canning CG. Balance and falls in Parkinson's disease: a meta-analysis of the effect of exercise and motor training. Mov Disord. 2011;26(9):1605–15.
13. Tinetti ME, Baker DI, McAvay G, Claus EB, Garrett P, Gottschalk M, et al. A multifactorial intervention to reduce the risk of falling among elderly people living in the community. N Engl J Med. 1994;331(13):821–7.
14. Salgado S, Williams N, Kotian R, Salgado M. An evidence-based exercise regimen for patients with mild to moderate Parkinson's disease. Brain Sci. 2013;3(1):87–100.
15. Volpe D, Giantin MG, Fasano A. A Wearable proprioceptive stabilizer (Equistasi®) for rehabilitation of postural instability in Parkinson's disease: a phase II randomized double-blind, double-dummy, controlled study. 2014 [cited 2016 Jan 10]; Available from: http://dx.plos.org/10.1371/journal.pone.0112065.
16. Ebersbach G, Ebersbach A, Edler D, Kaufhold O, Kusch M, Kupsch A, et al. Comparing exercise in Parkinson's disease—the Berlin BIG Study. Mov Disord. 2010;25(12):19028.
17. Lamotte G, Rafferty MR, Prodoehl J, Kohrt WM, Comella CL, Simuni T, et al. Effects of endurance exercise training on the motor and non-motor features of Parkinson's disease: a review. J Park Dis. 2015;5(1):21–41.
18. Chandola J. The effectiveness of exercise in people with Parkinson's disease. [cited 2016 Jan 10]; Available from: http://atp.uclan.ac.uk/buddypress/diffusion/?p=1758
19. Keus SH, Bloem BR, Hendriks EJ, Bredero-Cohen AB, Munneke M. Evidence-based analysis of physical therapy in Parkinson's disease with recommendations for practice and research. Mov Disord. 2007;22(4):451–60.
20. Ferrazzoli D, Fasano A, Maestri R, Bera R, Palamara G, Ghilardi MF, et al. Balance dysfunction in Parkinson's disease: the role of posturography in developing a rehabilitation program. Park Dis. 2015;2015:1.
21. Phillips B, Ball C, Sackett D, Badenoch D, Straus S, Haynes B, et al. Oxford centre for evidence-based medicine levels of evidence. Verfügbar Unter Httpwww Cebm Netlevelsofevidence Asp. 2001.
22. Verhagen AP, de Vet HC, de Bie RA, Kessels AG, Boers M, Bouter LM, et al. The Delphi list: a criteria list for quality assessment of randomized clinical trials for conducting systematic reviews developed by Delphi consensus. J Clin Epidemiol. 1998;51(12):1235–41.
23. de Morton NA. The PEDro scale is a valid measure of the methodological quality of clinical trials: a demographic study. Aust J Physiother. 2009; 55(2):129–33.
24. Protas EJ, Mitchell K, Williams A, Qureshy H, Caroline K, Lai EC. Gait and step training to reduce falls in Parkinson's disease. NeuroRehabilitation-Interdiscip J. 2005;20(3):183–90.
25. Conradsson D, Löfgren N, Nero H, Hagströmer M, Ståhle A, Lökk J, et al. The effects of highly challenging balance training in elderly with Parkinson's disease a randomized controlled trial. Neurorehabil Neural Repair. 2015;21:1545968314567150.
26. Allen NE, Canning CG, Sherrington C, Lord SR, Latt MD, Close JC, et al. The effects of an exercise program on fall risk factors in people with Parkinson's disease: a randomized controlled trial. Mov Disord. 2010;25(9):1217–25.
27. Schlenstedt C, Paschen S, Kruse A, Raethjen J, Weisser B, Deuschl G. Resistance versus balance training to improve postural control in Parkinson's disease: a randomized rater blinded controlled study. PLoS One. 2015;10(10):e0140584.
28. Cakit BD, Saracoglu M, Genc H, Erdem HR, Inan L. The effects of incremental speed-dependent treadmill training on postural instability and fear of falling in Parkinson's disease. Clin Rehabil. 2007;21(8):698–705.
29. Shen X, Mak MK. Technology-assisted balance and gait training reduces falls in patients with Parkinson's disease a randomized controlled trial with 12-month follow-up. Neurorehabil Neural Repair. 2014;29(2):103-11.
30. Klamroth S, Steib S, Devan S, Pfeifer K. Effects of exercise therapy on postural instability in Parkinson disease: a meta-analysis. J Neurol Phys Ther. 2016;40(1):3–14.

Muscle strength differences in healthy young adults with and without generalized joint hypermobility

Pranay Jindal[1*], Amitesh Narayan[2], Sailakshami Ganesan[2] and Joy C. MacDermid[1]

Abstract

Background: Generalized joint hypermobility (GJH), in the absence of symptoms, is a common clinical finding. The joint instability present due to excessive musculoskeletal flexibility in hypermobile joints impairs the external force production during muscle contraction. However, whether GJH is associated with muscle weakness is unclear. This study evaluated differences in upper and lower limb muscle strengths among asymptomatic young adults with and without GJH.

Methods: One hundred six young adults (53 hypermobile, i.e. 25 male (mean age 22 ± 1.8); 28 female (mean age 21 ± 1.8), and 53 non-hypermobile, i.e. 25 male (mean age 19 ± 1.06); 28 female (mean age 20 ± 1.4) were selected using a cut-off ≥ 4 on Beighton and Horan Joint Mobility Index. Isometric strength of elbow and knee extensors was measured using an isokinetic dynamometer. Independent sample t- tests were done to compare the muscle strengths of hypermobile and non-hypermobile participants. One-way ANCOVA was applied to control the effect of height and body mass on muscle strength.

Results: Male hypermobile participants had significantly less strength than non-hypermobile males in the right (71.7 Nm, SD = 23.1, vs 97.6 Nm, SD = 47.4, $p = 0.006$*) and left (74.8 Nm, SD = 24.3, vs 97.7 Nm, SD = 45.5, $p = 0.007$*) elbow extensors and right knee extensors (188.7 Nm, SD = 83.3, vs 228.3 Nm, SD = 106.7, $p = 0.03$*). In females, both elbow extensors (right: 51.9 Nm, SD = 16.2 vs 48.8 Nm, SD = 17.8, $p = 0.4$; left: 48.9 Nm, SD = 17.2, vs 44.7 Nm, SD = 15.1, $p = 0.2$) and knee extensors (right: 161.3 Nm, SD = 74.9 vs 145.5 Nm, SD = 75.8, $p = 0.3$; left: 155.2 Nm, SD = 73 vs 124.3 Nm, SD = 69.6, $p = 0.07$) strength were not statistically different between hypermobile and non-hypermobile participants.

Conclusion: The findings indicate that male participants with GJH have less isometric muscle strength in both elbow extensors and right knee extensors compared to non-hypermobile male participants. Female hypermobile participants did not show any significant differences in muscle strength compared to non-hypermobile female participants.

Keywords: Generalized joint hypermobility (GJH), Isometric Muscle Strength, BTe RS primus isokinetic dynamometer, Beighton and Horan Joint Mobility Index, India

* Correspondence: jindalp@mcmaster.ca
[1]McMaster University, Hamilton, ON, Canada
Full list of author information is available at the end of the article

Background

Generalized joint hypermobility (GJH) is defined as "a condition in which most of the individual's synovial joints move beyond the normal limits of the range of motion, taking into consideration the age, gender and ethnic background in otherwise healthy subjects" [1]. The genetic make-up of an individual determines the extent of GJH [2]. Ligamentous extensibility is a result of changes in the connective tissue like collagen, elastin, fibrillin, and tenascin [1, 2]. In females, hormones like relaxin also affect the ligament extensibility [3].

Epidemiologically 10 % of the Caucasian and 25 % of the African and Asian population has GJH [4–6]. Females are three times more likely to be hypermobile compared to males at any age [7–12], and hypermobility decreases with increasing age due to tissue stiffening [9, 11]. The reduction in joint hypermobility is more rapid during childhood, lesser in teenage years and very slow during adult life [13–15]. The non-dominant side (usually left) is typically more hypermobile than the dominant side (usually right) [7, 9].

Despite debate about the acceptability of the test maneuvers and components [16, 17], the Beighton and Horan Joint Mobility Index (BHJMI) is the most commonly used tool to measure GJH and has good to excellent reliability [16, 18]. The BHJMI defines hypermobility based on how many of the joints used in the index have a range of motion indicating hypermobility, resulting in a score between 0 and 9 [9, 18]. There are no universally accepted cut-off scores for diagnosing GJH [16, 17]; however, many define GJH as present if BHJMI score is ≥ 4 of 9 [7, 8, 19–24].

Many individuals with GJH have no symptoms or disability [25], and it may even serve as an advantage for professionals like ballet dancers [26] and musicians [27]. However, approximately 3.3 % women and 0.6 % men with GJH tend to develop pain in lower limbs and shoulder joints [10, 20, 25, 28]. Recent studies also suggest that young females with GJH have lower levels of physical fitness [29] and have decreased walking and jumping capacity [23]. Prospective cohort studies in pre-adolescent school-age children have shown that it takes 4 years for GJH to become symptomatic (painful) in lower limbs and shoulder joints [30, 31]. Studies also suggest that GJH in children can be a risk factor for developing joint pain later in adolescent years [32]. The symptomatic form of GJH is called benign joint hypermobility syndrome (BJHS). BJHS is characterized by generalized joint laxity with associated musculoskeletal complaints (arthralgia, recurrent subluxations or dislocations after an acute trauma, childbirth or change in physical activity) in the absence of any systemic, rheumatic, neurological, skeletal or metabolic disease [33]. Individuals with BJHS are found to have decreased physical fitness [34], poor joint proprioception [35] and muscle weakness [36]. Since BJHS is sequelae of GJH, it is possible that individual with GJH may also have muscle weakness and that this may place them at risk of future injury or disability.

There are limited studies and conflicting evidence on muscle strength in young asymptomatic hypermobile individuals [22, 24, 36–39]. All existing studies included only Caucasians [22, 24, 36–39], and most researchers [24, 36–39] have studied the pooled (right + left) muscle strength in the lower limb. Lower limb joints have more bony stability than upper limb joints, and there is less reliance on soft tissues for stability. Thus, effects of hypermobility may be more pronounced in upper limbs compared to lower limbs. Also, upper limbs are more mobile compared to lower limbs, and the impact of hypermobility coupled with decreased muscle strength could lead to work-related upper extremity disorders. Thus, the effects of hypermobility may differ between upper and lower limbs. The Dominant side is generally stronger [36, 40–43] and less hypermobile [7, 9], thus pooling the muscle strength of dominant and non-dominant side might have diminished the existing strength differences in dominant and nondominant extremities.

Asian and African populations with GJH have greater ranges of joint mobility as compared to Caucasians [9, 10, 44], and thus, might be more prone to injury and complications arising from GJH. However, there is a lack of literature assessing the effect of GJH on asymptomatic Asian young adults. Thus, an information gap exists whether there are muscle strength differences between hypermobile and non-hypermobile young Asian individuals in both the upper and lower limbs. Therefore, this study evaluated strength differences between individuals who exhibit GJH and those who do not in two key muscle groups (elbow and knee extensors) among age and gender matched healthy young adults, and controlling for the effect of height, body mass and limb dominance.

Methods

Institutional ethics committee (No. IEC/KMC/09/2007-2008) at KMC Mangalore, India, approved the study. All participants were recruited from a graduate student hostel in the southern part of India. After obtaining the written informed consent, 200 healthy volunteer participants aged 18–25 years were screened for GJH using BHJMI (Additional file 1). Using convenience sampling, we identified 53 hypermobile participants. We also recruited 53 non-hypermobile subjects of the same age. Exclusion criteria included: Involvement in more than 6 h per week of physical activities, any diagnosis of autoimmune disorders, connective tissue disorders, recent traumatic injury, musculoskeletal disorders, neurological disorders, as well as pain experienced currently or during the past 2 weeks.

The dominant upper limb was determined by asking participants about the preferred hand while writing. The dominant lower limb of the participants was determined by asking participants about the preferred lower limb while kicking a soccer ball [45]. In this study, a cut-off score of ≥ 4 on BHJMI was considered as hypermobile (for both males and females). A physiotherapist administered the protocol suggested by Juul-Kristensen [46] (Appendix 1) for screening. Both hypermobile and non-hypermobile participants were assessed for isometric muscle strength for right and left elbow extensors and knee extensors on Baltimore Therapeutic Equipment (BTe), Primus RS isokinetic dynamometer. The BTe RS primus isokinetic dynamometer was calibrated weekly during the testing. The same physiotherapist performed the hypermobility screening, testing and the strength evaluation in an out-patient setting.

A practice trial was provided to the participants to get accustomed to the testing maneuver. No verbal prompts were given during the strength testing. Participants were advised to stop the test immediately if they experienced any unusual pain or discomfort. As our participants were young and healthy, a 5-second rest was given between each trial to avoid fatigue. A 2 min rest was given after testing a muscle group or side, before testing the next muscle group. Ten minutes of rest was given after completing the testing procedure and participants were enquired for any pain or discomfort. The following sequence was followed for muscle strength testing: right elbow extensors, left elbow extensors, right knee extensors and left knee extensors. Standardized testing procedures and tool/pad number 701, as per the BTe RS Primus instruction manual, were used.

Test positions and procedure for Isometric muscle strength testing:

1. Test positions and procedure for elbow extension: Participants were asked to stand in front of the exercise head of the dynamometer with their feet shoulder width apart. Shoulders were in neutral rotation, flexion, and abduction. The Dynamometer axis was aligned with the lateral epicondyle of the elbow joint. The elbow was positioned in 90° flexion, with the forearm supinated, the wrist in a neutral position and the hand was placed centrally on the handle of the tool (Appendix 2, image 1). Participants were instructed to extend their elbow (exert pressure downwards on the pad) to exert a maximum contraction on the "Go" command of the examiner for 3 s.
2. Test position and procedure for knee extension: Participants were tested in a sitting position on a chair with a backrest. The anatomical axis of rotation of the knee joint was aligned with the dynamometer axis, and the pad of the tool was positioned centrally at the lower part of the shin of the tibia. The knee was kept at 90° flexion, the hip in neutral rotation and abduction, and the foot was positioned in plantar flexion. The hands were placed on the abdomen and the trunk, hips, and mid-thigh were stabilized on the chair by Velcro straps (Appendix 2, image 2). Participants were instructed to extend their knee (exert pressure upwards on the pad) and to exert a maximum contraction on the "Go" command of the examiner for 3 s.

Three criterion trials of maximum voluntary isometric contraction (MVIC) were made for elbow and knee extensor, and peak torque measurements were recorded in newton-meters (Nm). The largest value of three trials represented the participants' peak torque.

Statistical analysis

Data were entered and checked for quality by random re-checking of the original data against the electronic data file. Data were analyzed using SPSS v (21) software with p value set at 0.05. All statistical tests were two-tailed, and the statistical power was calculated post-hoc. Data were examined and accepted as being sufficiently normal if the skewness and kurtosis were within ±2 SD. The descriptive statistical analysis was done using independent samples t-test to obtain mean age (years), body mass (kg.), standing height (cms.), and Beighton scores for hypermobile and non-hypermobile participants. Gender and body size have an influence on muscle strength [47–49]; hence, the data were analyzed in two ways to help delineate factors associated with differences. First, the data for hypermobile and non-hypermobile participants were separated by gender, and independent sample t-tests were used to compare the subgroups for elbow and knee extensor strength. In the second analyses, one-way analysis of covariance (ANCOVA) was performed comparing hypermobile versus non-hypermobile strength scores across all participants, but controlling for the height and body mass (covariates). Analyzes were conducted separately for right and left elbow extensors and right and left knee extensors.

Results

One hundred six participants completed the testing without difficulty. All of the participants except one were right upper and lower limb dominant. None of the participants reported ambidexterity, any pain or discomfort during or after the strength testing. Table 1 shows the

Table 1 Description of study participants

Variables	Males ($n = 50$)		p	Females ($n = 53$)		p
	Hypermobile ($n = 25$)	Non-hypermobile ($n = 25$)		Hypermobile ($n = 28$)	Non-hypermobile ($n = 28$)	
Mean age (years)	22 ± 1.8	19 ± 1.06	0.01	21 ± 1.8	20 ± 1.4	0.7
Mean body mass (kg)	67.7 ± 11.4	61.4 ± 9.1	0.03	55.4 ± 6.4	55.2 ± 8.8	0.9
Mean standing height (cm)	170.4 ± 6.1	163.2 ± 22.2	0.1	160.4 ± 7.3	158.0 ± 5.9	0.1
Median BHJMI scores	5	0	NA	5	2	NA

descriptive statistics of body mass, height, and Beighton scores of both groups.

Independent sample t-tests showed that hypermobile males were significantly weaker compared to non-hypermobile males with respect to elbow extensor strength for both right ($p = 0.02$) and left ($p = 0.03$) extremities (Table 2, unadjusted mean strength). After controlling for height and body mass in ANCOVA analysis, there were large and statistically significant differences between male hypermobile and non-hypermobile participants for both right ($p = 0.006$) and left ($p = 0.007$) elbow extensors and the right knee extensors ($p = 0.03$) (Table 2, adjusted mean strength). Female participants did not have significant differences based on hypermobility, even after controlling for height and body mass. In males, height and body mass (covariates) accounted for 10 % of the variance in elbow strength and 9 % for right knee extensor strength (Table 2).

Discussion

In this study, among males, hypermobile participants demonstrated less isometric strength for right and left elbow extensors and right knee extensors than non-hypermobile participants. The differences were even more statistically significant after removing the influence of height and body mass as covariates. Controlling for these covariates increases our confidence that hypermobility underpinned the decreased elbow and knee extensor muscle strength. Amongst females, there were no statistically significant differences between hypermobile and non-hypermobile participants in elbow and knee extensor strength. Further, since this effect was retained after controlling for height and body mass, we are confident that there was no evidence of hypermobility compromising female extensor strength in this study.

The present study adds to the current knowledge as it establishes that males have weaker elbow extensors

Table 2 Comparison of isometric strength of elbow and knee extensors between Hypermobile (H) and Non-Hypermobile (NH) participants after one-way ANCOVA (height and body mass were selected as covariates)

Muscle group	Gender	Category	N	Unadjusted mean strength (Nm) ± SD (without controlling for covariates)	p value	Adjusted mean strength (Nm) (after controlling for covariates)	95 % CI		F	Partial eta squared
							Lower	Upper		
Elbow extensors right	Female	H	28	51.9 ± 16.2	$p = 0.4$	51.1	45	57.2	$p = 0.7$	0.002
		NH	28	48.8 ± 17.8		49.6	43.5	55.6		
	Male	H	25	71.7 ± 23.1	$P = 0.02$*	69	53.8	84.2	$p = 0.006$*	0.1
		NH	25	97.6 ± 47.4		100.3	85.1	115.5		
Elbow extensors left	Female	H	28	48.9 ± 17.2	$p = 0.26$	48	42.4	53.7	$p = 0.5$	0.007
		NH	28	44.7 ± 15.1		45.5	39.9	51.2		
	Male	H	25	74.8 ± 24.3	$p = 0.03$*	71.5	56.9	86.1	$p = 0.007$*	0.1
		NH	25	97.7 ± 45.5		101	86.4	115.7		
Knee extensors right	Female	H	28	161.3 ± 74.9	$p = 0.37$	158.2	130.8	185.5	$p = 0.6$	0.005
		NH	28	145.5 ± 75.8		148.6	121.2	175.9		
	Male	H	25	188.7 ± 83.3	$p = 0.13$	178.8	141	216.6	$p = 0.03$*	0.09
		NH	25	228.3 ± 106.7		238	200.3	276		
Knee extensors left	Female	H	28	155.2 ± 73	$p = 0.07$	152.3	126.3	178.4	$p = 0.1$	0.03
		NH	28	124.3 ± 69.6		127.1	101.1	153.1		
	Male	H	25	178.1 ± 96.2	$p = 0.23$	169.9	130.1	209.6	$p = 0.08$	0.06
		NH	25	212.9 ± 101.2		221.1	181.1	260.9		

* $p < 0.05$ denotes significant findings

strength in the presence of hypermobility. Scheper et al. [22] found decreased grip and shoulder abductor strength in healthy young adults with GJH. Since there is a higher risk of sports injuries in the upper limb in individuals with GJH [50], muscle weakness could be a contributing factor for increased risk of upper limb injuries during sports.

In this study, after controlling for body size, hypermobile males demonstrated less isometric strength of the right knee extensors compared to non-hypermobile males. Isometric strength of left knee extensors among hypermobile and non- hypermobile males, although it did not reach statistical significance ($p = 0.08$), the trend was in a similar direction as of right knee extensors. Our findings support a previous study showing that knee extensors are weak in hypermobile young males [22]. Our results are in contrast to studies by Jensen et al. [24], Stewart and Burden [37] and Kristensen et al. [38] who found no difference in knee extensor strength among hypermobile and non-hypermobile individuals. Stewart and Burden [37] included athlete males where sports participation might have influenced the muscle strength. Our sample was not actively involved in sports activities. Thus, it was easier to detect muscle strength differences that were not mitigated by sports specific training. Studies by Jensen et al. [24] and Kristensen et al. [38] included adult participants with knee joint pain, and Jensen et al. [24] found no differences in knee extensor strength in individuals with hypermobility. However, Kristensen et al. [38] found decreased knee extensor strength in adult females. Since males have high pain tolerance [51, 52], it could be possible that pain did not affect the muscle strength in males as compared to females who have less pain tolerance. Since our sample was young and asymptomatic, it could be possible that muscle strength differences are related to joint pain in hypermobile individuals. Studies by Jensen et al. [24] and Kristensen et al. [38] included adult males with mean age of 40.1 to 40.3 years. The extent of hypermobility decreases as age increases [9, 11], it could be possible that our sample of young adults (mean age 21 years) was more hypermobile and weaker compared to the adult population in Kristensen's and Jensen's study.

Jensen et al. [24] and Kristensen et al. [38] reported the pooled muscle strength in lower limbs, which might have influenced the strength differences in right and left extremities. Importantly, Kristensen et al. [38] compared the strength of hypermobile knee extensors (right or left) to dominant lower limb knee extensor strength in non-hypermobile adults. The effects of pain and dominance may have contributed to the variation that would have made it harder to detect the difference in muscle strength in earlier studies. Studies suggest that the dominant side has greater strength than the non-dominant side, [36, 40–43] and the dominant side has also been reported to be less hypermobile compared to the non-dominant side [7, 9]. Although our participants were healthy and young, decreased knee extensor strength at a young age could be of clinical relevance as they may be more prone to injuries. Recent studies show an increased risk of the knee joint injuries during contact sports in participants with GJH [53, 54].

In our study amongst females, there were no statistically significant differences between hypermobile and non-hypermobile participants with respect to right or left elbow and knee extensor strength. Our results are similar to studies by Jensen et al. [24], and Mebes et al. who found no difference in knee extensor strength among hypermobile and non-hypermobile females. Scheper et al. [22] reported decreased knee extension strength (pooled) in asymptomatic young females. Mebes et al. suggested that muscles in hypermobile women have a higher rate of force development as compared to non-hypermobile women. This higher rate of force development may counteract a lack of stability in hypermobile joints. Force development is an important factor for joint stabilization, and since individuals with GJH have less joint stability due to lax passive structures [55] they might be relying on neuromuscular mechanisms such as force development for more joint stability. We did not measure the rate of force development in our study, so we could not determine if this was used to counteract the impact of hypermobility on knee extensor strength in our sample. Our participants reported participated in less than 6 h of physical activity; however, we did not collect data on specific type and duration of physical activity participation. It could be possible that the type and duration of physical activity influenced the muscle strength among male and female participants.

Methodological and sampling issues in previous studies comparing the dominant side to the non-dominant side and pooling muscle strength values may have reduced the potential to find statistically significant differences in muscle strength among hypermobile and non-hypermobile participants compared to our study in which we have a younger sample that was controlled for gender and anthropometrics. Evidence suggests that with increasing age there is a decline in muscle strength [43, 56], and hypermobility [9, 11]. Given these trends, the impact of hypermobility may be more pronounced in younger individuals. We compared the right (dominant) side of hypermobile participants to the right side of non-hypermobile participants (dominant) and did the same for the left side which increased the likelihood of finding statistically significant differences.

A moderate statistical power due to small sample size in the present study ($N = 106$, 25–28 in each group) may have played a role in limiting the significance of some of the statistical comparisons conducted. On the post-hoc power analysis on the basis of between-groups means, and standard deviation observed in the present study, a sample size of approximately 50–70 participants per group would be needed to calculate 20 % difference in muscle strength (assuming 20 % difference in strength is clinically important).

There is sufficient evidence that hypermobility, particularly at the elbow, is associated with strength deficits in males. Reduced joint stability in combination with reduced muscle strength could be a major etiological factor in the development of upper extremity work-related disorders or sports injury and should be investigated further for prevention and management. Higher risk of upper limb [50] and lower limb sports injuries [53, 54, 57–59], pain [60] and decreased dynamic trunk stability [61] have been reported in individuals with GJH. These studies in combination with the findings of the present study suggest that a more detailed routine examination of GJH is needed during the investigation of musculoskeletal disorders.

Limitations

Our study findings should be considered in light of some inherent limitations. As our sample included only young participants, our results cannot be generalized to older adults. Secondly, we assessed only two different joints and the associated muscle strength thus we cannot generalize these findings to all upper extremity and lower extremity joints. Finally, the trends in the lower limb strength of males were consistent with the direction of the significant findings for the upper limb strength but were statistically significant only on one lower limb. It is possible that with a larger sample size these differences would have consistently reached statistical significance. We used a smaller rest period of 5 s between each strength testing trials for knee and elbow extensors, which might have influenced the muscle strength in our sample. Some statisticians suggest Bonferroni corrections to adjust for multiple p values; however, it is debatable [62]. Given our small sample size, we felt that to do a Bonferroni correction would unnecessarily increase type 2 errors. Our analytical approach did not use an overall omnibus tested which would have reduced the probability of Type 1 error, but rather performed sex-disaggregated and ANCOVA analyses which we used to provide additional insights into the nature of the differences between males and females with respect to hypermobility in different muscle groups.

Implications for future research

Large cross-sectional studies are needed to explore the effect of GJH in other muscle groups. These should include testing of multiple joints of the upper and lower limbs and should consider a broad age range, activity levels, and include dynamic strength testing in both genders. The effects of gender and limb dominance should be analyzed separately since differential effects may occur. Studies might also explore the relationship between severity of GJH and muscle strength, and could further investigate if there are differences between Caucasians and Asian strength taking into account their level of hypermobility. Future studies can also explore the relationships between participants' level and type of physical activity, hypermobility and muscle strength.

Conclusion

From the present study it can be concluded that Asian males with GJH have less isometric strength in both elbows and right knee extensors compared to non-hypermobile males. The impact of GJH in Asian females is not the same as for men and hypermobility appears to be a less important factor influencing muscular strength.

Consent to publish

Consent to publish the results was obtained from the participants.

Appendix 1

Test protocol for Beighton and Horan Joint Mobility Index testing

(1) Passive apposition of the thumb to the flexor side of the forearm (shoulder 90° flexed, elbow extended and hand pronated), tested on right and left side, is performed by the patient after the following procedure. The examiner performs the test and asks: 'Can you with a straight arm move your thumb down so it touches the lower part of the forearm?' If the test is negative, meaning no touch, the examiner asks: 'Have you been able to do this previously?'

(2) Passive dorsiflexion of the little finger > 90° (elbow flexed 90°, the forearm and hand pronated resting on a table), tested on the right and left side, is performed by the patient after the following procedure. The examiner performs the test and asks: 'Can you with the forearm resting on the table, move your little finger, so it is pointing a little bit backwards?' If the test is negative, the examiner asks: 'Have you been able to do this previously?'

(3) Passive hyperextension of the elbow >10° (shoulder 90° abducted and hand supinated), tested on the

right and left side, is performed by the patient after the following procedure. The examiner performs the test and asks: 'How much are you able to overstretch your elbow in this position (illustrated by the examiner) with your palm pointing towards the roof?' If the test is negative, meaning no overstretching, the examiner asks: 'Have you been able to overstretch the elbow previously?'

(4) Passive hyperextension of the knee >10° (standing), tested on right and left side, is performed by the patient after the following procedure. The examiner performs the test and asks: 'How much are you able to overstretch your knee when you are standing straight up?'

If the test is negative, meaning no overstretching, the examiner asks: 'Have you been able to overstretch the knee previously?'

(5) Forward flexion of the trunk, with knees straight, so that the palms of the hands rest easily on the floor, is performed by the patient after the following procedure. The examiner performs the test and asks: 'Can you with straight knees bend your body forward and place both palms easily on the ground?' If the test is negative, meaning no touch on the ground with the whole palm of the hands, the examiner asks: 'Have you been able to do this previously?'

Appendix 2

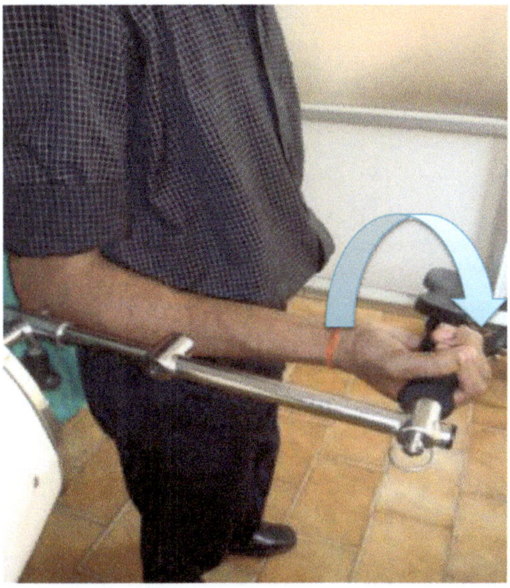

Fig. 1 Testing position for elbow extensors

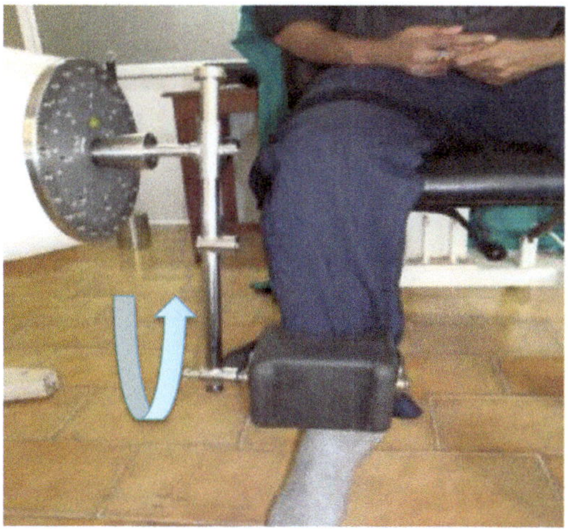

Fig. 2 Testing position for knee extensors

Additional files

Additional file 1: Beighton and Horan Joint Mobility Index. (DOCX 24 kb)

Additional file 2: Additional data file number 2. (XLS 39 kb)

Competing interests

The authors declare that they have no competing interests.

Authors' contributions

All authors have read and approved the final version of the manuscript. PJ did the literature review, data collection, data analysis and interpretation, coordinated with various people involved and prepared the final version of the manuscript. AN helped in conceptualizing and designing the study protocol. He also contributed towards revisions of the manuscript. SG—intellectually contributed towards refining the ideas and developing the methodology. JM—helped in multiple revisions of the final manuscript and intellectually contributed towards the analysis and discussion section.

Acknowledgements

Thanks to Mrs. Charu Eapen for helping in getting acquainted with the BTe RS Primus dynamometer. Thanks to all the volunteer participants for generously devoting their time to this study.

Author details

[1]McMaster University, Hamilton, ON, Canada. [2]Kasturba Medical College, Mangalore, Karnataka, India.

References

1. Beighton P, Grahame R, Bird H. Musculoskeletal Features of Hypermobility and Their Management. Hypermobility of Joints. 4th ed. London: Springer; 2012. p. 65–99.
2. Grahame R. Joint hypermobility and genetic collagen disorders: are they related? Arch Disabl Child. 1999;80:188–91.
3. Stanley P. Brown, Wayne C. Miller JME. Female-specific issues. In: exercise physiology: basis of human movement in health and disease. Lippincott Williams & Wilkins; 2006. p. 405–28.
4. Schweitzer G. Laxity of metacarpophalangeal joints of fingers and interphalangeal joint of the thumb: a comparative inter-racial study. S Afr Med J. 1970;44:246–9.

5. Harris H, Joseph J. Variation in extension of the metacarpophalangeal and interphalangeal joints of the thumb. Bone Jt Surg Br Vol. 1949;31:547–59.
6. Engelbert RH, Kooijmans FT, Van Riet AM, Feitsma TM, Uiterwaal CS, Helders PJ. The relationship between generalized joint hypermobility and motor development. Pediatr Phys Ther. 2005;17:258–63.
7. Al-Rawi Z, Al-Aszawi A, Al-Chalabi T. Joint mobility among university students in Iraq. Br J Rheumatol. 1985;24:326–31.
8. Bulbena A, Duro J, Porta M, Faus S, Vallescar R, Martin-Santos R. Clinical assessment of hypermobility of joints: assembling criteria. J Rheumatol. 1992;19:115–22.
9. Beighton P. Articular mobility in an African population. Ann Rheum Dis. 1973;32:413–8.
10. Hakim A. Joint hypermobility. Best Pract Res Clin Rheumatol. 2003;17:989–1004.
11. Larsson LG, Baum J, Mudholkar GS. Hypermobility: features and differential incidence between the sexes. Arthritis Rheum. 1987;30:1426–30.
12. Jansson A, Saartok T, Werner S, Renstrom P. General joint laxity in 1845 Swedish school children of different ages: age- and gender-specific distributions. Acta Paediatr. 2004;93:1202–6.
13. Kirk JA, Ansell BM, Bywaters EG. The hypermobility syndrome. Musculoskeletal complaints associated with generalized joint hypermobility. Ann Rheum Dis. 1967;26:419–25.
14. Gulbahar S, Azahin E, Baydar M, Bircan C. Hypermobility syndrome increases the risk for low bone mass. Clin Rhematol. 2006;25:511–4.
15. Adib N, Davies K, Grahame R. Joint hypermobility syndrome in childhood. A not so benign multisystem disorder? Rheumatology. 2005;44:744–50.
16. Remvig L, Jensen DV, Ward RC. Are diagnostic criteria for general joint hypermobility and benign joint hypermobility syndrome based on reproducible and valid tests ? a review of the literature. J Rheumatol. 2007;34:798–803.
17. Remvig L, Flycht L, Christensen KB, Juul-Kristensen B. Lack of consensus on tests and criteria for generalized joint hypermobility, ehlers-danlos syndrome: hypermobile type and joint hypermobility syndrome. Am J Med Genet Part A. 2014;164:591–6.
18. Boyle K. Intrarater and interrater reliability of the beighton and horan joint mobility index. J Athl Train. 2003;38:281–5.
19. Van der Giessen L, Liekens D, Rutgers KJ, Hartman A, Mulder P, Oranje A. Validation of beighton score and prevalence of connective tissue signs in 773 Dutch children. J Rheumatol. 2001;28:2726–30.
20. Rikken-Bultman D, Wellink L, Dongen P. Hypermobility in two Dutch school populations. Eur J Obs Gynecol. 1997;73:189–92.
21. Birrell F, Adebajo A, Hazleman BL, Silman A. High prevalence of joint laxity in West Africans. Br J Rheumatol. 1994;33:56–9.
22. Scheper M, De Vries J, Beelen A, De Vos R, Nollet F, Engelbert R. Generalized joint hypermobility , muscle strength and physical function in healthy adolescents and young adults. Curr Rheumatol Rev. 2014;10:1–9.
23. Scheper MC, de Vries JE, Juul-Kristensen B, Nollet F, Engelbert RH. The functional consequences of generalized joint hypermobility: a cross-sectional study. BMC Musculoskelet Disord. 2014;15:243.
24. Jensen BR, Olesen AT, Pedersen MT, Kristensen JH, Remvig L, Simonsen EB, et al. Effect of generalized joint hypermobility on knee function and muscle activation in children and adults. Muscle Nerve. 2013;48:762–9.
25. Grahame R. The hypermobility syndrome. Ann Rheum Dis. 1990;49:199–200.
26. Grahame R, Jenkins JM. Joint hypermobility - asset or liability? A study of joint mobility in ballet dancers. Ann Rheum Dis. 1972;31:109–11.
27. Larsson L, Baum J. Benefits and disadvantages of joint hypermobility among musicians. N Engl J Med. 1993;329:1079–82.
28. Wordsworth P, Ogilvie D, Smith R, Sykes B. Joint mobility with particular reference to racial variation and inherited connective tissue disorders. Br J Rheumatol. 1987;26:9–12.
29. Scheper MC, de Vries JE, de Vos R, Verbunt J, Nollet F, Engelbert RHH. Generalized joint hypermobility in professional dancers: a sign of talent or vulnerability? Rheumatology. 2013;52:651–8.
30. El-Metwally A, Salminen JJ, Auvinen A, Kautiainen H, Mikkelsson M. Lower limb pain in a preadolescent population: prognosis and risk factors for chronicity-a prospective 1- and 4-year follow-up study. Pediatrics. 2005;116:673–81.
31. Tobias JH, Deere K, Palmer S, Clark EM, Clinch J. Joint hypermobility is a risk factor for musculoskeletal pain during adolescence: findings of a prospective cohort study. Arthritis Rheum. 2013;65:1107–15.
32. Sohrbeck-Nohr O, Kristensen JH, Boyle E, Remvig L, Juul-Kristensen B. Generalized joint hypermobility in childhood is a possible risk for the development of joint pain in adolescence: a cohort study. BMC Pediatr. 2014;14:1–9.
33. Grahame R, Bird H, Child A. The revised (Brighton 1998) criteria for the diagnosis of benign joint hypermobility syndrome (BJHS). J Rheumatol. 2000;27:1777–9.
34. Engelbert R, Van Bergen M, Henneken T, Helders PJM, Takken T. Exercise tolerance in children and adolescents with musculoskeletal pain in joint hypermobility and joint hypomobility syndrome. Pediatrics. 2006;118:690–6.
35. Smith TO, Jerman E, Easton V, Bacon H, Armon K, Poland F, et al. Do people with benign joint hypermobility syndrome (BJHS) have reduced joint proprioception? a systematic review and meta-analysis. Rheumatol Int. 2013;33:2709–16.
36. Sahin N, Baskent A, Ugurlu H, Berker E. Isokinetic evaluation of knee extensor/flexor muscle strength in patients with hypermobility syndrome. Rheumatol Int. 2008;28:643–8.
37. Stewart DR, Burden SB. Does generalised ligamentous laxity increase seasonal incidence of injuries in male first division club rugby players? Br J Sports Med. 2004;38:457–60.
38. Juul-Kristensen B, Hansen H, Simonsen EB, Alkjær T, Kristensen JH, Jensen BR, et al. Knee function in 10-year-old children and adults with generalised joint hypermobility. Knee. 2012;19:773–8.
39. Mebes C, Amstutz A, Luder G, Ziswiler H, Stettler M, Villiger PM, et al. Isometric rate of force development, maximum voluntary contraction, and balance in women with and without joint hypermobility. Arthritis Rheum. 2008;59:1665–9.
40. Stoll T, Huber E, Seifert B, Michel BA, Stucki G. Maximal isometric muscle strength: normative values and gender- specific relation to age. Clin Rhematol. 2000;19:105–13.
41. Incel N, Ceceli E. Grip strength: effect of hand dominance. Singapore Med J. 2002;43:234–7.
42. Jacobs C, Uhl T, Seeley M. Strength and fatigability of the dominant and nondominant hip abductors. J Athl Train. 2005;40:203–6.
43. Hunter SK, Thompson MW, Adams RD. Relationships among age-associated strength changes and physical activity level, limb dominance, and muscle group in women. J Gerontol A Biol Sci Med Sci. 2000;55:B264–73.
44. Remvig L, Jensen DV, Ward RC. Epidemiology of general joint hypermobility and basis for the proposed criteria for benign joint hypermobility syndrome: Review of the literature. J Rheumatol. 2007;34:804–9.
45. Hoffman M, Schrader J, Applegate T, Koceja D. Unilateral postural control of the functionally dominant and nondominant extremities of healthy subjects. J Athl Train. 1998;33:319–22.
46. Juul-Kristensen B, Rogind H, Jensen D, Remvig L. Inter-examiner reproducibility of tests and criteria for generalized joint hypermobility and benign joint hypermobility syndrome. Rheumatology. 2007;46:1835–41.
47. Jaric S. Role of body size in the relation between muscle strength and movement performance. Exerc Sport Sci Rev. 2003;31:8–12.
48. Aouichaoui C, Trabelsi Y, Bouhlel E, Tabka Z, Dogui M, Richalet J, et al. The relative contributions of anthropometric variables to vertical jumping ability and leg power in tunisian children. J Strength Cond Res. 2012;26:777–88.
49. Jaric S. Muscle strength testing use of normalisation for body size. Sport Med. 2002;32:615–31.
50. Chahal J, Leiter J, McKee MD, Whelan DB. Generalized ligamentous laxity as a predisposing factor for primary traumatic anterior shoulder dislocation. J Shoulder Elb Surg. 2010;19:1238–42.
51. Woodrow K, Friedman G, Siegelaub A, Collen M. Pain tolerance: differences according to age, sex and race. Psychosom Med. 1972;34:548–56.
52. Wise EA, Price DD, Myers CD, Heft MW, Robinson ME. Gender role expectations of pain: relationship to experimental pain perception. Pain. 2002;96:335–42.
53. Pacey V, Nicholson LL, Adams RD, Munn J, Munns CF. Generalized joint hypermobility and risk of lower limb joint injury during sport: a systematic review with meta-analysis. Am J Sports Med. 2010;38:1487–97.
54. Konopinski MD, Jones GJ, Johnson MI. The effect of hypermobility on the incidence of injuries in elite-level professional soccer players: a cohort study. Am J Sports Med. 2012;40:763–9.
55. Simmonds JV, Keer RJ. Hypermobility and the hypermobility syndrome. Man Ther. 2007;12:298–309.
56. Fisher M, Birren J. Age and strength. J Appl Psychol. 1947;31:490–7.
57. Nicholas J. Injuries to Knee Ligaments relationship to looseness and tightness in football players. JAMA. 1970;212:2236–9.
58. Bin Abd Razak HR, Bin Ali N, Howe TS. Generalized ligamentous laxity may be a predisposing factor for musculoskeletal injuries. J Sci Med Sport. 2013; 17:474–8.

59. Myer GD, Ford KR, Paterno MV, Nick TG, Hewett TE. The effects of generalized joint laxity on risk of anterior cruciate ligament injury in young female athletes. Am J Sports Med. 2008;36:1073–80.
60. Mulvey MR, Macfarlane GJ, Beasley M, Symmons DPM, Lovell K, Keeley P, et al. Modest association of joint hypermobility with disabling and limiting musculoskeletal pain: results from a large-scale general population-based survey. Arthritis Care Res. 2013;65:1325–33.
61. Falkerslev S, Baago C, Alkjaer T, Remvig L, Halkjaer-Kristensen J, Larsen PK, et al. Dynamic balance during gait in children and adults with generalized joint hypermobility. Clin Biomech. 2013;28:318–24.
62. Perneger TV. What's wrong with Bonferroni adjustments. BMJ. 1998;316:1236–8.

21

Ultrasound assessment of fascial connectivity in the lower limb during maximal cervical flexion: technical aspects and practical application of automatic tracking

Carlos Cruz-Montecinos[1,2], Mauricio Cerda[3], Rodolfo Sanzana-Cuche[4], Jaime Martín-Martín[5,6] and Antonio Cuesta-Vargas[6,7,8*]

Abstract

Background: The fascia provides and transmits forces for connective tissues, thereby regulating human posture and movement. One way to assess the myofascial interaction is a fascia ultrasound recording. Ultrasound can follow fascial displacement either manually or automatically through two-dimensional (2D) method. One possible method is the iterated Lucas-Kanade Pyramid (LKP) algorithm, which is based on automatic pixel tracking during passive movements in 2D fascial displacement assessments. Until now, the accumulated error over time has not been considered, even though it could be crucial for detecting fascial displacement in low amplitude movements. The aim of this study was to assess displacement of the medial gastrocnemius fascia during cervical spine flexion in a kyphotic posture with the knees extended and ankles at 90°.

Methods: The ultrasound transducer was placed on the extreme dominant belly of the medial gastrocnemius. Displacement was calculated from nine automatically selected tracking points. To determine cervical flexion, an established 2D marker protocol was implemented. Offline pressure sensors were used to synchronize the 2D kinematic data from cervical flexion and deep fascia displacement of the medial gastrocnemius.

Results: Fifteen participants performed the cervical flexion task. The basal tracking error was 0.0211 mm. In 66 % of the subjects, a proximal fascial tissue displacement of the fascia above the basal error (0.076 mm ± 0.006 mm) was measured. Fascia displacement onset during cervical spine flexion was detected over 70 % of the cycle; however, only when detected for more than 80 % of the cycle was displacement considered statistically significant as compared to the first 10 % of the cycle (ANOVA, $p < 0.05$).

Conclusion: By using an automated tracking method, the present analyses suggest statistically significant displacement of deep fascia. Further studies are needed to corroborate and fully understand the mechanisms associated with these results.

Keywords: Fascia, Connective tissue, Myofascial, Tracking motion, Rehabilitation

* Correspondence: acuesta@uma.es; acuesta.var@gmail.com
[6]Departamento de Fisioterapia, Facultad de Ciencias de la Salud, Instituto Investigacion Biomedica de Málaga (IBIMA), Universidad de Málaga, Andalucia Tech, Cátedra de Fisioterapia y DiscapacidadGrupo de Clinimetria (FE-14), Málaga, Spain
[7]School of Clinical Science, Faculty of Health Sciences at Queensland University Technology, Brisbane, Australia
Full list of author information is available at the end of the article

Background

Fascia provides and transmits forces for connective tissues, thereby regulating human posture and movement [1]. Fascial tissue is of great interest to areas such anatomy, biomechanics, and musculoskeletal rehabilitation [2–4]. In regards to rehabilitation research, special interest in the concept of myofascial chains has grown in recent years [4] due to the application of soft tissue manipulation for gaining flexibility and, importantly, decreasing pain [5]. From the perspective of biomechanics, fascia plays important roles in movement restriction and proprioception [2, 6]. This restriction has been observed in fascial connectivity models, such as between the pelvis and deep fascia of the medial gastrocnemius (MG) [2], and has been reinforced by observations in cadaveric models, which suggest posterior fascial connectivity between the thoracolumbar spine, pelvis, and feet [4].

In the context of rehabilitation, various techniques apply the concept of myofascial connectivity to treat musculoskeletal disorders [7], thus highlighting the clinical importance of assessing the degrees of fascial connectivity throughout different regions of the human body. Among the widely used therapies, the fascial release technique assumes that fascial tissue is a continuous layer that spreads throughout the body [7]. Therefore, when fascial tissue is stretched in one area, it can cause tension, restriction, or pain in another area of the body [7]. In terms of general connectivity, while the connection between the thoracolumbar spine, pelvis, and feet is accepted [2, 4], cervical spine flexion should not increase MG tension [8]. However, *in situ* fascial tissue behavior has not been evaluated.

There are two possible pathways through which cervical spine flexion could cause MG fascial displacement. The first is through the posterior lamina of the thoracolumbar fascia, which is one of the main dorsal pathways of force transmission that directly connects to the gluteus maximus and hamstring fascia [9]. The second is through the neurodynamic response of the sciatic nerve [10]. Specifically, Johnson and Chiarelo [11] reported that cervical spine flexion, medial rotation of the hip, and ankle dorsiflexion exert neural mechanical tensions that are transmitted through the spinal cord, spinal dura, and lumbosacral roots to the sciatic nerve. Importantly, peripheral neural tissue has a close relationship with the surrounding fascia by means of the epineurum [10]; so forces transmitted through the neural structures could easily be transferred into fascial tissues. This point is particularly relevant when considering that previous studies have observed increased hamstring flexibility following the release of the suboccipital muscles [12, 13]. While the mechanism associated with this effect is uncertain, it could be due to an interaction between myofascial connections of the hamstring tendons and suboccipital muscle with a neural system that passes through the spinal dura [12–14].

One way to assess the myofascial interaction between the cervical region and lower leg is a fascia ultrasound recording. Ultrasound can follow fascial displacement either manually [15] or automatically through two-dimensional (2D) [2, 16] and three-dimensional (3D) methods [17]. Despite these diverse methods, previous studies have found that during active movements, fascia behaves in a longitudinal and transversal manner, but during passive uniaxial traction, fascia has longitudinal deformations [18]. One possible alternative for tracking of fascia, is the iterated Lucas-Kanade Pyramid (LKP) algorithm, which is based on automatic pixel tracking during passive movements in 2D fascial displacement assessments [2]. This algorithm presents great potential for facilitating dynamic studies of fascia. Nevertheless, the technical aspects derived from evaluation must be determined, since this algorithm has a proven accordance of 0.034 mm with manual tracking [2] and a precision of 0.2 mm in regards to a known distance [19].

Until now, the accumulated error over time has not been considered, even though it could be crucial for detecting fascial displacement in low amplitude movements. This accumulated error occurs as a result of displacement over time, which corresponds to the difference between a set of points and the original positions. If mistakes occur in the tracking between two frames, this will also be reflected as a displacement error that will propagate forward over time, i.e. a basal error. Determining the myofascial interaction between the cervical spine and lower body during postures associated with neural tension would help clarify the possible mechanisms associated with neurodynamic techniques and their interaction with myofascial chains.

Therefore, the main objective of the present study was to determine the basal error of LKP tracking and subsequently assess the MG fascial displacement using an ultrasound with automatized LKP tracking during maximal cervical spine flexion in a maximal kyphotic posture with the knees extended and ankles fixed at 90°.

Methods

Participants

Young males were recruited following authorization by and the guidelines of the Ethical Committee of the Northern Metropolitan Health Service of Santiago, Chile. The study complied with the ethical principles of the Declaration of Helsinki.

Before the measurement and the beginning of the study, each participant was given all information about the test and the purpose of the study. Participants had to sign an informed consent form in order to participate in the study. Participation in the study was voluntary and participants could discontinue their involvement at any time. The inclusion criteria for sedentary subjects considered less than 150 minutes per week of moderate physical activity [20]. Subjects were excluded if they presented a history of any musculoskeletal pain in the last six months, pathological conditions of the vertebral column, neurological diseases, respiratory diseases, a systemic rheumatic condition, heritable connective tissue disorders, and/or any previous abdominal surgery.

Procedure

A 5–10 MHz linear array transducer was used SonoSite TITAN® (Sonosite Inc., Bothell, WA, USA). Ultrasound images were taken at a depth of 39 mm, and video was recorded (Pinnacle Dazzle® DVD Recorder HD, Corel Corp., Ottawa, ON, Canada) at a rate of 30 frames per second and a resolution of 720 × 480 pixels.

Video-photogrammetric analysis was performed using the GoPro Hero3 camera (GoPro Inc, San Mateo, CA, USA) at a rate of 60 frames per second and a resolution of 1440 × 1440 pixels. Offline pressure sensors were used to synchronize the 2D kinematic data from cervical flexion and deep fascia displacement of the MG. To determine cervical flexion, an established 2D marker protocol was implemented (Fig. 1a) [21].

The transducer of the ultrasound system was placed on the extreme dominant belly of the MG by attaching a clamping device composed of a thermoplastic polymer and two elastic bands with velcro (Fig. 1b).

All signals and video processing was analyzed with a programing language in Matlab software (MathWorks Inc, Natick, Massachusetts, USA). Lucas–Kanade affine template tracking was used to automatically track the markers of interests [2]. Prior to applying the algorithms, an exploratory consistency assay was performed to evaluate angular variation against the Gold Standard, which is based on the infrared SMART-D 140® recoding system (BTS BioEngineering, Milan, Italy). A 2D angular variation curve of movement determined by a goniometer with three markers was compared at 60 frames per second on a frontal plane with the GoPro. Lin's concordance correlation coefficient was 0.999, and the average difference between the two methods was 0.360°, with threshold values of 1.0736–1.7946 (95 % confidence interval). The algorithm presented high precision and alignment with the Gold Standard. Finally, the angular variation curves of cervical flexion were processed using a 6 Hz low-pass filter [2].

A previously published methodology for automatic tracking was used to detect deep fascia displacement in the MG (Fig. 1c) [2]. From the automatically selected pixels to be used in tracking, the Euclidean distance (d)

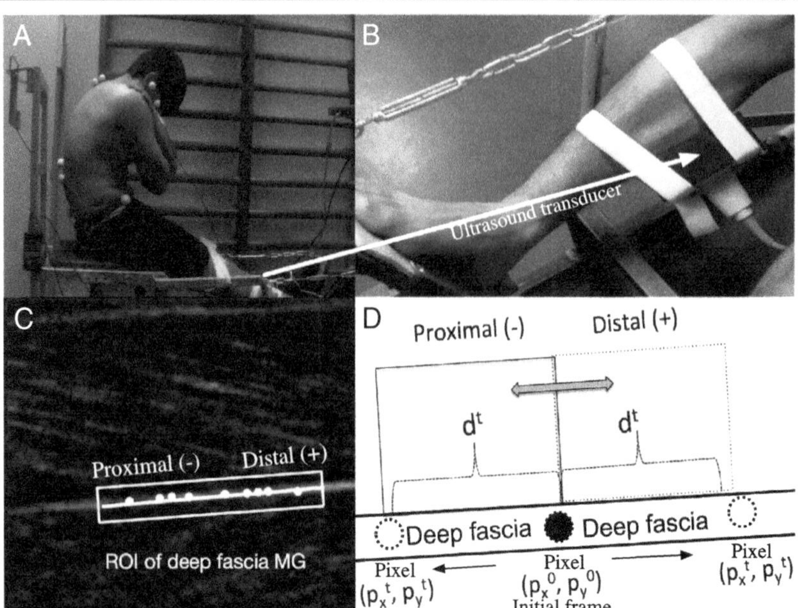

Fig. 1 **a** Example setup for kinematic analysis and location of the ultrasound. **b** Colocation of the ultrasound transducer in the medial gastrocnemius (MG). **c** Region of Interest (ROI) and automatic selection of pixels in the deep fascia of the MG. **d** Representation of one pixel in ROI for calculated Euclidean distance (d^t) between the position in time t (p_x^t, p_y^t) and the initial frame (p_x^0, p_y^0)

was calculated between the positions in time (t), (p_x^t, p_y^t) and in the initial frame (p_x^0, p_y^0).

$$d^t = \sqrt{\left(p_x^0 - p_x^t\right)^2 + \left(p_y^0 - p_y^t\right)^2}$$

Formula 1. Calculation for Euclidean distance (d^t).

The initial position on the axis (x) defined displacement in such a way that the distal end was positive and the proximal end negative (Fig. 1d). Since there are no prior reports for a time-related accumulation error for LKP tracking, an additional control experiment was performed in subjects that remained static during an ultrasound video recording of the deep fascia in the MG. This allowed for an evaluation of the basal tracking error in a temporal series. To ensure that subjects remained static, they were asked to suspend their breathing and hold a prone position for 4 s. This length of time was chosen as it was the average time recorded in experimental subjects from the start of movement to the end of the task. The basal tracking error was determined in two healthy men within the set ranges of the experimental groups. From the nine automatically selected tracking points, the Euclidean distance (d^t) was calculated. There was an average difference of 0.0063 mm in d^t (0.0664 pixels) between two consecutive frames, and the maximum standard deviation (max) (σ^t) was 0.0211 mm (0.2230 pixels) during the 4 s assay (total of 120 frames). This final error was defined as the basal tracking error (Fig. 2)

$$\max(\sigma^t) = \max\left(\sqrt{\sum_{k=1}^{9}\left(d_k^t - \sum_{p=1}^{9} d_p^t * \frac{1}{9}\right)^2 * \frac{1}{9}}\right)$$

Formula 2. Calculation for the basal tracking error.

To establish a reflex muscle contraction in the MG, the amplitude of muscle activity was recorded by surface electromyography at a sampling rate of 1000 Hz (Artoficio®, EMG VIII, Santiago, Chile). The skin was cleaned and the electrodes were positioned according to SENIAM recommendations [22]. To obtain a signal, a pass-band (20–450 Hz; Butterworth fourth order) and a band-stop filter (50 Hz; Butterworth fourth order) were used. Following this, the root mean square was applied with a 250 ms window. To assess electrical activity during the task, basal muscular activity was determined based on the average between a second before initiating the task and a second at the end of cervical spine flexion.

The task was practiced for 5 min prior to measurements, starting with the neck in a neutral position, as achieved by maintaining horizontal sight and keeping the other corporal segments relaxed and without any movement, and moving towards cervical spine flexion. Each subject was asked to perform each task three times. Each execution was standardized with a metronome so that the subject would finish each execution within 4 s. Maximal cervical flexion was performed in a sitting position with the lumbar and dorsal spine locked in maximal kyphosis and the knee fixed at full extension by a strap across the patella, which was adjusted as tightly as possible without causing pain or irritation for the subject. Ankles were locked at 90° by resting the foot on a static platform. Cervical flexion started from a neutral position to one of maximal flexion (Fig. 3). The task was considered successful if movement was only recorded for the cervical spine and, if this condition was not met, the test was nulled.

Data management and statistical analysis

Preliminary values were obtained from a pilot study in six subjects. The values of fascia displacement in the first 10 % of the cycle and those at the end of the cervical spine flexion were considered for sample size analysis. Since a statistical power of 90 %, an alpha of 5 %, and a loss rate 30 % were used to detect differences equal to or above 0.037 mm and with a standard deviation of 0.027 mm, the calculated sample size for the experimental condition was a minimum of 10 subjects.

Final average displacement was determined such that it would be above the basal LKP tracking error, thus

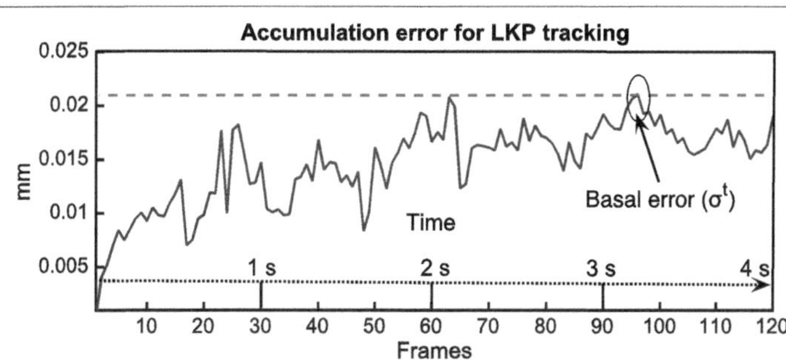

Fig. 2 Basal tracking error of Lucas-Kanade Pyramid (LKP). The maximum standard deviation (σ^t) during the 4 s assay (total of 120 frames)

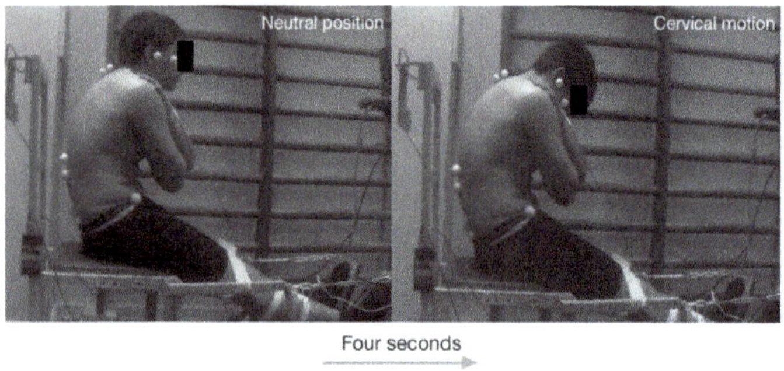

Fig. 3 Active cervical flexion starting in a neutral position and moving until maximum flexion

determining the existence of deep fascia displacement of the MG. All data were analyzed with the SPSS for Windows 22.0 software package (IBM Corp, Armonk, New York, USA). A value of $p < 0.05$ was considered statistically significant. To determine normal distribution, the Shapiro-Wilk test was used. All data were normally distributed. To assess average MG fascial displacement, ANOVA testing was used, and readings from every 10 % of the cycle were compared against the first 10 % of the cycle.

Results

All participants were male and dominantly right-handed in the inferior train. Fifteen participants were chosen to perform the cervical flexion task. The characteristics of the participants were as follows: an age of 23 ± 2.3 years, height of 1.75 ± 0.06 m, and body mass index (kg/m^2) of 24.21 ± 1.31.

Proximal fascial tissue displacement was observed in 66 % of the participants. Total displacement after subtracting the basal error was 0.076 ± 0.006 mm (Fig. 4). The onset of fascia displacement during cervical spine flexion was detected over 70 % of the cycle; however, only when detected for more than 80 % of the cycle, the displacement was significantly greater than the first 10 % of the cycle (ANOVA, $p < 0.05$) (Fig. 5). The onset of fascia displacement occurred at 36° of cervical spine flexion, equivalent to 76 % of maximal cervical spine flexion. The MG electromyography increased 2.6 % in regards to the basal value, but this was not statistically significant ($p = 0.452$).

Discussion

Deep fascia displacement of the MG was observed in 66 % of the subjects over 76 % of the final range of motion in cervical spine flexion. This displacement, which was above the basal error, showed an average proximal displacement of 0.076 mm. The same LKP tracking method was previously used in another report, obtaining distal fascia displacement of 1.50 mm in the MG during pelvic anteversion with the knees blocked in full extension and

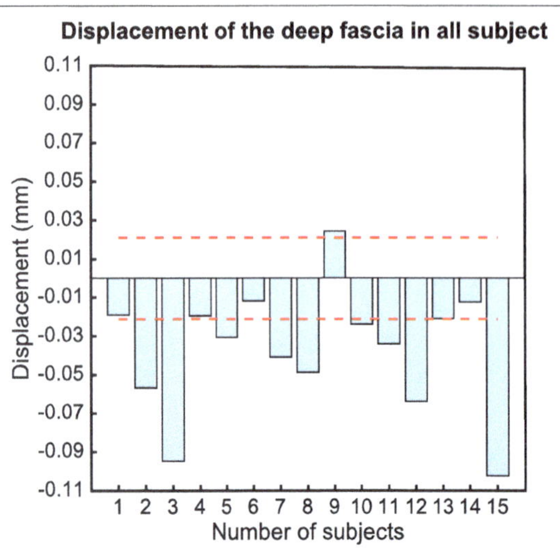

Fig. 4 Total deep fascia displacement of the medial gastrocnemius in all subjects. Red dotted line indicates the basal tracking error

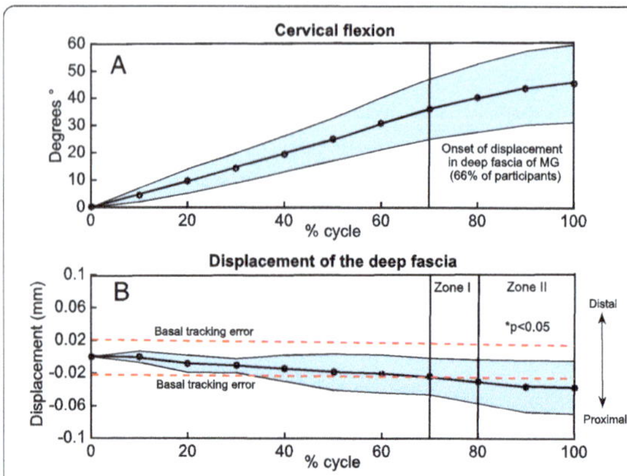

Fig. 5 a Range of motion of cervical spine flexion. **b** Medial gastrocnemius (MG) deep fascia displacement. Zone I shows the onset of MG deep fascia displacement. Zone II shows the cycle percentage where fascia displacement was greater than 10 % of the movement cycle with $p < 0.05$

the ankles at 90° [2]. Even though displacement in the present study was slight, it is relatable to previous studies that have detected minimal displacement of the sciatic nerve at the thigh during cervical spine flexion in a sitting position [23].

Since peripheral neural tissue has a close relationship with the surrounding fascia through the epineurium, force transmission might not only be through fascial tissue, but also through neural tissue [24]. During cervical flexion, the facial pathway may be transmitted through the posterior lamina of the thoracolumbar fascia, which is one of the main dorsal pathways of force transmission that directly connects to the gluteus maximus and hamstring fascia [9]. The neural pathway, which involves the spinal cord, spinal dura, and lumbosacral roots, creates tension in the sciatic nerve with different types of joint movements, including cervical spine flexion [10, 11]. In the hamstring, the fascial tissue and sciatic nerve have a connection through the epineurium.

A previous study showed different amounts of nerve excursion with different types of neural mobilization techniques, showing that slider mobilization creates greater longitudinal nerve displacement than tension or single joint mobilization [23]. In clinical practice, the interaction between suboccipital musculature inhibition and hamstring flexibility has been empirically evaluated [12, 13]. This effect can be explained by a connection of the hamstring tendons with the suboccipital muscle through a neural system that passes through the spinal dura, part of the posterior myofascial chain [12–14].

Until now, only one study has reported on the effects of the myofascial release technique with manual follow-up and manual tracking in ultrasound videos [15]. Regarding the tracking of fascia, this methodology can be used in future research to more fully explore aspects related to the transmission of myofascial force in different musculoskeletal and neurological pathological conditions. Specifically in manual therapy, there is great potential in assessing the effects of myofascial release techniques locally or over a distance by using automatized tracking methods.

The proximal displacement of the MG reported in this study might be a result of interactions between the neural and fascial tissues, especially considering that the cervical spine flexion test used in this study resembles the Slump test [25]. From a practical point of view, the results reported in this study provide new perspectives on the ultrasound assessment of fascial tissue, particularly for determining slight displacements and in providing new in vivo perspectives to apply and reinforce the concept of myofascial connectivity over a distance with a neurodynamic approach.

Nevertheless, further analyses of these results are needed, especially when considering that a recent study found cervical flexion to produce a non-significant sciatic nerve excursion during the slump test, as compared with upright-sitting and slump-sitting [26]. These differing results may be due to the use of a standardized 45 cm diameter ball in the present study for maintaining a slump position. When maximal cervical flexion in a maximal kyphotic posture is assessed, different results can be produced as compared to a standardized posture for all subjects. This would consequently produce different myofascial and nerve tensions.

Nevertheless, further studies are needed to compare different automatic tracking methods in fascial displacement assessments. For example, neural tissue assessments have used the cross correlation method that is based on the follow-up of a region of interest between two consecutive images [23, 26]. The precision between the cross correlation method and LKP tracking for neural and fascial tissue follow-up remains to be evaluated.

Study limitations

Regarding the limitations of this study, the slight facial displacement observed during cervical spine flexion was only evaluated in one position in the spine and hip. To fully determine the possible influence of spine position in myofascial transmission, further research that assesses different degrees of kyphosis is necessary. Furthermore, the methodology only considered the assessment of fascia in a relaxed position. Due to this, it was not possible to assess how different levels of trunk activation may induce fascia displacement. Moreover, this study focused only on men, and future research should consider comparative studies between genders, particularly regarding gender hormone differences that influence muscle flexibility and joint laxity [27, 28].

Moreover, future studies should additionally consider a simultaneous assessment of neural and fascial tissues and determine the anthropometric influence of facial displacement. Finally, while the present results show a certain tendency towards MG fascia displacement during cervical spine flexion, more studies are needed to corroborate this finding.

Conclusion

In conclusion, by using an automated tracking method, the present analyses evidence statistically significant displacement of deep fascia. These results suggest myofascial connectivity between the cervical spine and lower limbs. Further studies are needed to understand the mechanisms associated with these results.

Abbreviations

2D, two-dimensional; 3D, three-dimensional; LKP, Lucas-Kanade Pyramid; MG, medial gastrocnemius

Acknowledgements

The authors would like to thank the Programa de Anatomía y Biología del Desarrollo, Faculty of Medicine, University of Chile, Santiago, Chile. MC is funded by grants FONDECYT 3140447, ICM P09-015-F and the Latin American Cancer Research Network (US-LACRN).

Authors' contributions

C C-M participated in the conception and design of the study, in the data collection, analysis, interpretation of data and helped to draft the manuscript. M C participated in conception, analysis, interpretation of data and drafted the manuscript. R S-C participated analysis, interpretation of data and drafted the manuscript. J M-M participated analysis, interpretation of data and drafted the manuscript. A C-V participated in the conception and design of the study, analysis, interpretation of data and helped to draft the manuscript. All authors read and approved the final manuscript.

Competing interests

The authors state that no conflicts of interest have been reported by the authors or by any individual in control of the content of this article. This information has not been presented previously.

Consent for publication

The authors consent to publish the manuscript in current format. Any individual persons data contained in this manuscript.

Ethics approval and consent to participate

Ethical Committee of the Northern Metropolitan Health Service of Santiago, Chile.

Author details

[1]Department of Physical Therapy, Faculty of Medicine, University of Chile, Santiago, Chile. [2]Laboratory of Biomechanics, San José Hospital, Santiago, Chile. [3]SCIAN-Lab, Programa de Anatomía y Biología del Desarrollo, ICBM, University of Chile, Santiago, Chile. [4]Departamento de Ciencias Morfológicas, Facultad de Ciencia, Universidad San Sebastián, Santiago, Chile. [5]Escuela de Terapia Ocupacional, Facultad de Salud, Deporte y Recreación, Universidad Bernardo O Higgins, Santiago, Chile. [6]Departamento de Fisioterapia, Facultad de Ciencias de la Salud, Instituto Investigacion Biomedica de Málaga (IBIMA), Universidad de Málaga, Andalucia Tech, Cátedra de Fisioterapia y DiscapacidadGrupo de Clinimetria (FE-14), Málaga, Spain. [7]School of Clinical Science, Faculty of Health Sciences at Queensland University Technology, Brisbane, Australia. [8]Facultad de Ciencias de la Salud, Universidad de Málaga, Av. Arquitecto Peñalosa s/n (Teatinos Campus Expansion), 29009 Málaga, Spain.

References

1. Schleip R, Klingler W, Lehmann-Horn F. Active fascial contractility: Fascia may be able to contract in a smooth muscle-like manner and thereby influence musculoskeletal dynamics. Med Hypotheses. 2005;65:273–7.
2. Cruz-Montecinos C, González A, López D, Cerda M, Sanzana-Cuche R, Cuesta-Vargas A. In vivo relationship between pelvis motion and deep fascia displacement of the medial gastrocnemius: anatomical and functional implications. J Anat. 2015;227:665–72.
3. Langevin HM, Fox JR, Koptiuch C, Badger GJ, Greenan-Naumann AC, Bouffard NA, Konofagou EE, Lee W-N, Triano JJ, Henry SM. Reduced thoracolumbar fascia shear strain in human chronic low back pain. BMC Musculoskelet Disord. 2011;12:203.
4. Wilke J, Krause F, Vogt L, Banzer W. What is evidence-based about myofascial chains? A systematic review. Arch Phys Med Rehabil. 2015. doi: 10.1016/j.apmr.2015.07.023.
5. Ajimsha MS, Al-Mudahka NR, Al-Madzhar JA. Effectiveness of myofascial release: Systematic review of randomized controlled trials. J Bodyw Mov Ther. 2015;19:102–12.
6. Schleip R. Fascial plasticity–a new neurobiological explanation: Part 1. J Bodyw Mov Ther. 2003;7:11–9.
7. McKenney K, Elder AS, Elder C, Hutchins A. Myofascial release as a treatment for orthopaedic conditions: A systematic review. J Athl Train. 2013;48:522–7.
8. Andrade RJ, Lacourpaille L, Freitas SR, McNair PJ, Nordez A. Effects of hip and head position on ankle range of motion, ankle passive torque, and passive gastrocnemius tension. Scand J Med Sci Sports. 2016;26:41–7.
9. Vleeming A, Pool-Goudzwaard AL, Stoeckart R, van Wingerden JP, Snijders CJ. The posterior layer of the thoracolumbar fascia. Its function in load transfer from spine to legs. Spine. 1995;20:753–8.
10. Butler DS, Jones MA. Mobilisation of the Nervous System. 1st ed. New York: Churchill Livingstone; 1991.
11. Johnson EK, Chiarello CM. The slump test: the effects of head and lower extremity position on knee extension. J Orthop Sports Phys Ther. 1997;26:310–7.
12. Cho SH, Kim SH, Park DJ. The comparison of the immediate effects of application of the suboccipital muscle inhibition and self-myofascial release techniques in the suboccipital region on short hamstring. J Phys Ther Sci. 2015;27:195–7.
13. Aparicio ÉQ, Quirante LB, Blanco CR, Sendín FA. Immediate Effects of the Suboccipital Muscle Inhibition Technique in Subjects With Short Hamstring Syndrome. J Manipulative Physiol Ther. 2009;32:262–9.
14. Kahkeshani K, Ward PJ. Connection between the spinal dura mater and suboccipital musculature: Evidence for the myodural bridge and a route for its dissection-A review. Clin Anat. 2012;25:415–22.
15. Ichikawa K, Takei H, Usa H, Mitomo S, Ogawa D. Comparative analysis of ultrasound changes in the vastus lateralis muscle following myofascial release and thermotherapy: A pilot study. J Bodyw Mov Ther. 2014;19:327–36.
16. Bojsen-Møller J, Hansen P, Aagaard P, Svantesson U, Kjaer M, Magnusson SP. Differential displacement of the human soleus and medial gastrocnemius aponeuroses during isometric plantar flexor contractions in vivo. J Appl Physiol Bethesda Md 1985. 2004;97:1908–14.
17. Condino S, Turini G, Parrini S, Stecco A, Busoni F, Ferrari V, Ferrari M, Gesi M. A semiautomatic method for in vivo three-dimensional quantitative analysis of fascial layers mobility based on 3D ultrasound scans. Int J Comput Assist Radiol Surg. 2015;10:1721–35.
18. Azizi E, Roberts TJ. Biaxial strain and variable stiffness in aponeuroses. J Physiol. 2009;587:4309–18.
19. Magnusson SP, Hansen P, Aagaard P, Brønd J, Dyhre-Poulsen P, Bojsen-Moller J, Kjaer M. Differential strain patterns of the human gastrocnemius aponeurosis and free tendon, in vivo. Acta Physiol Scand. 2003;177:185–95.
20. Bennett JA, Winters-Stone K, Nail LM, Scherer J. Definitions of sedentary in physical-activity-intervention trials: a summary of the literature. J Aging Phys Act. 2006;14:456.
21. Kuo YL, Tully EA, Galea MP. Video Analysis of Sagittal Spinal Posture in Healthy Young and Older Adults. J Manipulative Physiol Ther. 2009;32:210–5.
22. Hermens HJ, Freriks B, Merletti R, Stegeman D, Blok J, Rau G, Disselhorst-Klug C, Hägg G. European Recommendations for Surface ElectroMyoGraphy. Roessingh Res Dev. 1999;8–11.
23. Ellis RF. Comparison of Different Neural Mobilization Exercises Upon Longitudinal Sciatic Nerve Movement: An In-Vivo Study Utilizing Ultrasound Imaging. J Orthop Sports Phys Ther. 2012;42:667–75.
24. Huijing PA. Epimuscular myofascial force transmission: A historical review and implications for new research. International society of biomechanics Muybridge award lecture, Taipei, 2007. J Biomech. 2009;42:9–21.
25. Philip K, Lew P, Matyas TA. The inter-therapist reliability of the slump test. Aust J Physiother. 1989;35:89–94.
26. Ellis R, Osborne S, Whitfield J, Parmar P, Hing W. The effect of spinal position on sciatic nerve excursion during seated neural mobilisation exercises: an in vivo study using ultrasound imaging. J Man Manip Ther. 2015; doi:10.1179/2042618615Y.0000000020.
27. Youdas JW, Krause DA, Hollman JH, Harmsen WS, Laskowski E. The influence of gender and age on hamstring muscle length in healthy adults. J Orthop Sports Phys Ther. 2005;35:246–52.
28. Romani W, Patrie J, Curl LA, Flaws JA. The correlations between estradiol, estrone, estriol, progesterone, and sex hormone-binding globulin and anterior cruciate ligament stiffness in healthy, active females. J Womens Health. 2003;12:287–98.

Permissions

All chapters in this book were first published in SSMR, by BioMed Central; hereby published with permission under the Creative Commons Attribution License or equivalent. Every chapter published in this book has been scrutinized by our experts. Their significance has been extensively debated. The topics covered herein carry significant findings which will fuel the growth of the discipline. They may even be implemented as practical applications or may be referred to as a beginning point for another development.

The contributors of this book come from diverse backgrounds, making this book a truly international effort. This book will bring forth new frontiers with its revolutionizing research information and detailed analysis of the nascent developments around the world.

We would like to thank all the contributing authors for lending their expertise to make the book truly unique. They have played a crucial role in the development of this book. Without their invaluable contributions this book wouldn't have been possible. They have made vital efforts to compile up to date information on the varied aspects of this subject to make this book a valuable addition to the collection of many professionals and students.

This book was conceptualized with the vision of imparting up-to-date information and advanced data in this field. To ensure the same, a matchless editorial board was set up. Every individual on the board went through rigorous rounds of assessment to prove their worth. After which they invested a large part of their time researching and compiling the most relevant data for our readers.

The editorial board has been involved in producing this book since its inception. They have spent rigorous hours researching and exploring the diverse topics which have resulted in the successful publishing of this book. They have passed on their knowledge of decades through this book. To expedite this challenging task, the publisher supported the team at every step. A small team of assistant editors was also appointed to further simplify the editing procedure and attain best results for the readers.

Apart from the editorial board, the designing team has also invested a significant amount of their time in understanding the subject and creating the most relevant covers. They scrutinized every image to scout for the most suitable representation of the subject and create an appropriate cover for the book.

The publishing team has been an ardent support to the editorial, designing and production team. Their endless efforts to recruit the best for this project, has resulted in the accomplishment of this book. They are a veteran in the field of academics and their pool of knowledge is as vast as their experience in printing. Their expertise and guidance has proved useful at every step. Their uncompromising quality standards have made this book an exceptional effort. Their encouragement from time to time has been an inspiration for everyone.

The publisher and the editorial board hope that this book will prove to be a valuable piece of knowledge for researchers, students, practitioners and scholars across the globe.

List of Contributors

Sebastian Ulsamer, Christoph Alexander Rüst and Thomas Rosemann
Institute of General Practice and for Health Services Research, University of Zurich, Zurich, Switzerland

Romuald Lepers
INSERM U1093, Faculty of Sport Sciences, University of Burgundy, Dijon, France

Beat Knechtle
Facharzt FMH für Allgemeinmedizin, Vadianstrasse 26, Gesundheitszentrum St. Gallen, St. Gallen, Switzerland

Anthony Barnett
School of Exercise and Nutrition Sciences, Deakin University, 221 Burwood Highway, Burwood, VIC 3125, Australia
Institute for Health & Ageing, Australian Catholic University, Melbourne, VIC 3000, Australia

Ester Cerin
School of Exercise and Nutrition Sciences, Deakin University, 221 Burwood Highway, Burwood, VIC 3125, Australia
School of Public Health, The University of Hong Kong, Pokfulam, Hong Kong SAR

Corneel Vandelanotte
Centre for Physical Activity Studies, Central Queensland University, Rockhampton, QLD 4702, Australia

Aya Matsumoto
Baker IDI Heart and Diabetes Institute, 75 Commercial Road, Melbourne, VIC 3004, Australia

David Jenkins
School of Human Movement and Nutrition Sciences, The University of Queensland, Brisbane, QLD 4072, Australia

Christoph A Rüst, Thomas Rosemann and Matthias A Zingg
Institute of Primary Care, University of Zurich, Zurich, Switzerland

Beat Knechtle
Institute of Primary Care, University of Zurich, Zurich, Switzerland
Gesundheitszentrum St. Gallen, Vadianstrasse 26, 9001 St. Gallen, Switzerland

Linda Ooms
Netherlands Institute for Health Services Research (NIVEL), PO Box 1568, 3500 BN Utrecht, The Netherlands

Cindy Veenhof
Physical Therapy Research, Program in Clinical Health Sciences & Department of Rehabilitation, Nursing Science and Sport, Brain Center Rudolf Magnus, University Medical Center Utrecht, PO Box 85500, 3508 GA Utrecht, The Netherlands

Nicolette Schipper-van Veldhoven
Netherlands Olympic Committee and Netherlands Sports Federation (NOC*NSF), PO Box 302, 6800 AH Arnhem, The Netherlands

Dinny H. de Bakker
Netherlands Institute for Health Services Research (NIVEL), PO Box 1568, 3500 BN Utrecht, The Netherlands
Scientific Center for Transformation in Care and Welfare (Tranzo), Tilburg University, PO Box 90153, 5000 LE Tilburg, The Netherlands

Maremka Zwinkels and Olaf Verschuren
Center of Excellence for Rehabilitation Medicine and Brain Center Rudolf Magnus, De Hoogstraat Rehabilitation and University Medical Center Utrecht, Utrecht, the Netherlands
Partner of Shared Utrecht Pediatric Exercise Research (SUPER) Lab, Utrecht, the Netherlands

Kristel Lankhorst, Karin van der Ende-Kastelijn and Janke de Groot
Partner of Shared Utrecht Pediatric Exercise Research (SUPER) Lab, Utrecht, the Netherlands
Research Group Lifestyle and Health, Institute of Human Movement Studies, University of Applied Sciences, Utrecht, the Netherlands

Frank Backx
Department of Rehabilitation, Nursing Science and Sports, University Medical Center Utrecht, Utrecht, the Netherlands

Anne Visser-Meily
Center of Excellence for Rehabilitation Medicine and Brain Center Rudolf Magnus, De Hoogstraat Rehabilitation and University Medical Center Utrecht, Utrecht, the Netherlands
Department of Rehabilitation, Nursing Science and Sports, University Medical Center Utrecht, Utrecht, the Netherlands

Tim Takken
Partner of Shared Utrecht Pediatric Exercise Research (SUPER) Lab, Utrecht, the Netherlands
Child Development and Exercise Center, University Medical Center Utrecht, Wilhelmina Children's Hospital, P.O. Box 850903508AB, Utrecht, the Netherlands

Åsa Fomin, Mattias Ahlstrand and Anders Gabrielsen
Department of Medicine, Unit of Cardiology, Karolinska University Hospital, Stockholm, Sweden

Cristina Da Silva
Department of Cardiology, Karolinska University Hospital, Stockholm, Sweden
School of Technology and Health, RoyalInstitute of Technology, Stockholm, Sweden

Anders Sahlén, Lars Lund and Marcus Stahlberg
Department of Cardiology, Karolinska University Hospital, Stockholm, Sweden

Aristomenis Manouras
Department of Cardiology, Karolinska University Hospital, Stockholm, Sweden
School of Technology and Health, RoyalInstitute of Technology, Stockholm, Sweden
Department of Clinical Physiology and Cardiology, Karolinska University Hospital Huddinge, SE-141 86 Stockholm, Sweden

Tiina Freimann
Tartu University Hospital, Puusepa 8, Tartu 51014, Estonia
Department of Public Health, Medical Faculty, University of Tartu, Ravila 14a, Tartu 50411, Estonia

Eda Merisalu
Institute of Technology, Estonian University of Life Sciences, Kreuzwaldi 56, Tartu 51014, Estonia

Mati Pääsuke
Institute of Exercise Biology and Physiotherapy, University of Tartu, Ravila 14a, Tartu 50411, Estonia

Beat Knechtle
Gesundheitszentrum St. Gallen, Vadianstrasse 26 9001, St. Gallen, Switzerland
Institute of Primary Care, University of Zurich, Zurich, Switzerland

Thomas Rosemann and Christoph A. Rüst
Institute of Primary Care, University of Zurich, Zurich, Switzerland

Jakob Kümmel, Julian Bergmann, Andreas Kramer and Markus Gruber
Sensorimotor Performance Lab, Department of Sport Science, University of Konstanz, 78476 Konstanz, Germany

Olaf Prieske and Urs Granacher
Division of Training and Movement Sciences, Faculty of Human Sciences, University of Potsdam, 14469 Potsdam, Germany

Birinder S Cheema
School of Science and Health, University of Western Sydney, Locked Bag 1797, Penrith, 2751 Campbelltown, New South Wales, Australia
The National Institute of Complementary Medicine, University of Western Sydney, Campbelltown, NSW 2650, Australia

Timothy B Davies, Matthew Stewart and Shona Papalia
School of Science and Health, University of Western Sydney, Locked Bag 1797, Penrith, 2751 Campbelltown, New South Wales, Australia

Evan Atlantis
School of Nursing and Midwifery, University of Western Sydney, Campbelltown, New South Wales, Australia
School of Medicine, University of Adelaide, Adelaide, South Australia, Australia

Amaya M Singh, Robin E Duncan, Jason L Neva and W Richard Staines
Department of Kinesiology, University of Waterloo, 200 University Avenue West, Waterloo, ON N2L 3G1, Canada

Roberto Zambelli, João Murilo Brandão Magalhães, Fernando Araujo Silva Lopes and Rodrigo Simões Castilho
Orthopedic Department, Hospital Mater Dei, Belo Horizonte, Minas Gerais, Brazil

Rafael Z. Pinto
Pain Management Research Institute, University of Sydney at the Royal North Shore Hospital, Sydney, Australia
Departamento de Fisioterapia, Faculdade de Ciências e Tecnologia, Universidade Estadual Paulista (UNESP), Presidente Prudente, São Paulo, Brazil

Daniel Baumfeld
Orthopedic Department, Hospital Felício Rocho, Belo Horizonte, Minas Gerais, Brazil

Thiago Ribeiro Teles dos Santos
Department of Physical Therapy, School of Physical Education, Physical Therapy and Occupational
Therapy, Universidade Federal de Minas Gerais (UFMG), Belo Horizonte, MG, Brazil

Nicola Maffulli
Department of Musculoskeletal Disorders, University of Salerno School of Medicine and Surgery, Salerno, Italy
Centre for Sports and Exercise Medicine, Queen Mary University, Mile End Hospital, London, UK

Monique AM Gignac
Institute for Work and Health; Division of Health Care & Outcomes Research, Arthritis Community Research and Evaluation Unit, Toronto Western Research Institute; Dalla Lana School of Public Health, University of Toronto, Toronto, Canada

Xingshan Cao
Arthritis Community Research and Evaluation Unit, Toronto Western Research Institute, Toronto, Canada

Subha Ramanathan
Postdoctoral Fellow, Faculty of Kinesiology and Physical Education, University of Toronto, Toronto, Canada

Lawrence M White
Joint Department of Medical Imaging, Faculty of Medicine, University Health Network, Mount Sinai Hospital, Women's College Hospital, University of Toronto, Toronto, Canada

Mark Hurtig
Ontario Veterinary College, University of Guelph, Guelph, Canada

Monica Kunz
Division of Orthopaedic Surgery, Sunnybrook Health Sciences Centre, Toronto, Canada

Paul H Marks
Division ofOrthopaedic Surgery, Faculty of Medicine, Sunnybrook Health Sciences Centre, University of Toronto, Toronto, Canada

Stefanie Wild, Christoph Alexander Rüst and Thomas Rosemann
Institute of General Practice and for Health Services Research, University of Zurich, Zurich, Switzerland

Beat Knechtle
Institute of General Practice and for Health Services Research, University of Zurich, Zurich, Switzerland
Gesundheitszentrum St. Gallen, Vadianstrasse 26, 9001 St. Gallen, Switzerland

Ben Serrien and Jonathan Blondeel
Department Biomechanics, Vrije Universiteit Brussel, Brussels, Belgium

Ron Clijsen
Department Biomechanics, Vrije Universiteit Brussel, Brussels, Belgium
Thim Van Der Laan University College, Landquart, Switzerland
Department Health Sciences, University of Applied Sciences and Arts of Southern Switzerland, Landquart, Switzerland

Maggy Goossens
Thim Van Der Laan University College, Landquart, Switzerland
University of Antwerp, ICT-electronics, Antwerp, Belgium

Jean-Pierre Baeyens
Department Biomechanics, Vrije Universiteit Brussel, Brussels, Belgium
Thim Van Der Laan University College, Landquart, Switzerland
University of Antwerp, ICT-electronics, Antwerp, Belgium

E Paul Zehr
Rehabilitation Neuroscience Laboratory, University Victoria, PO Box 3010 STN CSC, Victoria, BC V8W 3P1, Canada
Human Discovery Science, International Collaboration on Repair Discoveries (ICORD), Vancouver, BC, Canada
Centre for Biomedical Research, University of Victoria, Victoria, BC, Canada
Division of Medical Sciences, University of Victoria, Victoria, BC, Canada

Tsuyoshi Nakajima
Department of Integrative Physiology, Kyorin University School of Medicine, 6-20-2 Shinkawa, Mitaka, Japan

Trevor Barss and Taryn Klarner
Rehabilitation Neuroscience Laboratory, University Victoria, PO Box 3010 STN CSC, Victoria, BC V8W 3P1, Canada
Human Discovery Science, International Collaboration on Repair Discoveries (ICORD), Vancouver, BC, Canada
Centre for Biomedical Research, University of Victoria, Victoria, BC, Canada

Stefanie Miklosovic
Rehabilitation Neuroscience Laboratory, University Victoria, PO Box 3010 STN CSC, Victoria, BC V8W 3P1, Canada

Rinaldo A Mezzarane
Laboratory of Signal Processing and Motor Control, College of Physical Education, University of Brasília, Brasília, Brazil
Biomedical Engineering Laboratory, EPUSP, PTC, University of São Paulo, São Paulo, Brazil
Department of Health and Sports Sciences, Faculty of Education, Chiba University, Chiba, Japan

Matthew Nurse
Nike Sport Research Laboratory, Beaverton, OR, USA

Tomoyoshi Komiyama
Department of Health and Sports Sciences, Faculty of Education, Chiba University, Chiba, Japan

Fabian Stöcker and Christoph Von Oldershausen
Center for Teaching and Learning, Technische Universität München, Connollystraße 32, 80809 München, Germany

Florian Kurt Paternoster
Department for Biomechanics in Sports, Technische Universität München, München, Germany

Thorsten Schulz and Renate Oberhoffer
Department for Preventive Pediatrics, Technische Universität München, München, Germany

Tina Junge
Department of Physiotherapy, University College Lillebaelt, Odense, Denmark
Health Sciences Research Centre, University College Lillebaelt, Odense, Denmark
Department of Sports Science and Clinical Biomechanics, University of Southern Denmark, Odense, Denmark

Peter Henriksen
Health Sciences Research Centre, University College Lillebaelt, Odense, Denmark
Department of Sports Science and Clinical Biomechanics, University of Southern Denmark, Odense, Denmark

Heidi Lund Andersen, Linette Dyg Byskov and Hans Kromann Knudsen
Department of Physiotherapy, University College Lillebaelt, Odense, Denmark

Birgit Juul-Kristensen
Department of Sports Science and Clinical Biomechanics, University of Southern Denmark, Odense, Denmark
Institute of Occupational Therapy, Physiotherapy and Radiography, Bergen University College, Bergen, Norway

Asmare Yitayeh
Department of Physiotherapy, School of Medicine, College of Medicine and Health Sciences, University of Gondar, Gondar, Ethiopia

Amare Teshome
Department of Dentistry, School of Medicine, College of Medicine and Health Sciences, University of Gondar, Gondar, Ethiopia

Pranay Jindal and Joy C. MacDermid
McMaster University, Hamilton, ON, Canada

Amitesh Narayan and Sailakshami Ganesan
Kasturba Medical College, Mangalore, Karnataka, India

Carlos Cruz-Montecinos
Department of Physical Therapy, Faculty of Medicine, University of Chile, Santiago, Chile
Laboratory of Biomechanics, San José Hospital, Santiago, Chile

Mauricio Cerda
SCIAN-Lab, Programa de Anatomía y Biología del Desarrollo, ICBM, University of Chile, Santiago, Chile

Rodolfo Sanzana-Cuche
Departamento de Ciencias Morfológicas, Facultad de Ciencia, Universidad San Sebastián, Santiago, Chile

Jaime Martín-Martín
Escuela de Terapia Ocupacional, Facultad de Salud, Deporte y Recreación, Universidad Bernardo O Higgins, Santiago, Chile
Departamento de Fisioterapia, Facultad de Ciencias de la Salud, Instituto Investigacion Biomedica de Málaga (IBIMA), Universidad de Málaga, Andalucia Tech, Cátedra de Fisioterapia y DiscapacidadGrupo de Clinimetria (FE-14), Málaga, Spain

Antonio Cuesta-Vargas
Departamento de Fisioterapia, Facultad de Ciencias de la Salud, Instituto Investigacion Biomedica de Málaga (IBIMA), Universidad de Málaga, Andalucia Tech, Cátedra de Fisioterapia y DiscapacidadGrupo de Clinimetria (FE-14), Málaga, Spain
School of Clinical Science, Faculty of Health Sciences at Queensland University Technology, Brisbane, Australia
Facultad de Ciencias de la Salud, Universidad de Málaga, Av. Arquitecto Peñalosa s/n (Teatinos Campus Expansion), 29009 Málaga, Spain

Index